OPERATING ROOM SKILLS

Fundamentals for the Surgical Technologist

NANCY N. DANKANICH, RN, BSN, MA, CNOR

Program Director and Clinical Coordinator, Surgical Technology

Faculty, Surgical Technology and Nursing Programs

Frederick Community College

Frederick, Maryland

PEARSON

Boston Columbus Indianapolis New York San Francisco Upper Saddle River Amsterdam
Cape Town Dubai London Madrid Milan Munich Paris Montreal Toronto Delhi Mexico City
Sao Paulo Sydney Hong Kong Seoul Singapore Taipei Tokyo

Publisher: Julie Levin Alexander
Publisher's Assistant: Regina Bruno
Editor in Chief: Mark Cohen
Executive Editor: John Goucher
Assistant Editor: Nicole Ragonese
Editorial Assistant: Erica Viviani
Director of Marketing: David Gesell
Executive Marketing Manager: Katrin Beacom
Marketing Coordinator: Michael Sirinides
Senior Managing Editor: Patrick Walsh
Project Manager: Christina Zingone-Luethje
Senior Operations Supervisor: Ilene Sanford

Operations Specialist: Lisa McDowell
Senior Art Director: Jayne Conte
Cover Designer: Bruce Kenselaar
Cover Photo: Lasse Kristensen/Shutterstock
Media Editor: Amy Peltier
Lead Media Project Manager: Lorena Cerisano
Full-Service Project Management: Bruce Hobart, Laserwords, Maine
Composition: Laserwords
Printer/Binder: Quad/Graphics
Cover Printer: Lehigh-Phoenix Color/Hagerstown
Text Font: Garamond 11/13.5

Compass Illustration: Angela Jones/Shutterstock

Credits and acknowledgments for content borrowed from other sources and reproduced, with permission, in this textbook appear on appropriate page within text.

Library of Congress Cataloging-in-Publication Data
Dankanich, Nancy N.
   Operating room skills : fundamentals for the surgical technologist / Nancy N. Dankanich.
     p. ; cm.
   Includes bibliographical references and index.
   ISBN-13: 978-0-13-509378-8
   ISBN-10: 0-13-509378-3
   I. Title.
   [DNLM: 1. Operating Room Nursing—education.   2. Operating Room Technicians—education.   3. Clinical Competence.
4. Operating Room Nursing—methods.   5. Operating Rooms—standards.   6. Surgical Procedures, Operative—standards. WY 18.2]
   617'.0231—dc23

                                                                                                2012002442

10 9 8 7 6 5 4 3 2 1

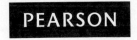

ISBN 10:   0-13-509378-3
ISBN 13: 978-0-13-509378-8

Dedication

This lab manual is written for my students and colleagues,
who make a difference in the lives they touch.

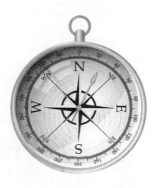

Past, Present, and Future
Foundational Values, Abundant Love, and Blissful Hope

Joseph and Margaret, Alexander and Mary
Alex, Alexis, Nicholas, and Andrew

Each of you enriches my life, and I am most truly blessed!

Contents

Preface

Stakeholders in our modern teaching-learning process for surgical technology education demand graduates with the perfect blend of cognitive, affective, and psychomotor skills. The education system and the student are equally responsible for meeting these expectations. The surgeon, the patient, employers, and team members expect students and program graduates to display professionalism, specific interpersonal skills, and hands-on prowess. In addition, graduates of accredited surgical technology programs must sit for the national certification examination in surgical technology. Surgical technology education offers challenges and opportunities for all involved.

Operating Room Skills: Fundamentals for the Surgical Technologist focuses on essential skills needed to perform safely and competently in the operating room environment, as an integral team member. This lab manual and accompanying video exhibit a unique format which follows the role of the surgical technologist in conjunction with the movement of the patient through the surgical experience. New learners are prompted to organize their responsibilities in an uninterrupted sequence, which begin in the locker room and conclude through room turnover. Active learning is promoted when students demonstrate the skills presented in each chapter in the risk-free laboratory setting. Role-playing, face-to-face communication, small group scenarios and simulations, teamwork, and problem solving are encouraged as precise performance and critical thinking are developed. Once skill competence is evaluated and verified by using the competency assessments found in each chapter, students progress into the clinical setting where they apply skills during actual invasive surgical procedures. Laboratory or preclinical training is an integral and essential portion of an entire education in surgical technology. This lab manual is envisioned to be a complimentary tool, used in conjunction with other resources.

The skill sequences and instructions in this lab manual highlight best practices advocated by a cadre of professional and government organization, including OSHA, CDC, ECRI, JC, AHA, AST, AORN, and the AST's sixth edition of the *Core Curriculum for Surgical Technology,* and examples from practicing certified surgical technologists, registered nurses, first assistants, surgeons, and educators. Foundational concepts pertaining to communication, accountability, aseptic technique, safety, and critical thinking are integrated into each chapter along with the psychomotor skills. Educators are encouraged to supplement the content with their own hospital's policies as they use the lab manual, competencies, discussion questions, and video to facilitate student success.

Operating Room Skills: Fundamentals for the Surgical Technologist is organized to support the role of the student functioning in the nonsterile and sterile team member roles including first scrub, second assisting or second scrub, and assistant circulator. There are 25 chapters which integrate theory and clinical practice. *Unit I: Prepare for Surgery* includes Chapters 1 through 18. This section presents concepts and skills related to infection control, aseptic technique, counting, medications, vital signs, urinary catheterization, fire safety awareness, and safe practice parameters. *Unit II: Surgery Fundamentals* includes Chapters 19 through 22. Foundational concepts for the first and second scrub roles are presented for interfacing with the surgeon; identifying and passing instruments, suture, and free ties; the care of specimens; identifying and correcting contamination errors; preparing wound drains and dressings; and facilitating post anesthesia care. *Unit III: Essentials after Surgery* includes Chapters 23 and 24 and accentuates the importance of following a protocol for cleaning the room in between procedures, preventing cross-contamination among patients, furniture, and personnel, and the proper readying of the room for the next procedure. *Unit IV: Minimally Invasive Surgery* includes Chapter 25. Essential mechanical components and the affiliated skills are presented in a step-by-step format for the novice learner.

Key features include:

- 600 full-color illustrations and tables
- Supplement to any fundamental operating room textbook
- Team member roles
- Principles for practice—professional and governmental
- Learner objectives
- Skill Sequences—instructions and illustrations
- Teamwork—transform modern social networking into face-to-face communication
- Competency Assessments—lab and clinical settings
- Discussion Questions—recall, application, and analysis
- Companion Website: www.myhealthprofessionskit.com
  - View interactive video segments and clips
  - Refer to appendices and answer keys
  - Transition into the clinical setting
  - Document student surgical case participation according to AST's guidelines
  - Customize tools for evaluation and documentation

Anyone affiliated with the OR will attest to the value of visualization and repetition when first learning these complex skills. The accompanying interactive video facilitates instruction and review of skills taught in the lab manual. The sequence and logical progression of the skills will be appreciated by learners who are new to the OR setting. The student can select to view:

- The Complete Perioperative Process
- The Laparoscopic Process
- Individual Skills
- Introduction to Anesthesia

Precise skill performance is an essential component in health care education. The competency assessments found in each chapter provide a framework to evaluate the student's ability to integrate theory into practice and to demonstrate precise, professional skills required to work successfully with stakeholders. The assessments may be used in the lab or clinical setting by instructors, preceptors, and students. Once the skill has been introduced by the instructor in the lab setting, students benefit from small group practice where they teach, observe, and critique each other. Personalization of the competency assessment allows educators to select grading rubrics and to formulate plans for improvement along with the student.

All skills have mutual components which are grouped and evaluated in each competency assessment. The *Mutual Professional and Scholastic Criteria* include:

AFFECTIVE DOMAIN

1. Demonstrates initiative, self-direction, and accountability
2. Accepts responsibility; does not blame others
3. Enthusiastic; respects efforts of faculty and staff supporting educational opportunities
4. Completes assignments and incorporates appropriate patient information
5. Consistently communicates precisely and professionally with peers, instructors, OR staff, and patients
6. Exhibits respect and a pleasant demeanor to all affiliates
7. Follows directions; acts on constructive evaluations
8. Adheres to program, hospital, and OR policies
9. Respects the property of others
10. Preserves patient confidentiality

COGNITIVE DOMAIN

1. Applies theory to lab or clinical practice
2. Demonstrates critical thinking, sound judgment, and appropriate independence
3. Blends previous career skills with the practice of surgical technology
4. Exhibits a surgical conscience

PSYCHOMOTOR DOMAIN

1. Punctual; consistent in time management
2. Exhibits manual dexterity and physical stamina
3. Introduces self and role to instructors, OR personnel, and the patient
4. Consistently performs hand hygiene
5. Dons appropriate OR attire and PPE; securely wears ID badge
6. Verifies surgeon's preference card then selects ordered supplies and equipment
7. Assists OR team to verify function of equipment
8. Applies and maintains aseptic technique; nonsterile and sterile roles

9. Identifies the patient and explains the procedure, as appropriate
10. Participates in the surgical pause
11. Performs safely; makes infrequent minor errors, and prevents injuries to self and others
12. Participates in surgical procedures with increasing complexity according the latest edition of AST's *Core Curriculum for Surgical Technology*
13. Documents, as appropriate
14. Notifies appropriate personnel of malfunctioning equipment

Operating Room Skills: Fundamentals for the Surgical Technologist presents operating room concepts and skills in a sequential real-time format. The lab manual is patient-centered and student-focused, and supports the development of precise performance and critical thinking demanded by stakeholders. Safe patient care incorporates recommendations and best practices from professional and government organizations, industry, and practicing OR personnel. Educators and students will use this lab manual, Companion Website, and videos to prepare for entry into the operating room as a team member. Later these same tools will be useful during preparation for the national certification examination in surgical technology.

Acknowledgments

This lab manual may not have been possible without the question first posed by Mr. Leslie Thompson in February, 2006: "Why don't you make your own?" Thank you, Les, for asking the question.

My colleagues, Richard Schellenberg and Jason Santelli, are gifted professionals in the field of video and digital technology. They worked countless hours over many weekends to help me realize my quest for developing a skills DVD that my students could use at home or in the classroom. Originally, I had no idea how video production worked or how tedious and exacting editing can be. Our collaboration has given me a newfound respect for their industry. Thank you; you are really awesome!

I am grateful to all of the staff members at Pearson Education for their vision, faith, sage advice, energy, guidance, and cheerleading. My first contact was with Alice Barr, the college book representative, who promptly referred me to Mark Cohen, the acquisitions editor. Thank you, for this gift and opportunity to set new goals. Appreciation is also extended to all of the affiliates: your expertise and guidance gave this opportunity a richer dimension.

Colleagues, I appreciate your enthusiasm, dedication to lifelong learning, editorial comments, and willingness to share your clinical expertise.

Marina Bartgis, CST
Susie Benner, MS, RNFA
Marissa Case, BA, CST
Regina Castor, CST
Cathleen Corcoran, CST
Lois Covati, CNOR, RNFA
Kelly Drury, CST
Meghan Fleagle, CST
Stephanie Friend, CST
Jessica Huff, CST
Ashley Hyrkas, CST
Karen Kendall, BA, CST
Claudia King, BS, CNOR RNFA
Ericca Knowlden, AAS, CST
Shirley Lee, AAS, CST
Jessica Lertora, BA, CST
Vanessa Lovato, MS, RN

James McClellan, DVM, CST
Angie Meyer, BA, CST
Keith Mull, PA, CST
Paula Neiderberger, CST
Carolyn Poston, CST
Kimberly Reese, CST
Christine Rhyner, CST
Sara Smith, BA, CST
Eric Strange, BA, CST
Neal Summers, CST
Leslie Thompson, CST
Paul Webster, Ed.D, PA
Cheryl Wilmer, CNOR RNFA
Roger Wilmer, M.Div., CST
Karen Yanus, CNOR RN
Thomas Yewell, BA, CST

About the Author

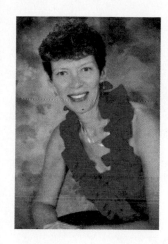

Nancy Dankanich is the Surgical Technology Program Director at Frederick Community College in Frederick, Maryland. During the 15 years in this position, she has facilitated the development of the program by implementing national standards, negotiating contracts with numerous clinical sites, and overseeing growth in the number of qualified program applicants. She has taught in health care for over 25 years—surgical technology theory, laboratory, and clinical—and in the registered nurse and practical nurse programs. Additional teaching responsibilities include online documentation training for nurses, electronic medication administration record-training for nurses, and American Heart Association CPR for the Healthcare Provider. Service to the college includes participation on numerous college-wide committees: scholarship, peer evaluation, emergency preparedness, international education, academic master planning, and academic program review. As the recipient of several innovation and summer grants from the college, she has networked with colleagues to develop and implement strategies that promote student success. The author has collaborated on the development of surgical instrument training products, including a general surgery instrument CD and general surgery applications for the iPhone and iPad.

Broad interests and experience in acute care, intensive care, operating room, pediatrics, home health, and long-term care complement the author's teaching experience. She holds a bachelor's degree with high honors in nursing from the University of Maryland, and a master's degree, summa cum laude, from Hood College. Professional memberships are held in Phi Kappa Phi, Sigma Theta Tau, AST, and AORN. Volunteer activities include Maryland Responds Disaster Nurse Volunteer program, and participation in Stephen's Ministry through her local church congregation. Dedication to lifelong learning is evidenced by attendance at national conferences; completion of several peer reviews for medical publications; the accumulation of continuing education hours in medical, surgical, and educational topics; and the establishment of the Joseph and Margaret Droll Memorial Student Scholarship fund through the Frederick Community College Foundation, Inc.

The dearest of all moments are spent at home with her husband Alex, of 34 years, with her three children—Alexis, Nicholas, and Andrew—and with her pets—Mojo and Tiffany.

Lab Manual Features

1. EVERY CHAPTER OPENS WITH A VISUAL OF THE TEAM MEMBER'S ROLE.

Team Member	Type of Role		Timing		
	Nonsterile	Sterile	Preop	Intraop	Postop
Surgical Technologist		X	X		
Assistant Circulator					
Operating Room Team		X	X		

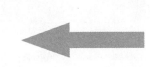

2. THE INTRODUCTION PROVIDES LEARNERS AND INSTRUCTORS WITH AN OVERVIEW AND INSTRUCTIONS FOR DEMONSTRATION IN THE LAB AND CLINICAL SETTINGS.

INTRODUCTION

The fluid-resistant sterile gown and two pairs of sterile gloves provide barriers which protect the patient and the health care worker from blood-borne pathogens during invasive surgical procedures. In this chapter you will practice donning the gown and gloves that you set up in Chapter 4.

- Before performing the following skill, your lab instructor will discuss some of the principles for practice and objectives involved in this chapter as well as the importance of following the skill sequence and instructions.
- Use the closed-gloving method to don your gloves, and practice this skill frequently until your perfect it. Work with your lab partner. Encourage and critique

each other. Your instructor will offer strategies for success. Appendix E highlights the value of teaching others as a component of active learning strategies. Refer to Appendix C for an overview of the chapter.
- The lab instructor will advise you of any additional criteria to be evaluated. At a designated time, demonstration of these skills will be evaluated and graded by your lab instructor using the competency assessment tool.
- When in the clinical setting, your instructor may once again assess your performance using the same tool. Refer to Appendix A for clinical evaluation and documentation.

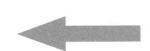

3. THE PRINCIPLES FOR PRACTICE SECTION PROMOTES ADDITIONAL RESEARCH INTO THE RATIONALE FOR THE SKILLS.

 ### Principles for Practice

The foundation and rationale for our practice, in the perioperative environment, stem from evidence provided by professionals, organizations, and governmental agencies. Refer to the Bibliography, Glossary of Terms, and the following documents or developmental agencies:

- Manufacturers' product guidelines
- Operating room policies

- American College of Surgeons (ACS)
- American Association of Orthopedic Surgeons (AAOS)
- Occupational Safety and Health Administration (OSHA)
- Centers for Disease Control and Prevention (CDC)
- Association of Surgical Technologists (AST)
- Association of periOperative Registered Nurses (AORN)

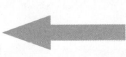

4. OBJECTIVES PROVIDE A FRAMEWORK FOR THE INSTRUCTOR AND LEARNER.

OBJECTIVES

The learner will demonstrate this skill with 100 percent accuracy each time entering the operating room:

1. Maintain aseptic technique when relating to the sterile field and supplies on the Mayo stand.
2. Dry hands and arms thoroughly by using the sterile towel upon completion of the traditional, water-surgical scrub.
3. Allow hands and arms to air-dry upon completion of the waterless scrub.
4. Don a sterile surgical gown.
5. Double glove using the closed-gloving method.

5. A STEP-BY-STEP FORMAT IS PRESENTED ALONG WITH FIGURES TO EMPHASIZE THE SEQUENCE.

SKILL SEQUENCE AND INSTRUCTIONS

1. Enter the OR suite.
   - Maintain the position of your scrubbed hands and arms between your waist and midchest level.
   - Keep hands and arms in front of you, with elbows bent and away from your face mask. Refer to Chapter 5.
   - Do not touch nonsterile surfaces.
   - Monitor the movement of other team members and avoid them (see Figure 6.1).
2. Approach the front of your Mayo stand.
   - Reach into your sterile field on the Mayo stand, and pinch up the drying towel by an exposed corner or central area only.
   - Do not drip water onto your gown or gloves, and do not touch them with your hand.
   - Move into an open area nearby, but away from the Mayo stand (see Figure 6.2).

3. Unfold the towel, and dry your hands and arms while keeping both hands elevated.
   - Hold the towel by the superior edge, and dry your opposite hand and arm.
   - Move the towel with a blotting motion as you proceed from your fingertips to your elbow.
   - Bend forward at the waist to increase the distance between your OR attire and the towel.
   - Do not touch the towel onto your top or pants.
   - Switch to the lower half of the towel, and dry your opposite hand and arm.
   - Drop the drying towel into a receptacle. Keep your hands elevated (see Figure 6.3).

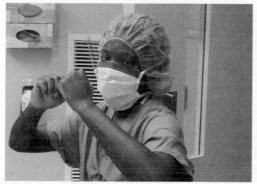

FIGURE 6.1 Enter OR.

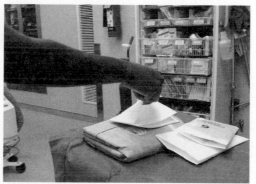

FIGURE 6.2 Lift towel in the center.

6. EVALUATE PERFORMANCE USING THE COMPETENCY ASSESSMENT, FOUND IN EACH CHAPTER. FEATURES ALLOW FOR INDIVIDUALIZATION.

COMPETENCY ASSESSMENT

STUDENT'S NAME: _____

CHAPTER 6 GOWN AND GLOVE SELF— CLOSED-GLOVING METHOD

PERFORMANCE RANK:

S or √ = Satisfactory: Competent—safe, accurate, sequential, and timely
U = Unsatisfactory: Unsafe—inaccurate and unprepared

PERFORMANCE RATING:

5	Independent: Expert—safe, confident, seamless performance; mentors others
4	Minimally monitored: Intermediate—safe, self-corrects few errors
3	Competent: Novice—safe, revises with evaluator cues, few errors
2	Remedial: Unsafe—critical errors, unable to implement evaluator cues consistently
1	Dependent: Unsafe—unacceptable, requires multiple evaluator interventions

PERFORMANCE CRITERIA	Performance Rank	Performance Rating
1. Perform Mutual Professional and Scholastic Criteria as appropriate (see Preface or Appendix A).		1 2 3 4 5
2. Approach the Mayo stand and retrieve drying towel; bend over at waist.		1 2 3 4 5
3. Unfold towel held by superior edge.		1 2 3 4 5
4. Dry first hand, arm, and elbow with blotting motion.		1 2 3 4 5
5. Switch towel to inferior edge and dry second side.		1 2 3 4 5
6. Dispose of towel.		1 2 3 4 5
7. Retrieve gown at neckline, orient it, allow it to unfold, and insert arms; keep hands inside sleeves.		1 2 3 4 5
8. Retrieve right glove with your left hand; position and don it.		1 2 3 4 5
9. Retrieve left glove with your right hand; position and don it.		1 2 3 4 5
10. Retrieve and don second pair of sterile gloves; adjust fit.		1 2 3 4 5
11. Prepare waist tag and tie; turn and tie with circulator.		1 2 3 4 5
12. Hold hands in sterile zone.		1 2 3 4 5

7. REINFORCE LEARNING WITH APPENDICES, AND ACTIVITIES AND DISCUSSION QUESTIONS FOUND IN EACH CHAPTER. VIEW APPENDICES AND ANSWER KEYS ON WWW.MYHEALTHPROFESSIONSKIT.COM.

ACTIVITIES AND DISCUSSION QUESTIONS

Activities

1. View the Complete Perioperative Process and Focus on Skills video, Skill #6 (video can be found at www.myhealthprofessionskit.com).
2. Observe the instructor perform the skill.
3. Practice the skill in the lab, with your lab partner or in small groups.
4. Select one skill, teach a classmate, and observe and critique the performance.

Discussion Questions

1. List the critical steps in performing this skill.
2. Define closed-gloving.
3. Compare closed-gloving with open-gloving. (You will need to look ahead in the lab manual to Chapter 15.)
4. What do you do to prevent contamination of the sterile drying towel? Name at least two tasks.
5. List two ways you can contaminate your gown when you are putting it on.

8. VIEW OPERATING ROOM SKILLS ON WWW.MYHEALTHPROFESSIONSKIT.COM. SELECT FULL LENGTH SCENARIOS OR INDIVIDUAL SKILLS IN VIDEO CLIPS.

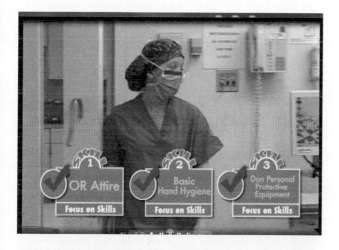

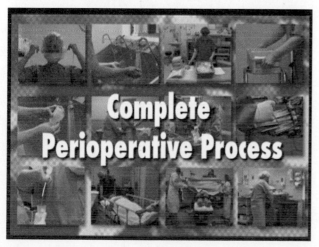

9. COMPANION WEBSITE REINFORCES LABORATORY EXERCISES, AND TRANSITIONS STUDENTS INTO THE CLINICAL SETTING. GO TO WWW.MYHEALTHPROFESSIONSKIT.COM TO VIEW:

- Appendices
- AST's guidelines for student participation during surgical cases
- Forms to document and tally student participation in 14 surgical specialties
- Competency assessment tools, with options to customize

PEARSON
myhealthprofessionskit™

Use this address to access the Companion Website created for this textbook. Simply select "Surgical Technology" from the choice of disciplines. Find this book and log in using your username and password to access interactive activities, videos, and much more.

Introduction

As a new student member of the surgical team in the operating room, your goal is to promote a positive surgical outcome for the patient while working with the other team members. During surgery, many professionals educated in various disciplines gather. Each has a unique focus; all perform within their scope of practice. All converge as prepared individuals, and all are advocates for the patient. Patient and team member safety are, by design, built into the foundations of practice. As a new surgical team member, if you use three broad concepts as your compass, you will perform professionally, safely, and confidently. These concepts are communication, anticipation, and passion. An acronym, CAP, will help you remember these fundamental concepts.
Communication–Anticipation–Passion

COMMUNICATION

The first compass concept is communication. This concept is a major thread that permeates professional practice in the entire perioperative environment. Good communication is more than just our spoken language. Communication includes preparation, adherence to a dress code, time management, initiative, nonverbal communication, respect, and teamwork. All methods of communication promote safety and success. However, it is not a surprise that a majority of competencies, daily student evaluations, job interview questions, and annual employer evaluations refer to one's performance as a participant on a team. For years, healthcare providers have recognized the value of communication in the form of teamwork.

In January 2009 the New England Journal of Medicine published a study performed by the World Health Organization. The study reported that improved communication among team members occurred when a surgical safety checklist was implemented during a pause in the work flow. Ultimately, the patient benefited from the fluidity in communication: precision was enhanced, and death and complications were reduced. One of the leaders of the WHO's Safe Surgery Saves Lives program, Atul Gawande, MD, describes the development of the program in his book, *The Checklist Manifesto: How to Get Things Done Right*. In it he states that just ticking off boxes on a list is not the ultimate goal. Rather we are to "embrace a culture of teamwork and discipline" (Gawande, 2009). Giving and receiving messages are successful when we place value in the communication process and award power to it.

ANTICIPATION

The second compass concept is anticipation. The surgeon and the patient depend on your ability to anticipate. This concept is evident in the perioperative environment through the following: aseptic technique, surgical conscience, performance parameters, application of knowledge, efficiency, consistency, safety, and critical thinking. Incorporating the fundamental skills, the ones that you use during each procedure, must become second nature during your training. You must perfect the basic, core skills. Focus on the fundamentals and demonstrate consistency.

During the 2010 Winter Olympics in Vancouver, British Columbia, American, Evan Lysack won the Men's Figure Skating Gold Medal. He gave a flawless performance described as being strong from start to finish. During a televised interview, Lysack credits this success to relentless practice of the basics. Strategically, he focused on practice that would give his foundational moves in figure skating an "easy" appearance. Lysack's strategy demonstrated his ability to anticipate. He recognized what he needed to do to reach his goal.

The importance of anticipation is also evident in a presentation entitled, "Going from Good to Great," given by Steven Brand, MD, on April 13, 2011 to a class of graduating surgical technologists. During this enlightening and informative session, Dr. Brand asks the class if performing at 99.9 percent—almost perfect—is acceptable. He further dazzles the students with a few statistics related to performing at 99.9 percent. At this almost perfect rate, the following would occur: the IRS would lose two million documents per year; there would be one major airplane crash every three days; the banking industry would experience almost 40,000 ATM errors per hour; 12 moms and dads would leave the hospital with someone else's child each day; cardiac pacemakers would be placed incorrectly in 291 patients; and over 107 erroneous surgical procedures would be performed each day. The students received the message, loud and clear. No, 99.9 percent is not good enough! Anticipate, prepare, and know the case as performed by the surgeon because the patient and the team depend on you.

PASSION

The third compass concept is passion. A Google search describes passion as a powerful feeling. Other sources describe passion as a strong liking or enthusiasm for a subject or activity. Your role is to demonstrate the passion you have for becoming an outstanding surgical team member. Let those around you recognize that you are interested, focused, attentive, prepared, and eager to learn. Demonstrate your passion, embrace the adventure, and appreciate the knowledge of those surrounding you. Think of your training or clinical time as an opportunity for a long job interview. Furthermore, your passion will encourage preceptors and educators to fashion learning experiences that match your energy level.

One chief of surgery stated that he is the consumer of the OR team's skills, in particular, those of the surgical technologist. Attentiveness, responsiveness, preparation, and interest are expected. When the ST is not interested, this surgeon would rather see them leave and allow others to scrub in. The surgeon further stated that he gives 200 percent and, therefore, expects the same from all team members. Even though you are new to the operating room environment, you are expected to convey a passion for your role. Your attitude conveys respect and appreciation for the patient and for those who are teaching you.

Passion for performing as a valuable operating room team member does not stop with your student role. As a professional, you want to connect with others in your area of expertise. Professional organizations such as the Association of Surgical Technologists and the Association of PeriOperative Registered Nurses offer a plethora of opportunities for networking and education. As a professional, you will to validate your knowledge and skill level by sitting for a professional certification. The National Board of Surgical Technology and Surgical Assisting (NBSTSA) offers the national certifying examination for surgical technologists, and the Competency and Credentialing Institute (CCI) offers the certification examination for operating room nurses. As a professional, you will offer your expertise to future new graduates and colleagues. You will also become a mentor and preceptor in years to come. Passion for your vocation is displayed when you are a student and, later, when you are employed.

ASK KEY QUESTIONS

The fundamental concepts of performing as an outstanding team member are communication, anticipation, and passion, or CAP. This lab manual has been designed to incorporate these fundamental concepts into the fundamental, or core, skills that you need to be successful as you begin your training. Later, at the end of your training, you should refer to the fundamental skills again and review the key components as you study for the certifying examination.

At the start of your day, ask yourself a few key questions related to these fundamental concepts: "How can I demonstrate my eagerness to learn and my passion for this opportunity? What do I need to communicate to my instructor, preceptor, surgeon, and patient? How can I anticipate so that I meet the needs of the patient, the surgeon, and the team?" Be accountable to yourself and to the team. Communication, anticipation, and passion will catapult you into a successful student experience and into a new career where you will be a respected colleague.

STUDENT-GENERATED INITIATIVE

In the spring of 2006, I asked my surgical technology students to assist me in selecting new instructional materials for the next class. During the course of their training, some students had expressed a few concerns. They had not seen enough materials that showcased in an organized format all of the skills the faculty wanted them to learn. The Internet presented many new options, but the class had not identified any one product that was useful. I obtained a few DVDs for preview, and the class watched along with me. None of the products seemed to meet their needs, and I had to concur. There were many good products for one skill or another, or there were products that took hours to complete because of the interspersed activities or tests. One of my students, Leslie Thompson, said to me, "Mrs. Dankanich, why can't you make your own?"

Through affiliations and collaboration, I did produce a surgical technology skills DVD which follows the uninterrupted sequence of the surgical experience for the patient and the surgical technologist. Sterile and nonsterile team member roles intertwine to represent the actual sequence of events. In 2008 new audio, and video footage, and a new design generated yet another DVD which continues to be updated. Over the past five years, students and educators have offered many positive comments, and they love having a visual product they can use at home. Some students practice skills while they are viewing the DVD. (Perform skills such as loading and unloading a knife handle only in the lab setting with instructors present.) In class, students enjoy sharing how they practice at home and how they are proud to demonstrate what they are learning to their friends or family members.

This lab manual was written for students who are learning fundamental operating room skills. It is a supplement for any operating room textbook and corresponds with the original vision found in the DVD. Authors spend countless hours developing content that will assist students along their journey of becoming outstanding new team members. Instructors present core concepts and skills in the classroom and lab settings. Testing performance of core skills is essential before students enter the operating room. The fundamental skills are assessed in this lab manual by using competency assessments found in each chapter. Finally, students progress into the OR where they are paired with preceptors, and their education continues. I sincerely hope the information provided in this lab manual and in the Web-based visual media will bring success and confidence as you prepare for your new career.

Unit I

Surgery Preparation

Don Operating Room Attire

1

INTRODUCTION

Aseptic technique is a foundational concept which begins at home and continues in the perioperative environment. Infection control and prevention of surgical site infections are imbedded in this skill. Wash your hands, and don clean hospital-laundered operating room (OR) attire, a disposable surgical cap, and shoe covers.

- Before performing the following skill, your lab instructor will discuss some of the principles for practice and objectives involved in this chapter as well as the importance of following the skill sequence and instructions.
- In the privacy of a locker room, change out into OR attire.

- Offer suggestions to your lab partner. Your instructor will offer strategies for success. Appendix E highlights the value of teaching others as a component of active learning strategies. Refer to Appendix C for an overview of the chapter.
- The lab instructor will advise you of any additional criteria to be evaluated. At a designated time, demonstration of this skill will be evaluated and graded by your lab instructor using the competency assessment tool.
- When in the clinical setting, your instructor may once again assess your performance using the same tool. Refer to Appendix A for clinical evaluation and documentation.

Team Member	Type of Role		Timing		
	Nonsterile	Sterile	Preop	Intraop	Postop
Surgical Technologist	X		X		
Assistant Circulator	X		X		
Operating Room Team	X		X		

OBJECTIVES

The learner will demonstrate the following skill with 100 percent accuracy each time the perioperative environment is entered.

1. Demonstrate a professional work ethic.
2. Use clear verbal, nonverbal, and written communication.
3. Perform hand hygiene in the unrestricted area or locker room.
4. Don hospital-laundered OR attire (a scrub outfit) and personal protective equipment (PPE), such as the surgical cap and shoe covers.
5. Respect shared space in the locker room.

Principles for Practice

The foundation and rationale for our practice, in the perioperative environment, stem from evidence provided by professionals, organizations, and governmental agencies. Refer to the Bibliography, Glossary of Terms, and the following documents or developmental agencies:

- Occupational Safety and Health Administration (OSHA)
- Centers for Disease Control and Prevention (CDC)
- Association of Surgical Technologists (AST)
- Association of periOperative Registered Nurses (AORN)

SKILL SEQUENCE AND INSTRUCTIONS

1. Dress in appropriate street clothing and undergarments, perform personal hygiene, and attach to your person proper identification (ID) before entering the hospital clinical setting.

   - Do not wear nail polish, artificial applications to the nails, perfume, or after shave.
   - Do not wear any jewelry, including body-piercing jewelry.
   - Cover visible tattoos.
   - Demonstrate a positive attitude and a professional work ethic. Refer to the Glossary of Terms for a detailed definition of appropriate communication etiquette.
   - Wash your hands upon entering the locker room or unrestricted perioperative area. Refer to Chapter 2 and Appendix D for detailed information on hand washing (see Figure 1.1).

2. Obtain hospital-laundered scrub top and pants, disposable hat, and shoe covers (as required by your facility).
   - Select from tops and pants arranged by various sizes on shelves or access an automated valet system (see Figures 1.2 and 1.3).

3. Store your street clothing on hangers or in designated lockers.
   - Respect the personal space of facility employees (see Figure 1.4).

4. Don the disposable cap, then your scrub top and pants.
   - Contain all hair under the cap.
   - Conceal all allowable undergarments under the OR attire.
   - Think of the acronym CAP (communication, anticipation, and passion) each time you don your OR cap. CAP represents key concepts for success in the surgical technology role. Refer to the Introduction for additional information (see Figure 1.5).

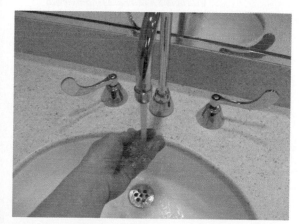

FIGURE 1.1 Wash your hands.

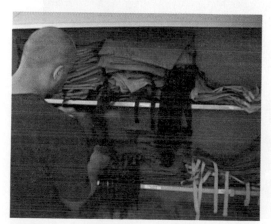

FIGURE 1.2 Colored-ties assist with size selection.

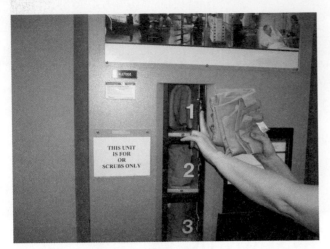

FIGURE 1.3 Automated valet system.

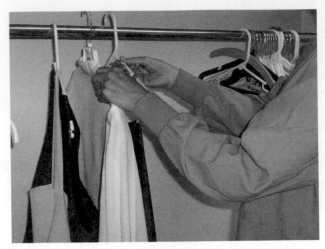

FIGURE 1.4 Store your street clothing.

5. Wear comfortable, protective, and dedicated OR shoes.

- Noncloth athletic-style shoes are acceptable.
- Shoes should enclose your toes, and heels should be low.
- Wear support-style hose for ladies or socks for men, which will help prevent leg fatigue (see Figure 1.6).

6. Don disposable shoe covers over your OR shoes per hospital policy (see Figure 1.7).
7. Tuck your top into your pants, and tuck in the draw stings (see Figure 1.8).

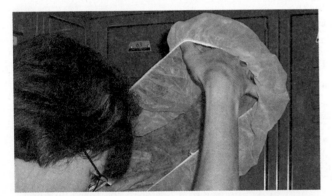

FIGURE 1.5 Don disposable cap.

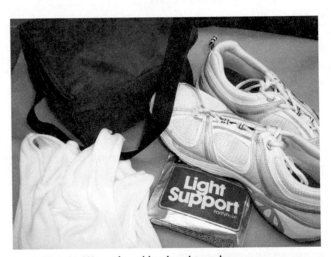

FIGURE 1.6 Wear closed heel and toe shoes.

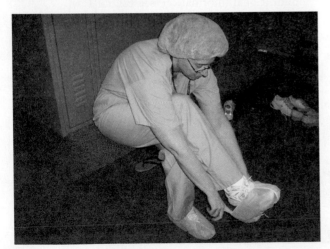

FIGURE 1.7 Wear shoe covers.

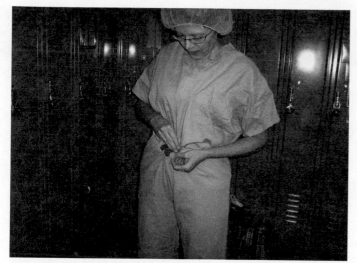

FIGURE 1.8 Tuck in top and drawstrings.

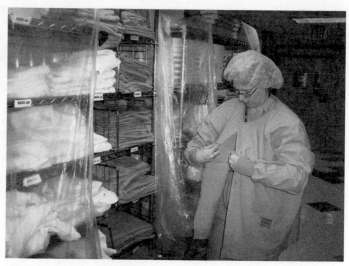

FIGURE 1.9 Don jacket.

8. Wear a long-sleeved snap-up jacket when in the nonsterile role, which prevents skin and microbe shedding into the OR environment.

   • Secure all snap closures.
   • Remove and store the jacket prior to scrubbing at the sink when preparing for the sterile role. The jacket's use is optional at many facilities (see Figure 1.9).

9. Wear proper identification at all times; secure ID badge into the top scrub suit pocket to prevent contamination of any sterile field. Store a small note pad and pen in the back pocket of your scrub pants, if you might need to take notes.

10. Change into new OR attire whenever it becomes visibly soiled or wet in order to prevent cross-contamination of microorganisms.

STUDENT'S NAME: _____

CHAPTER 1 DON OPERATING ROOM ATTIRE

PERFORMANCE RANK:

S or √ = Satisfactory: Competent—safe, accurate, sequential, and timely
U = Unsatisfactory: Unsafe—inaccurate and unprepared

PERFORMANCE RATING:

5   Independent: Expert—safe, confident, seamless performance; mentors others
4   Minimally monitored: Intermediate—safe, self-corrects, few errors
3   Competent: Novice—safe, revises with evaluator cues, few errors
2   Remedial: Unsafe—critical errors, unable to implement evaluator cues consistently
1   Dependent: Unsafe—unacceptable, requires multiple evaluator interventions

PERFORMANCE CRITERIA	Performance Rank	Performance Rating
1. Perform Mutual Professional and Scholastic Criteria as appropriate (See the Preface or Appendix A).	*n/a*	1 2 3 4 5
2. Demonstrate home preparation: personal care, natural nails, and no jewelry, aftershave, or perfume		1 2 3 4 ⑤
3. Enter locker room; wash hands; gather attire *supplies ✓*		1 2 3 4 ⑤
4. Secure personal effects; respect space of others		1 2 3 4 ⑤
5. Don OR cap; assess for stray hair and correct		1 2 3 4 ⑤
6. Don hospital-laundered attire; tuck in top and draw strings		1 2 3 4 ⑤
7. Don dedicated OR shoes; use shoe covers per policy		1 2 3 4 ⑤
8. Don and snap jacket for nonsterile role per policy	*n/a*	1 2 3 4 5
9. Wear and secure ID badge		1 2 3 4 ⑤
10. State two conditions for donning fresh OR attire		1 2 3 4 ⑤

ADDITIONAL COMMENTS _____

PERFORMANCE EVALUATIONS AND RECOMMENDATIONS   *50/50*

☑ PASS: Satisfactory Performance
    ☑ Demonstrates professionalism
    ☑ Exhibits critical thinking
    ☑ Demonstrates proficient clinical performance appropriate for time in the program
☐ FAIL: Unsatisfactory Performance
    ☐ Critical criteria not met (See Performance Rank or Rating Above)
    ☐ Professionalism not demonstrated.
    ☐ Critical thinking skills not demonstrated.
    ☐ Skill performance unsafe or not demonstrated.
☐ REMEDIATION:
    ☐ Schedule lab practice. Date: _____
    ☐ Reevaluate by instructor. Date: _____
☐ DISMISS from lab or clinicals today.
☐ Program director notified. Date: _____

SIGNATURES

Date _9/30/13_____   Evaluator _____   Student _____

ACTIVITIES AND DISCUSSION QUESTIONS

Activities

1. View the Complete Perioperative Process and Focus on Skills video, Skill #1 (video can be found at www.myhealthprofessionskit.com).
2. Observe the instructor perform the skill.
3. Practice the skill in the lab, with your lab partner or in small groups.
4. Teach this skill to a classmate and observe and critique the performance.
5. Refer to your ST (Surgical Technology) textbook and this lab manual to answer the Discussion Questions (see next column).
6. Review the video and the information in this lab manual when you prepare for your certification examination.

Discussion Questions

1. List the essential steps of this skill in order.
2. Why do we use OR attire?
3. Why do you change into fresh, hospital-laundered attire?
4. When do you change into OR attire?
5. What do AST and AORN recommend concerning the use of home-laundered OR attire?
6. Once you graduate, what will you tell a new student entering the semirestricted area about jewelry and watches?
7. You had a manicure five days ago, and the clear nail polish looks unchipped. What principle will guide your next action? What will be your next action?
8. What does professional communication mean to you?
9. Make notes here for clarification or discussion with your instructor or preceptor.

PEARSON
myhealthprofessionskit™

Use this address to access the Companion Website created for this textbook. Simply select "Surgical Technology" from the choice of disciplines. Find this book and log in using your username and password to access interactive activities, videos, and much more.

Perform Basic Hand Hygiene

2

INTRODUCTION

According to the Centers for Disease Control and Prevention, hand hygiene is the single most effective method used to prevent the spread of disease. And it is an essential component of aseptic technique and infection control.

- Before performing the following skill, your lab instructor will discuss some of the principles for practice and objectives involved in this chapter as well as the importance of following the skill sequence and instructions.
- Practice the skill with your lab partner. Encourage and critique each other. Your instructor will offer strategies for success. Appendix E highlights the value of teaching others as a component of active learning strategies. Refer to Appendix C for an overview of the chapter.
- The lab instructor will advise you of any additional criteria to be evaluated. At a designated time, demonstration of these skills will be evaluated and graded by your lab instructor using the competency assessment tool.
- When in the clinical setting, your instructor may once again assess your performance using the same tool. Refer to Appendix A for clinical evaluation and documentation.

Team Member	Type of Role		Timing		
	Nonsterile	Sterile	Preop	Intraop	Postop
Surgical Technologist	X		X		X
Assistant Circulator	X		X		X
Operating Room Team	X		X		X

OBJECTIVES

The learner will demonstrate the following skill with 100 percent accuracy each time it is performed in the perioperative environment.

1. Prevent cross-contamination due to direct or indirect contact with pathogenic microbes.
2. Perform hand hygiene with soap and water or with waterless solutions provided by the clinical facility.

Principles for Practice

The foundation and rationale for our practice, in the perioperative environment, stem from evidence provided by professionals, organizations, and governmental agencies. Refer to the Bibliography, Glossary of Terms, and the following documents or developmental agencies:

- Operating room policies
- Food and Drug Administration (FDA)
- Occupational Safety and Health Administration (OSHA)
- Centers for Disease Control and Prevention (CDC)
- Association of Surgical Technologists (AST)
- Association of periOperative Registered Nurses (AORN)

SKILL SEQUENCE AND INSTRUCTIONS

1. Prepare for the basic hand wash, or prewash.

   - Inspect your skin for weeping cuts, scrapes, or lesions. Notify your manager or instructor if your skin is not intact. You will then be given an alternate assignment.
   - Roll up your sleeves.
   - Clean under your nails with a fingernail pick, if the subungual area is visibly soiled.
   - Use the hand- or knee-activated lever or movement sensor to turn on the faucet.
   - Wet your hands and arms to approximately two inches above your elbows.
   - Refer to Chapter 1 for preparatory duties related to jewelry and nails. (see Figure 2.1).

2. Dispense FDA-approved liquid soap into your palms according to the manufacturer's instructions. You are not to use a product intended for use in the home or brought from home (see Figures 2.2 and 2.3).

3. Adjust the water temperature until warm.
   - Use soap and friction while interlacing and rubbing your fingers, finger tips, and web spaces (see Figure 2.4).

4. Use friction and soap to wash all planes of your hands, forearms, and arms up to two inches above the elbows for a minimum of 15 seconds, according to your OR policy.
   - Refer to Appendix D (see Figures 2.5 and 2.6).

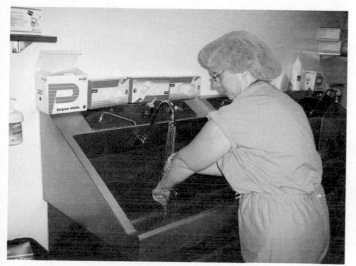

FIGURE 2.1   Inspect and wet.

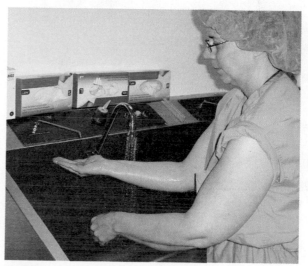

FIGURE 2.2   Use liquid soap at the scrub sink.

5. Rinse hands and arms thoroughly with warm water.
   - Fingers and hands are pointed downward for the rinse.
   - Make sure the water is off.
   - Use a paper towel to turn off manually operated faucets (see Figure 2.7).

6. Dry your hands and arms with a disposable paper towel.
   - Apply hand moisturizer, as provided by your facility, to maintain skin integrity and prevent drying or cracking (see Figure 2.8).

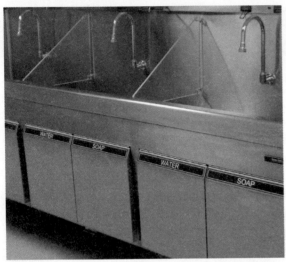

FIGURE 2.3 Dispense soap with a knee-activated pad option.

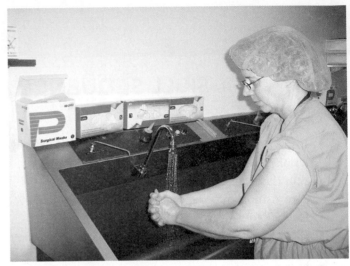

FIGURE 2.4 Interlace fingers.

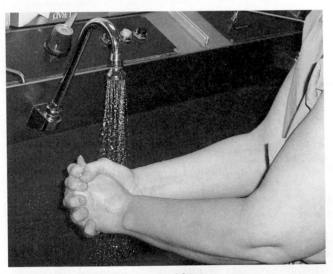

FIGURE 2.5 Wash with soap and friction.

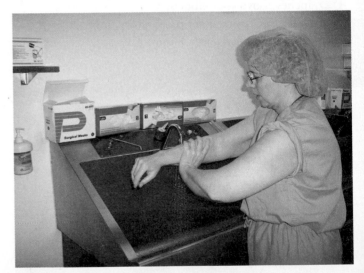

FIGURE 2.6 Wash all planes.

7. Wash your hands throughout the day including during the following:

- Before performing the surgical hand scrub.
- Before and after eating or using the restroom.
- At any time when potentially hazardous materials, equipment, or fluids are touched.
- Refer to Diagram 2.1 and Appendix D.

8. When in the clinical setting, proceed to the assignment board or report room to obtain your assignment for the day. Follow guidelines for upholding patient confidentiality and professionalism; refer to Chapter 24 (see Figure 2.9).

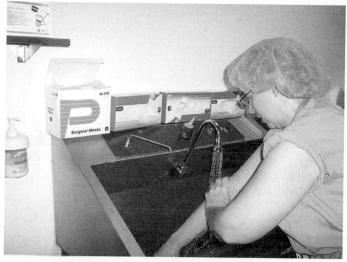

FIGURE 2.7   Rinse.

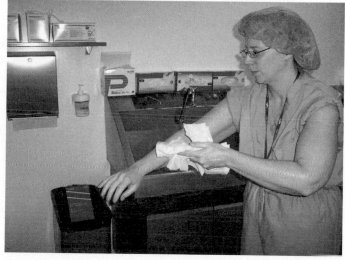

FIGURE 2.8   Dry.

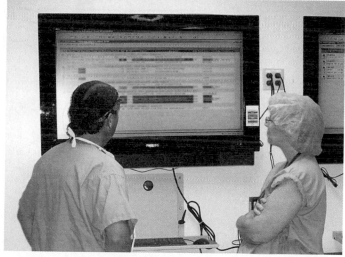

FIGURE 2.9   Receive assignment.

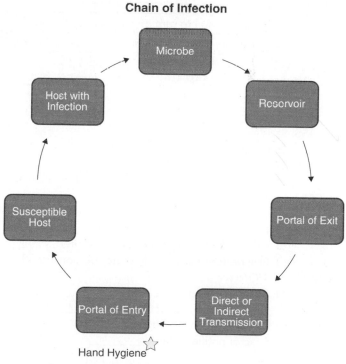

DIAGRAM 2.1   Complex Process of Infection.

STUDENT'S NAME: _____

CHAPTER 2 PERFORM BASIC HAND HYGIENE

PERFORMANCE RANK:

S or √ = Satisfactory: Competent—safe, accurate, sequential, and timely

U = Unsatisfactory: Unsafe—inaccurate and unprepared

PERFORMANCE RATING:

5   Independent: Expert—safe, confident, seamless performance; mentors others

4   Minimally monitored: Intermediate—safe, self-corrects, few errors

3   Competent: Novice—safe, revises with evaluator cues, few errors

2   Remedial: Unsafe—critical errors, unable to implement evaluator cues consistently

1   Dependent: Unsafe—unacceptable, requires multiple evaluator interventions

PERFORMANCE CRITERIA	Performance Rank	Performance Rating
1. Perform Mutual Professional and Scholastic Criteria as appropriate. (See the Preface or Appendix A.)	N/a	1 2 3 4 5
2. Prepare for basic hand wash; wet hands and arms; use warm water and soap; conserve water per policy.		1 2 3 4 (5)
3. Use fingernail pick if subungual areas contain debris.		1 2 3 4 (5)
4. Apply friction with soap and water for at least 15 seconds.		1 2 3 4 (5)
5. Rinse areas with warm water, and remove lather.		1 2 3 4 (5)
6. Dry hands and arms with disposable towel.		1 2 3 4 (5)
7. Use disposable towel to turn off hand-controlled faucet.		1 2 3 4 (5)
8. State at least four situations where hand washing is required.		1 2 3 4 (5)

ADDITIONAL COMMENTS _____

PERFORMANCE EVALUATIONS AND RECOMMENDATIONS

40/40

☑ PASS: Satisfactory Performance

     ☑ Demonstrates professionalism

     ☑ Exhibits critical thinking

     ☑ Demonstrates proficient clinical performance appropriate for time in the program

☐ FAIL: Unsatisfactory Performance

     ☐ Critical criteria not met (see Performance Rank or Rating Above)

     ☐ Professionalism not demonstrated.

     ☐ Critical thinking skills not demonstrated.

     ☐ Skill performance unsafe or not demonstrated.

☐ REMEDIATION:

     ☐ Schedule lab practice. Date: _____

     ☐ Reevaluate by instructor. Date: _____

☐ DISMISS from lab or clinicals today.

☐ Program director notified. Date: _____

SIGNATURES

Date 9-30-13   Evaluator _____   Student _____

ACTIVITIES AND DISCUSSION QUESTIONS

Activities

1. View the Complete Perioperative Process and Focus on Skills video, Skill #2 (video can be found at www.myhealthprofessionskit.com).
2. Observe the instructor perform the skill.
3. Practice the skill in the lab, with your lab partner or in small groups.
4. Discuss why this is a foundational skill in the application of aseptic technique.
5. Teach this skill to a classmate and observe and critique the performance.
6. Refer to your ST textbook and this lab manual to answer the Discussion Questions (see next column).
7. Review the video and the information in this lab manual when you prepare for your certification examination.

Discussion Questions

1. List the essential steps of this skill in sequential order.
2. Why do we perform a basic hand wash?
3. When do we perform a basic hand wash?
4. Discuss the importance of this skill outside of the OR environment.
5. Which federal agency regulates the types of surgical hand soaps and scrubs that are used in the OR environment?
6. Once you graduate, what will you tell a new student about the basic hand wash?
7. Note here any questions you have that you need your instructor to clarify.

PEARSON
myhealthprofessionskit™

Use this address to access the Companion Website created for this textbook. Simply select "Surgical Technology" from the choice of disciplines. Find this book and log in using your username and password to access interactive activities, videos, and much more.

Don and Doff Personal Protective Equipment

3

INTRODUCTION

The Occupational Safety and Health Administration (OSHA) requires health care workers to protect themselves from potentially infectious or hazardous materials by wearing appropriate personal protective equipment, or PPE. In the operating room, PPE routinely includes the surgical scrub cap, face mask, eye protection, liquid-resistant gown, fluid-resistant shoe covers, and gloves. You will don a face mask and eye protection for this lab session.

- Before performing the following skill, your lab instructor will discuss some of the principles for practice and objectives involved in this chapter as well as the importance of following the skill sequence and instructions.

- Practice the skill with your lab partner. Encourage and critique each other. Appendix E highlights the value of teaching others as a component of active learning strategies. Refer to Appendix C for an overview of the chapter.
- The lab instructor will advise you of any additional criteria to be evaluated. At a designated time, demonstration of these skills will be evaluated and graded by your lab instructor using the competency assessment tool.
- When in the clinical setting, your instructor may once again assess your performance using the same tool. Refer to Appendix A for clinical evaluation and documentation.

Team Member	Type of Role		Timing		
	Nonsterile	Sterile	Preop	Intraop	Postop
Surgical Technologist	X		X	X	X
Assistant Circulator	X		X	X	X
Operating Room Team	X		X	X	X

OBJECTIVES

The learner will demonstrate the following skill with 100 percent accuracy each time when preparing to encounter potentially infectious or hazardous materials.

1. Select and don a face mask and eye protection as appropriate for the procedure and risk of exposure.

2. Remove the surgical face mask at the end of the procedure by grasping only the tie strings.
3. Select and use nonsterile gloves.
4. Remove gloves to prevent self-contamination.
5. Select and use case-specific protection against injury, such as wearing a lead apron to shield gamma radiation.

Principles for Practice

The foundation and rationale for our practice, in the perioperative environment, stem from evidence provided by professionals, organizations, and governmental agencies. Refer to the Bibliography, Glossary of Terms, and the following documents or developmental agencies:

- Manufacturers' product instructions
- Operating room policies
- Radiation safety officer guidelines
- Occupational Safety and Health Administration (OSHA)
- Centers for Disease Control and Prevention (CDC)
- Association of Surgical Technologists (AST)
- Association of periOperative Registered Nurses (AORN)

SKILL SEQUENCE AND INSTRUCTIONS

1. Select an appropriate surgical face mask and eye protection from the supply boxes. Prescription glasses used to correct vision are not acceptable eye protection.

   - Wear a mask and eye protection during invasive procedures when splashing or spraying of potentially hazardous fluid is possible, as required by OSHA for your protection against cross-contamination.
   - Wear a mask when in the restricted OR areas, including when standing at the scrub sink, opening sterile supplies, and entering designated center core areas (see Figure 3.1).

2. Don the mask by pinching the flexible nose band over the bridge of your nose.
   - Secure the upper ties behind your head (see Figure 3.2).

3. Fold and tuck lower edge of mask under your chin to cover your nose and mouth (see Figure 3.3).

4. Secure lower ties behind your head.
   - Prevent venting of the sides (gaps) of the mask. The mask must filter your exhaled breath to afford protection to the patient.
   - Practice wearing the mask for extended periods of time, as you will in the OR (see Figure 3.4).

5. Wear nonsterile disposable gloves for protection including:
   - When using cleaning supplies to wipe off surfaces in between procedures.
   - When handling potentially infectious or hazardous material, such as specimen containers or soiled linens.
   - When performing care on all patients (see Figures 3.5, 3.6, and 3.7).

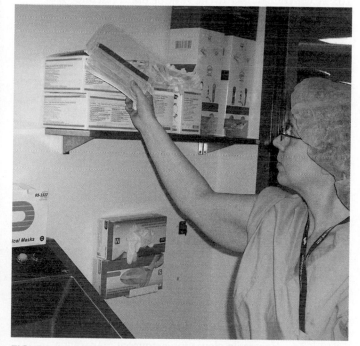

FIGURE 3.1   Select mask.

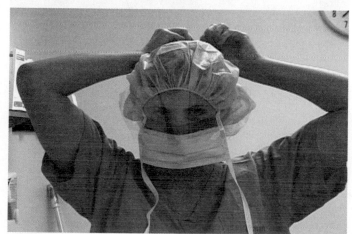

FIGURE 3.2   Secure upper ties.

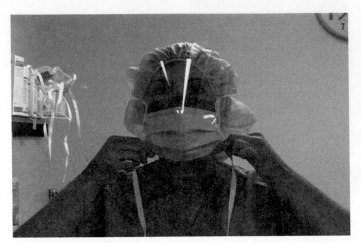

FIGURE 3.3 Secure under chin.

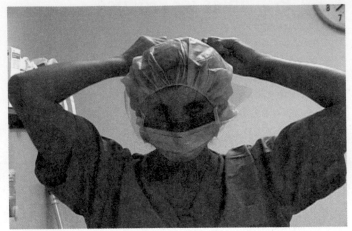

FIGURE 3.4 Secure lower ties.

6. Select and don additional appropriate protection.
   - Wear a protective lead apron and thyroid shield in the nonsterile or sterile role when radiography is used in the OR.
   - Secure an assigned dosimeter, or x-ray badge, to your scrub top sleeve, according to instructions from the laser safety officer. Store the dosimeter as designated. Do not take it home.
   - Wear attenuating gloves when assisting to position the patient during radiography, in a nonsterile role.
   - Wear special goggles to protect your retina from exposure during procedures where LASERS are in use (see Figure 3.8).

7. Remove gloves so that your skin does not touch the outer, used, or contaminated surfaces of the gloves.
   - Remove the gloves following the sequence of touching glove to glove, then touching skin to skin (see Figures 3.9 and 3.10).
8. Remove the face mask.
   - Grasp the mask by the tie strings for removal.
   - Do not touch the front, filter portion of the mask (see Figure 3.11).
9. Dispose of the mask in the proper trash receptacle (see Figure 3.12).
10. Wash your hands at the sink or use an alcohol-based product; follow manufacturer's instructions.

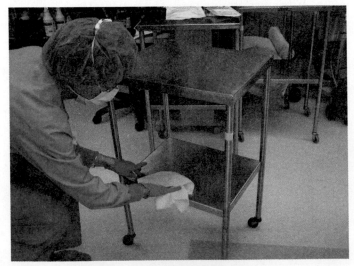

FIGURE 3.5 Nonsterile gloves for cleaning.

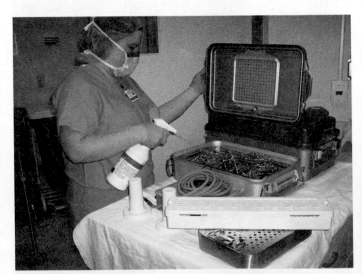

FIGURE 3.6 Nonsterile gloves for instrument preparation.

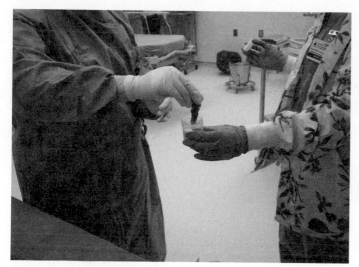

FIGURE 3.7 Nonsterile gloves, right.

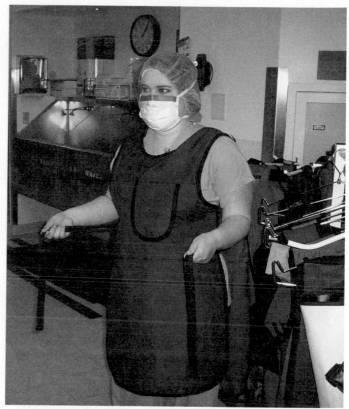

FIGURE 3.8 Lead apron protection.

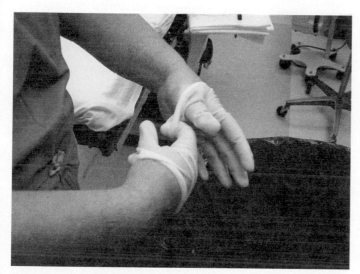

FIGURE 3.9 Touch "glove to glove."

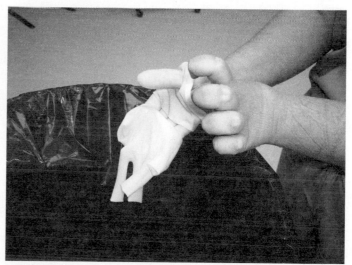

FIGURE 3.10 Touch "skin to skin."

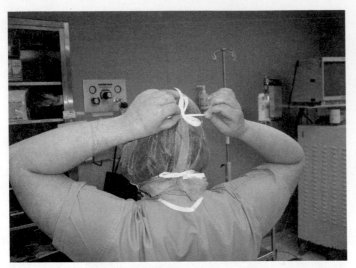

FIGURE 3.11 Remove (doff) mask by ties.

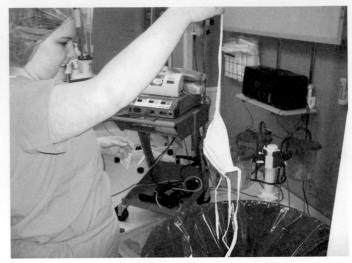

FIGURE 3.12 Dispose of mask.

COMPETENCY ASSESSMENT

STUDENT'S NAME: _____

CHAPTER 3 DON AND DOFF PERSONAL PROTECTIVE EQUIPMENT

PERFORMANCE RANK:

S or √ = Satisfactory: Competent—safe, accurate, sequential, and timely
U = Unsatisfactory: Unsafe—inaccurate and unprepared

PERFORMANCE RATING:

5   Independent: Expert—safe, confident, seamless performance; mentors others
4   Minimally monitored: Intermediate—safe, self-corrects, few errors
3   Competent: Novice—safe, revises with evaluator cues, few errors
2   Remedial: Unsafe—critical errors, unable to implement evaluator cues consistently
1   Dependent: Unsafe—unacceptable, requires multiple evaluator interventions

PERFORMANCE CRITERIA	Performance Rank	Performance Rating
1. Perform Mutual Professional and Scholastic Criteria as appropriate (see Preface or Appendix A).	N/A	1 2 3 4 5
2. State the conditions for donning the mask and eye protection.		1 2 3 4 ⑤
3. Select appropriate surgical facial mask.		1 2 3 4 ⑤
4. Don mask using appropriate technique, and enclose the mouth and nose.		1 2 3 4 ⑤
5. State conditions for donning nonsterile gloves.	cleaning/prep OK	1 2 3 4 ⑤
6. Select and don nonsterile gloves.		1 2 3 4 ⑤
7. Doff nonsterile gloves; prevent self-contamination and dispose.		1 2 3 4 ⑤
8. Remove the surgical mask; touch only the strings and dispose.		1 2 3 4 ⑤
9. Perform hand hygiene.		1 2 3 4 ⑤

ADDITIONAL COMMENTS _____

PERFORMANCE EVALUATIONS AND RECOMMENDATIONS

☑ PASS: Satisfactory Performance
    ☑ Demonstrates professionalism
    ☑ Exhibits critical thinking
    ☑ Demonstrates proficient clinical performance, appropriate for time in the program
☐ FAIL: Unsatisfactory Performance
    ☐ Critical criteria not met (see Performance Rank or Rating Above)
    ☐ Professionalism not demonstrated.
    ☐ Critical thinking skills not demonstrated.
    ☐ Skill performance unsafe or underdeveloped.
☐ REMEDIATION:
    ☐ Schedule lab practice. Date: _____
    ☐ Reevaluate by instructor. Date: _____
☐ DISMISS from lab or clinicals today.
☐ Program director notified. Date: _____

45/45

SIGNATURES

Date 9 8 13   Evaluator _____   Student _____

ACTIVITIES AND DISCUSSION QUESTIONS

Activities

1. View the Complete Perioperative Process and Focus on Skills video, Skill #3 (video can be found at www.myhealthprofessionskit.com).
2. Observe the instructor perform the skill.
3. Practice the skill in the lab, with your lab partner or in small groups.
4. Select one skill, teach a classmate, and observe and critique the performance.
5. Refer to your ST textbook and this lab manual to answer the Discussion Questions (see next column).
6. Review the video and the information in this lab manual when you prepare for your certification examination.

Discussion Questions

1. When must you wear a face mask in the perioperative environment?
2. Can you give an example of when the face mask could be used outside of the OR environment?
3. Which federal agency advocates the use of face masks as personal protective equipment (PPE)?
4. Name the step that is considered the most important when donning the surgical face mask, and state why.
5. State why only the ties are handled when removing the mask.
6. When do you wear nonsterile gloves in the perioperative setting?
7. How do you remove the gloves after use?
8. Even though not useful in protecting against the transmission of communicable diseases, can you give an example of a protective device that protects the health care worker from injury?
9. Once you graduate, what will you tell a new student about the importance of using PPE throughout the day?
10. Note here any questions that you need your instructor to clarify.

4 Open Sterile Supplies

INTRODUCTION

Creating and maintaining a sterile field for each patient are critical components of aseptic technique and preventing surgical site infections.

- Before performing the following skill, your lab instructor will discuss some of the principles for practice and objectives involved in this chapter as well as the importance of following the skill sequence and instructions.
- Practice opening sterile supplies for a laparotomy procedure with your lab partner. Encourage and critique each other. Your instructor will offer strategies for success. Appendix E highlights the value of teaching others as a component of active learning strategies. Refer to Appendix C for an overview of the chapter.
- Use a timer as a guide to gauge improvement in efficiency. The lab instructor will advise you of any additional criteria to be evaluated. At a designated time, demonstration of this skill will be evaluated and graded by your lab instructor using the competency assessment tool.
- When in the clinical setting, your instructor may once again assess your performance using the same tool. Refer to Appendix A for clinical evaluation and documentation.

Team Member	Type of Role		Timing		
	Nonsterile	Sterile	Preop	Intraop	Postop
Surgical Technologist	X		X		
Assistant Circulator	X		X	X	
Operating Room Team	X		X		

OBJECTIVES

The learner will demonstrate the following skill set using aseptic technique with 100 percent accuracy each time sterile supplies, equipment, and instruments are opened.

1. Define aseptic technique.
2. Define a surgical conscience.
3. Use the surgeon's preference card to gather supplies and equipment for a selected procedure.
4. Introduce self to team members.
5. Arrange OR furniture to promote a safe traffic pattern.
6. Inspect and open plastic dust covers on packs.
7. Open the back table and basin packs.
8. Inspect and open envelope-style packs.
9. Inspect and open peel packs.
10. Inspect and open irregularly shaped supplies.
11. Inspect and prepare own gown pack and gloves.
12. Inspect and open instrument trays, or container systems.

Principles for Practice

The foundation and rationale for our practice, in the perioperative environment, stem from evidence provided by professionals, organizations, and governmental agencies. Refer to the Bibliography, Glossary of Terms, and the following documents or developmental agencies:

- Manufacturer's product instructions
- Operating room policies
- Surgeon's preference card

- The Surgical Care Improvement Project (SCIP)
- Federal Drug Administration (FDA)
- Centers for Disease Control and Prevention (CDC)
- Association for the Advancement of Medical Instrumentation (AAMI)
- Association of Surgical Technologists (AST)
- Association of periOperative Registered Nurses (AORN)

SKILL SEQUENCE AND INSTRUCTIONS

1. Observe and demonstrate all principles of aseptic technique.

    - Establish a new sterile field for each patient.
    - Refer to AST and AORN for a complete listing of principles and recommended practices.
    - A summary includes the following:

        ○ Establish, maintain, and monitor the sterile field, using approved methods.
        ○ Cover all nonsterile equipment, the patient, and all team members to be included in the sterile field with sterile drapes and in sterile attire.
        ○ Introduce only sterile items onto the sterile field.

2. Work collaboratively with the OR team to prepare the room by performing the following:

    - Apply a "surgical conscience" or moral compass to your practice. Refer to the Glossary of Terms.
    - Perform a basic hand wash and don appropriate OR attire and PPE. Refer to Chapters 1 through 3.
    - Introduce yourself and your role.
    - Damp dust or disinfect all equipment and flat surfaces in the room.
    - Rearrange furniture to support a safe traffic pattern, and bring any additional furniture into the room.
    - Arrange the back table, Mayo stand, prep stand, and ring stands so that sterile drapes can be opened with ease and without contamination (at least 1 foot from the wall).

    - Note the location of the OR door, and keep furniture to be draped away from the walkway.
    - Assess the function of the suction equipment.
    - Prepare the OR bed area for the patient according to the scheduled procedure, and arrange positioning aids, padding, warming blankets, and poles for solutions. Refer to Chapter 24.

3. Verify that the room may be prepared, or opened, by validating the in-house presence of the patient and the surgeon.

    - Obtain, sort, and open sterile supplies based on the surgeon's preference card, checking expiration dates for packs containing solutions, ointments, or degradable ingredients.
    - Inspect the integrity of all packages; sterility is event related. Refer to instruction 4.
    - Respect the environment and contain costs: follow OR policy regarding reserving selected items to be opened by the circulator later in the procedure (see Figures 4.1 and 4.2).

4. Inspect the plastic dust cover of the unopened back table pack for holes, tears, or moisture: these are considered to be the result of an "event" rendering the pack nonsterile. If any of those conditions are present, discard the pack. If the pack is secure, discard the cover and place the pack onto the back table (see Figure 4.3).

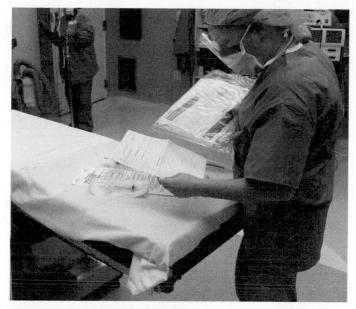

FIGURE 4.1 Preference card guide.

5. Orient then open the back table pack (see Figures 4.4 and 4.5).

- Tear open the tape seal and unfold the first flap of the drape away from you.
- Continue to unfold and grasp only the outer 1-inch margins of the drape.
- Cover the table top and cascade the drape over the sides. Do not reorient the drape once it has been opened.
- Work inside the 1-inch margins only when you are in the sterile role. Refer to Chapter 7.

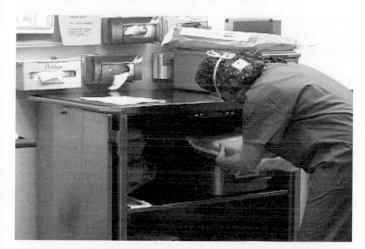

FIGURE 4.2 Case cart storage system.

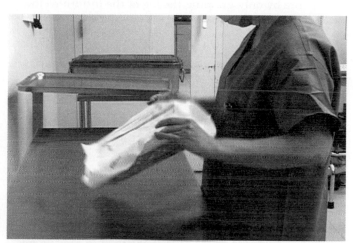

FIGURE 4.3 Inspect back table pack.

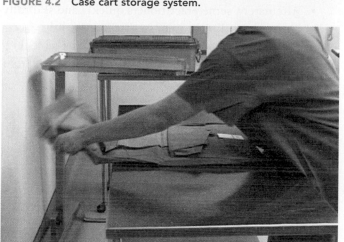

FIGURE 4.4 Unfold the drape.

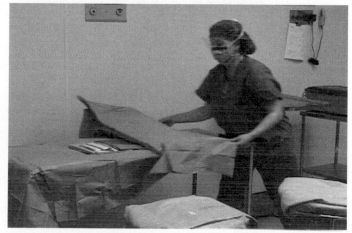

FIGURE 4.5 Sterile boundary; grasp 1-inch edge.

6. Open the ring stand basin cover using the same concepts. Inspect the integrity of the wrapper.

   - Observe the sterilization indicator tape for a color change indicating that the sterilization parameters have been met.
   - Nonsterile hands may only touch what will become the underside of the cover.
   - Open the first flap away from the body and the remaining three flaps using aseptic technique.
   - Once the drape edges have dropped below table level, they are no longer considered to be sterile. The inner contents are sterile.
   - Place the ring stand near the back table by grasping only the exposed metal leg under the drape. Do not lean over the basin.
   - Do not walk in between draped, sterile tables in your nonsterile attire.
   - A nonsterile team member may move draped furniture by only grasping the leg of the furniture close to the floor (see Figure 4.6).

7. Open the instrument pan pack, which is wrapped like an envelope.

   - Validate the indicator tape on the outside of the pack for a color change which indicates that the pack has undergone the sterilization process.
   - Assess for holes, tears, or moisture: if found, the pack may not be used.
   - Position the pack in your hands so that when you begin to open it, the first flap can be lifted out and away from your body (see Figure 4.7).
   - Lift the first flap out and away from your body. Carefully secure the tails of the flaps so they do not spring back onto the sterile area and contaminate it (see Figure 4.8).
   - Open the two side flaps sequentially, and grasp the tails in the palm of your nondominant hand.
   - Do not move your nonsterile arm over the sterile contents. (see Figure 4.9).
   - Grasp the edge of the fourth flap and pull it towards you. Secure it in your nondominant hand.
   - Make sure you have control and that there are no hanging wrapper edges or indicator strips (see Figure 4.10).

8. Place the sterile, small instrument pan onto the edge of the back table. If it is tossed, it may tear the back table drape and, therefore, contaminate it.

   - Maintain a 12-inch or greater distance from the back table (see Figure 4.11).
   - As an alternative, the circulator may open and present the pack at a later time to the ST in sterile attire; the ST can remove and transfer the inner sterile item to the sterile field. Refer to the companion website and Figure 4.16.

9. Add supplementary items to the sterile field. The primary sterile field is the back table cover. As an additional sterile area, a basin in the ring stand can be used to hold smaller sterile items.

   - Inspect peel packs and pouches for sterile processing indicators and for package integrity.
   - Add items in peel pouches to the field in such a way that the inner item remains sterile. The item cannot slide out over the opened edge, which is considered to be contaminated.
   - Grasp the package between your thumbs and forefingers and separate by pulling the edges apart approximately halfway down the package. Use a rolling motion to cuff the edges over your fingers and hands.
   - Remember to control the edges first; then, present the item onto the sterile field. If you do not have control, the item may become contaminated. The peel pack can act as a barrier as the sterile item is presented onto the field. Maintain at least a 12-inch distance from the field. This method is the "peel and shield" (see Figure 4.12).
   - Alternately, some practitioners quickly and skillfully pop, toss, or flip the item so that it is slightly airborne before it lands on the sterile back table or ring stand. Maintain at least a 12-inch distance from the field. This method is the "peel and pop" (see Figures 4.13 and 4.14).
   - AST and AORN guidelines instruct practitioners to present items onto the sterile field without contamination.

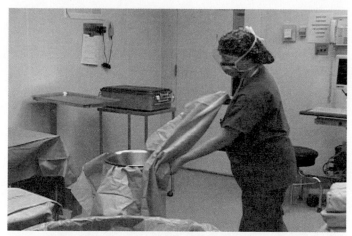
FIGURE 4.6 Open sterile basin pack in the ring stand.

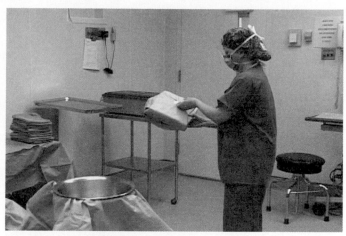
FIGURE 4.7 Assess indicator tape.

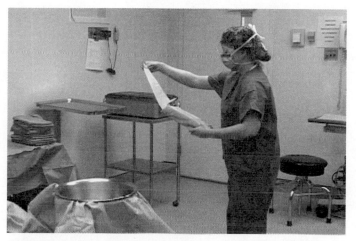
FIGURE 4.8 Open first flap away.

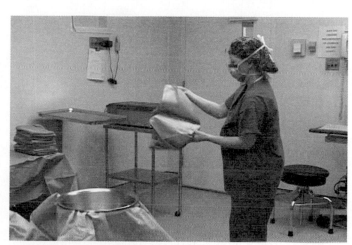
FIGURE 4.9 Sequentially open.

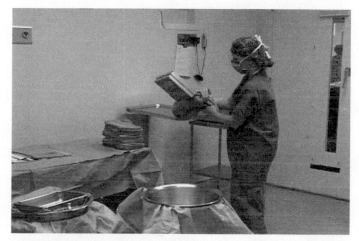
FIGURE 4.10 Contain wrap.

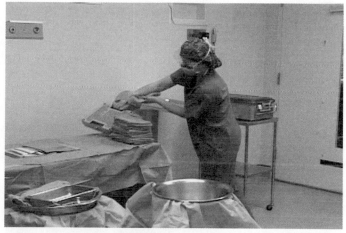
FIGURE 4.11 Place small pan.

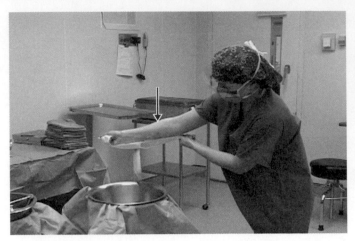

FIGURE 4.12 "Peel and shield" method.

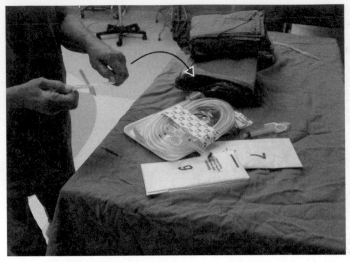

FIGURE 4.13 "Peel and pop" hypo.

10. Open light items in an envelope-style wrap sequentially and securely.

   - Maneuver or place the item inside onto the back table. Do not touch it with nonsterile hands.
   - Follow the facility's standard of practice regarding how items are introduced onto the sterile back table.
   - Select and open the surgeon's and surgical assistant's gowns and gloves onto the back table. Use the preference card as a guide.
   - The team member in Figure 4.15 is at least 1-foot from the field, and tosses the green OR towels onto the field while securely holding the blue wrap, which does not touch the sterile field. Aseptic technique is maintained (see Figure 4.15).

11. Open heavy items on a separate surface, preoperatively, and retrieve later when in sterile attire. The nonsterile team member may open irregularly shaped items and present them to the sterile team member.

   - Do not drop heavy or irregularly shaped items onto the back table because they may tear the back table cover and destroy its integrity (see Figure 4.16).

12. Prepare a sterile field for your own gown and gloves preoperatively on a bare Mayo stand using the gown and towel pack.

   - Inspect the gown pack; open and discard the dust cover.
   - Orient the pack so that the first flap will open away from you.
   - Place the pack at the front edge of the Mayo stand to ensure complete coverage of this edge during the draping sequence.

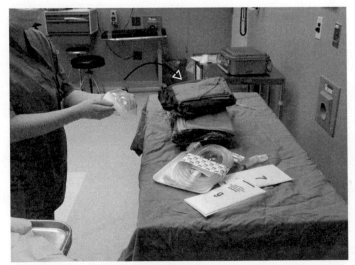

FIGURE 4.14 "Peel and pop" syringe.

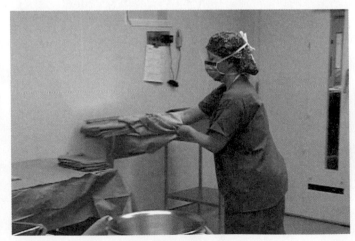

FIGURE 4.15 Toss light items in wrap.

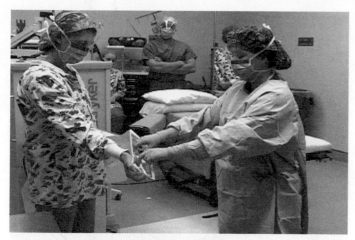
FIGURE 4.16 Grasp irregularly shaped item.

13. Open the gown and towel pack.
    - Open the first flap away from you (see Figure 4.17). Drape sizes vary among manufacturers. Compare Figure 4.17 with 4.22.
    - Open the second flap laterally, or to the left (see Figure 4.18).
    - Touch only the 1-inch margin of this drape while continuing to open and cover the Mayo stand.
    - Open the third flap laterally, or to the right (see Figure 4.19).
    - Use both hands to grasp and gently tug on the drape edges while preventing contamination of your sterile gown. The creases in this drape may cause the edges to return or spring back into the center, thereby contaminating your gown.

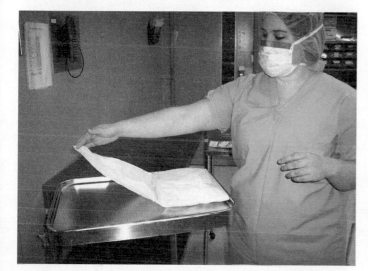
FIGURE 4.17 Orient and open first flap.

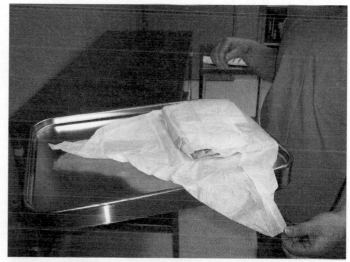
FIGURE 4.18 Open sides.

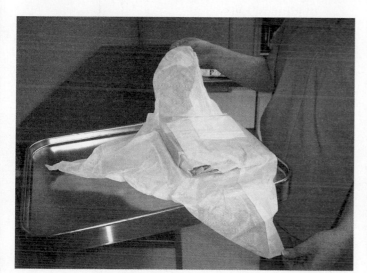
FIGURE 4.19 Control memory.

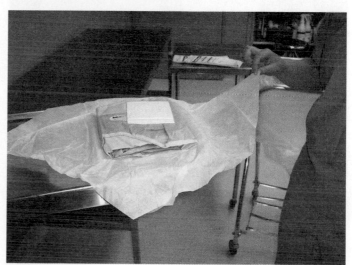
FIGURE 4.20 Open fourth flap.

- Open the fourth flap towards yourself (see Figure 4.20). Maintain at least a 12-inch distance from the open sterile drape.
- Evaluate coverage of the Mayo stand with the drape. Ask, "Can I place my sterile gloves here next? Can I gown and glove myself effectively from this surface?"

14. Select, open, and place gloves.

- Obtain two pairs of gloves according to your size preferences; sizes 6 through 9 are stocked on carts. Contact the facility's materials management department to obtain your size, if it is not on the OR cart.
- Inspect the glove package for integrity.
- Maintain a 12-inch distance, and dispense your sterile gloves onto the sterile field established on the Mayo stand. However, do not cover up your towel. You will need to reach the towel after you have performed the traditional surgical hand scrub.
- Peel open the pack, control the wrapper edges, then pop or flip the gloves onto the sterile field.
- Obtain a new package if the outer wrap tears or if the sterile gloves touch or slide over the open package edges.
- Place the smallest pair of gloves down first; follow with the pair one half-size larger.
- You will don the larger pair first, and it should be on the top (see Figures 4.21 and 4.22).

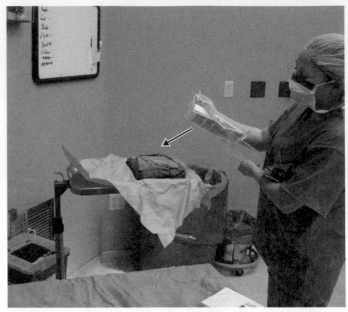

FIGURE 4.22   "Peel and shield" method.

15. Open the pan (container system) housing sterile instruments.

- Assess the integrity of the pan seals. Only use pans with intact seals.
- Remove and discard the pan seals (see Figure 4.23).
- Lift the lid up and away from the pan. Look inside the pan for moisture, or a visible sterilization indicator.
- Hold the lid away from the pan and assess the filters in the lid.
- The instruments may not be used in the following conditions:
  - moisture is present in the filters, lid, or tray
  - holes or tears appear in the filter
  - debris or hair is present on the instruments
- The nonsterile team member may not reach inside the instrument tray (see Figures 4.24 and 4.25).

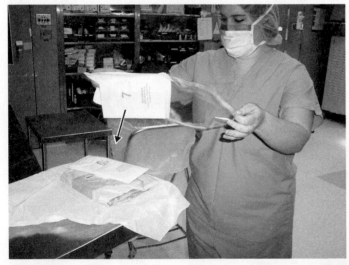

FIGURE 4.21   "Peel and pop" method.

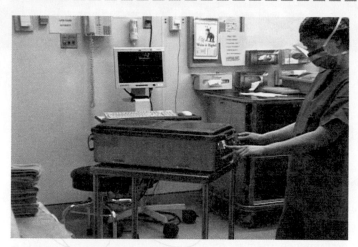

FIGURE 4.23 Assess tray seals.

16. The room has been prepared for the surgical procedure.
    • Inform the circulator that you are leaving the room to perform the surgical hand scrub. The circulator will meet the patient in the pre-op holding area. The anesthesia care provider and other OR staff members remain in the room preparing for their role in the procedure.

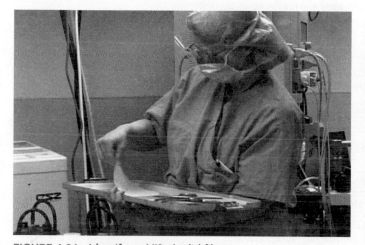

FIGURE 4.24 Identify and lift the lid filter.

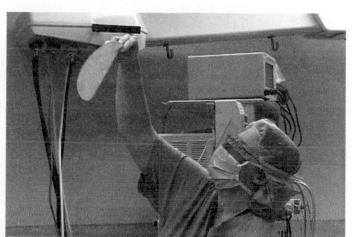

FIGURE 4.25 Assess the filter.

COMPETENCY ASSESSMENT

STUDENT'S NAME: _____

CHAPTER 4 OPEN STERILE SUPPLIES

PERFORMANCE RANK:

S or √ = Satisfactory: Competent—safe, accurate, sequential, and timely

U = Unsatisfactory: Unsafe—inaccurate and unprepared

PERFORMANCE RATING:

5   Independent: Expert—safe, confident, seamless performance; mentors others

4   Minimally monitored: Intermediate—safe, self-corrects, few errors

3   Competent: Novice—safe, revises with evaluator cues, few errors

2   Remedial: Unsafe—critical errors, unable to implement evaluator cues consistently

1   Dependent: Unsafe—unacceptable, requires multiple evaluator interventions

PERFORMANCE CRITERIA	Performance Rank	Performance Rating
1. Perform Mutual Professional and Scholastic Criteria as appropriate (see Preface or Appendix A).		1 2 3 4 (5)
2. Introduce self and role to OR staff.		1 2 3 4 (5)
3. Assess the surgeon's preference card; select and arrange equipment and furniture.		1 2 3 4 (5)
4. Inspect and open back table packs; use aseptic technique.		1 2 3 4 (5)
5. Inspect and open ring stand basin pack; use aseptic technique.		1 2 3 4 (5)
6. Inspect and open envelope-style wrapped items onto the sterile field; use aseptic technique.		1 2 3 4 (5)
7. Inspect and open peel-packaged items onto the sterile field; use aseptic technique.		1 2 3 4 (5)
8. Inspect and open large or heavy sterile, wrapped items. Open on a separate flat surface, such as a prep table; use aseptic technique.		1 2 3 4 (5)
9. Inspect and open own envelope-style wrapped gown onto the Mayo stand; use aseptic technique.	*remember grab flap & longer*	1 (2) 3 4 (5)
10. Inspect and open own glove packages onto the Mayo stand within the established sterile field; use aseptic technique.		1 2 3 4 (5)
11. Inspect outer pan, remove seals, and open instrument tray lid; lift lid away from tray; verify lid filters; place lid in designated nonsterile location; use aseptic technique.	*not over field* *sterile*	1 2 3 4 (5)

ADDITIONAL COMMENTS _____

PERFORMANCE EVALUATIONS AND RECOMMENDATIONS

☑ PASS: Satisfactory Performance

     ❑ Demonstrates professionalism

     ❑ Exhibits critical thinking

     ❑ Demonstrates proficient clinical performance appropriate for time in the program

❑ FAIL: Unsatisfactory Performance

     ❑ Critical criteria not met (see Performance Rank or Rating above)

     ❑ Professionalism not demonstrated.

❑ Critical thinking skills not demonstrated.

❑ Skill performance unsafe or underdeveloped.

❑ REMEDIATION:

❑ Schedule lab practice. Date: _____

❑ Reevaluate by instructor. Date: _____

❑ DISMISS from lab or clinicals today.

❑ Program director notified. Date: _____

SIGNATURES

Date _____   Evaluator _____   Student _____

ACTIVITIES AND DISCUSSION QUESTIONS

Activities

1. View the Complete Perioperative Process and Focus on Skills video, Skill #4 (video can be found at www.myhealthprofessionskit.com).
2. Observe the instructor perform the skill.
3. Practice the skill in the lab, with your lab partner or in small groups.
4. Select one skill, teach a classmate, and observe and critique the performance.
5. Select four or five aseptic technique errors, demonstrate them to your lab partner, and ask your partner to identify the errors. Discuss methods to prevent and correct the errors.
6. Refer to your ST textbook and this lab manual to answer the Discussion Questions (see next column).
7. Review the video and the information in this lab manual when you prepare for your certification examination.

Discussion Questions

1. Name at least two critical preparatory steps that you will take before opening a back table pack.
2. When opening the back table pack, how do you know where to begin?
3. Name at least two critical steps that you must take when opening the envelope style wrapper.
4. How do you gain control of the peel pack before introducing the sterile item onto the sterile field?
5. Name at least two visual indications of package integrity that are assessed externally before opening any pack.
6. Explain why debris or hair found in a sealed instrument tray will render the tray not sterile.
7. Note here any questions that you need your instructor to clarify.

5

Perform Surgical Hand Scrub

INTRODUCTION

The surgical hand scrub is a foundational aseptic technique skill, and it bridges the nonsterile and sterile roles. This scrub is effective in reducing the microbial colony count on the hands and forearms of the surgical team. Performed before donning the sterile gown and gloves, the hand scrub adds another layer of protection and decreases the risk of surgical site infections.

- Before performing the following skill, your lab instructor will discuss some of the principles for practice and objectives involved in this chapter as well as the importance of following the skill sequence and instructions.
- Practice the counted brush-stroke method and the waterless scrub method with your lab partner.

Encourage and critique each other. Your instructor will offer strategies for success. Appendix E highlights the value of teaching others as a component of active learning strategies. Refer to Appendix C for an overview of the chapter.

- Use a timer to gauge improvement in your efficiency. The lab instructor will advise you of any additional criteria to be evaluated. At a designated time, demonstration of this skill will be evaluated and graded by your lab instructor using the competency assessment tool.
- When in the clinical setting, your instructor may once again assess your performance using the same tool. Refer to Appendix A for clinical evaluation and documentation.

Team Member	Type of Role		Timing		
	Nonsterile	Sterile	Preop	Intraop	Postop
Surgical Technologist		X	X		
Assistant Circulator					
Operating Room Team		X	X		

OBJECTIVES

The learner will demonstrate the following with 100 percent accuracy each time performing the surgical hand scrub:

1. Present intact skin on hands, forearms, and cuticles; fingernails will be natural, short, and polish-free.
2. Present hands and arms, free of rings, watches, and bracelets.

 Principles for Practice

The foundation and rationale for our practice, in the peri-operative environment, stem from evidence provided by professionals, organizations, and governmental agencies. Refer to the Bibliography, Glossary of Terms, and the following documents or developmental agencies:

3. Perform a basic hand wash, or prewash.
4. Perform the counted brush-stroke method or timed method. (The counted-brush stroke method is used in this skill.)
5. State the appropriate corrective action due to a contamination error.
6. Perform a waterless surgical hand scrub.

- Manufacturers' product instructions
- Operating room policies
- Food and Drug Administration (FDA)
- Centers for Disease Control and Prevention (CDC)
- Association of Surgical Technologists (AST)
- Association of periOperative Registered Nurses (AORN)

SKILL SEQUENCE AND INSTRUCTIONS

1. Perform preparatory steps.

   - Inspect your hands and arms for cuts, abrasions, or weeping dermatitis. Poor skin integrity and fresh tattoos will prevent you from scrubbing and working in a surgical case. You may be given an alternative assignment or may be asked to go home until your skin is intact, based on hospital policy. Refer to Chapters 1 and 2.
   - Prepare your OR attire. Roll up your sleeves, and adjust your OR attire for comfort.
   - Don a face mask and eye protection before beginning the surgical hand scrub. Refer to Chapter 3.
   - Wash your hands and forearms, or perform a prewash. Refer to Chapter 2 (see also Figures 5.1 and 5.2).

2. Select a scrub brush packet and nail pick (see Figure 5.3).

3. Clean under your nails.

   - Open the packet and retrieve the fingernail pick.
   - Turn on the warm water. Stand approximately 6 inches away from the sink to keep your attire dry.
   - Run the fingernail pick under each nail while holding your nails under running water to remove debris.
   - Discard the used nail pick in the trash receptacle. Do not drop it into the sink (see Figures 5.4 and 5.5).

4. Begin the scrub starting at the nail tips.

   - Retrieve the sponge brush, discard the wrapper, and begin to scrub your fingernail tips using the bristle side of the sponge.
   - Use 30 strokes over the fingernails of one hand and repeat with the second hand.
   - Each stroke is one back and forth motion. Keep your hands slightly elevated to prevent water or soap from flowing toward your hands (see Figures 5.6 and 5.7).

5. Scrub the fingers, hands, and then the arms by anatomical divisions.

   - Use the sponge side of the brush, and scrub one hand and arm before moving to the next.
   - Use a circular motion when scrubbing your hands and arms.
   - Visually divide the fingers, hands, and forearms into four planes each.
   - Scrub each plane 10 times. Each back and forth motion over the plane is one count.
   - Scrub the web spaces between the fingers with 10 strokes, also.
   - Carefully include the most frequently missed areas during scrubbing: the thumb of the dominant hand, the backs of the hands, the fingertips, and the inner webs.

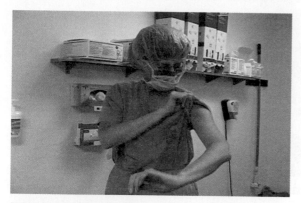

FIGURE 5.1 Prepare.

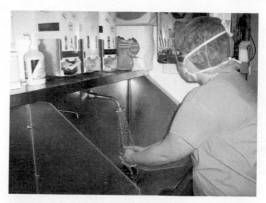

FIGURE 5.2 Perform prewash.

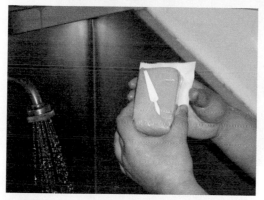

FIGURE 5.3 Select packet and nail pick.

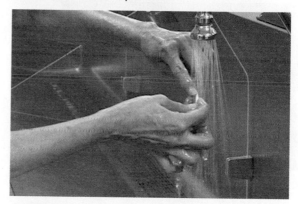

FIGURE 5.4 Clean under running water.

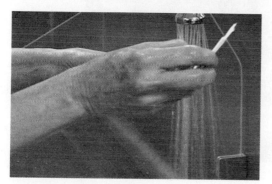

FIGURE 5.5 Discard nail pick.

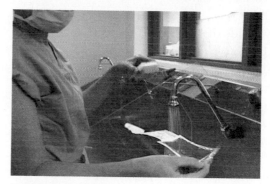

FIGURE 5.6 Retrieve sponge and discard wrapper.

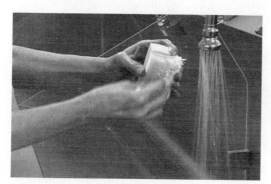

FIGURE 5.7 Scrub fingernails.

6. Scrub all fingers and the web spaces on the first hand with 10 strokes each.

   • Rewet the brush, as needed, to increase the amount of suds.

   • Do not rinse your hands at this time (see Figures 5.8 and 5.9).

7. Scrub the four planes on the hand.

   • Scrub each plane with 10 strokes each.

   • Do not touch the faucet, dividers, or other surfaces. If you do, you must begin the scrub over.

   • Keep fingers pointed upwards (see Figure 5.10).

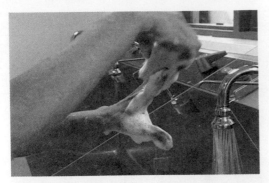

FIGURE 5.8 Scrub fingers.

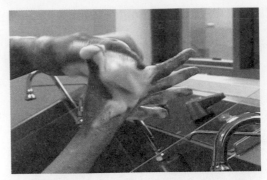

FIGURE 5.9 Scrub web spaces.

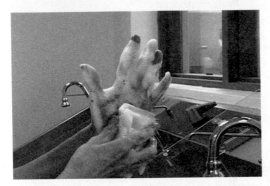

FIGURE 5.10 Scrub four planes or surfaces.

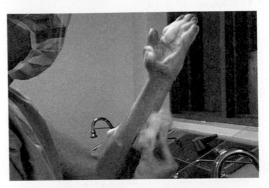

FIGURE 5.11 Scrub arm by sections.

8. Scrub the arm.

- Visually divide the arm into three sections. Each section has four planes, or surfaces.
- The first section on the arm is approximately the wrist area.
- The second section is the mid-forearm.
- The final section covers the arm up to two inches above the elbow.
- Rewet the brush as needed to revitalize the suds.
- Continue to keep the hand pointed upward and away from the faucet, and scrub each plane. Work distally to proximally.
- Larger-sized students may need to divide their arms into more planes to scrub all skin surfaces (see Figures 5.11 through 5.13).

9. Scrub your second hand and arm.

- Continue to use the sponge side of the brush.
- Move distally to proximally.
- Repeat the steps listed above for your second arm.

10. Dispose of the used scrub brush into the trash receptacle. Hold your hand at or above waist level as you discard the brush (see Figure 5.14).

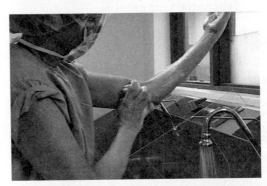

FIGURE 5.12 Scrub through two inches above the elbow.

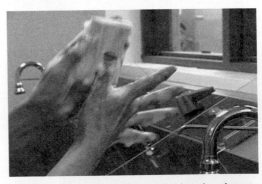

FIGURE 5.13 Repeat for second hand and arm.

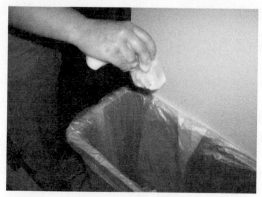

FIGURE 5.14   Dispose of brush.

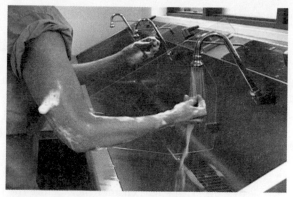

FIGURE 5.15   Rinse.

11. Rinse your hands and arms. Point hands upwards, and begin to rinse thoroughly one hand and arm.

- Use a scooping motion. Pass your fingers and hand under the water, then rinse your arm. Move slowly as the water rinses off the soap suds.
- Do not move your arm in a back and forth motion under the water. Only move forward.
- Your scrub attire should remain dry.
- Repeat the process with your opposite hand and arm.
- Hold your hands pointing upward, and allow the water to drip off of your elbows (see Figures 5.15 and 5.16).

12. Elevate your arms and hands in front of you.

- Hold your arms away from your OR attire as you walk to the OR.
- Open the door with your back or with a foot-operated device.
- Proceed to your Mayo stand where your sterile field is ready with your towel, gown, and gloves (see Figure 5.17).

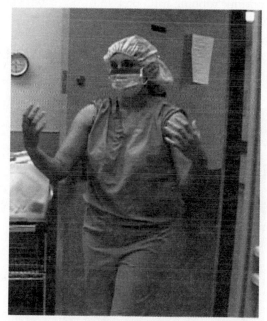

FIGURE 5.17   Keep hands within view.

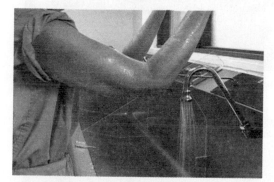

FIGURE 5.16   Allow water to drip into sink.

WATERLESS SURGICAL HAND SCRUB

1. Follow the manufacturer's recommendations for use. Containers of the solution are wall mounted, and instructions for use are on the container or posted nearby for reference. Sample instructions include the following steps:

   - Apply to clean, dry hands, and do not rinse off.
   - Clean nails with a nail cleaner/pick before the first case of the day.
   - Pump #1: Dispense about 2 ml of antiseptic hand prep into the palm of one hand.
   - Dip fingernails of the opposite hand into the hand prep and work it over the hand and up the arm to two inches above the elbow.
   - Pump #2: Dispense another 2 ml into the opposite palm, and repeat the procedure.
   - Pump #3: Dispense another 2 ml into either palm, and reapply to all aspects of both hands up to the wrist.
   - Continue rubbing hand prep into your hands until dry.
   - Walk into the OR.
   - When dry, don sterile gown and gloves.
   - Do not use a sterile towel to dry your hands and arms.

2. One suggestion for using the traditional and waterless hand scrubs instructs team members to perform a traditional hand scrub at the beginning of the shift, and again when returning from the lunchroom.

   - During the remainder of the shift, perform the waterless hand scrub before donning sterile attire (see Figures 5.18 through 5.21).

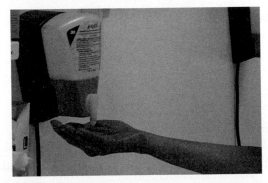

FIGURE 5.19 Pump into palm.

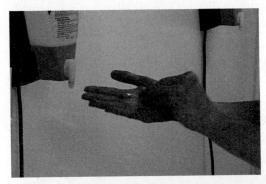

FIGURE 5.20 Rub fingers in scrub solution.

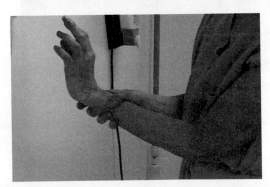

FIGURE 5.21 Rub solution to two inches above elbows.

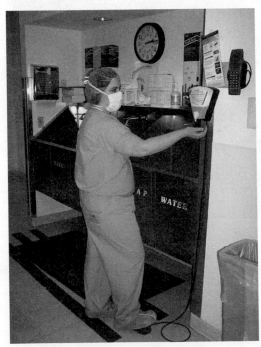

FIGURE 5.18 Waterless scrub solution.

COMPETENCY ASSESSMENT

STUDENT'S NAME: _____

CHAPTER 5 PERFORM SURGICAL HAND SCRUB

PERFORMANCE RANK:

S or √ = Satisfactory: Competent—safe, accurate, sequential, and timely
U = Unsatisfactory: Unsafe—inaccurate and unprepared

PERFORMANCE RATING:

5   Independent: Expert—safe, confident, seamless performance; mentors others
4   Minimally monitored: Intermediate—safe, self-corrects few errors
3   Competent: Novice—safe, revises with evaluator cues, few errors
2   Remedial: Unsafe—critical errors, unable to implement evaluator cues consistently
1   Dependent: Unsafe—unacceptable, requires multiple evaluator interventions

PERFORMANCE CRITERIA	Performance Rank	Performance Rating
1. Perform Mutual Professional and Scholastic Criteria as appropriate (see Preface or Appendix A).	N/A	1 2 3 4 5
2. State rationale for donning additional protective equipment, such as a lead apron and dosimeter badge. Refer to Chapter 3.		1 2 3 4 ⑤
3. Prepare scrub attire, don PPE- mask and eye protection.		1 2 3 4 ⑤
4. Collect supplies, open scrub brush packet, and secure its location.		1 2 3 4 ⑤
5. Regulate faucet water temperature and flow; stand at least 6 inches from sink.		1 2 3 4 ⑤
6. Perform basic hand wash, or prewash.		1 2 3 4 ⑤
7. Clean fingernails under running water with fingernail pick, and discard in trash.		1 2 3 4 ⑤
8. Grasp brush, discard package in trash, and wet the brush; rewet brush as needed throughout.		1 2 3 4 ⑤
9. Start time:_____ Use bristle side and scrub nails with 30 strokes on each hand.		1 2 3 4 ⑤
10. Switch to foam side and scrub using 10 strokes for each of the four planes of the hand, fingers, and web spaces.		1 2 3 4 ⑤
11. Scrub each of the four planes of the arm for each of the three arm sections; end the scrub two inches above elbow.		1 2 3 4 ⑤
12. Repeat scrub for the second hand and arm.		1 2 3 4 ⑤
13. Stop time:_____ Approximately 5 minutes.		1 2 3 4 ⑤
14. Correct self and begin the scrub again in the event of contamination.		1 2 3 4 ⑤
15. Discard the brush in the trash.		1 2 3 4 ⑤
16. Rinse each hand, arm, and elbow with a forward motion; begin with fingertips; maintain elevation of hands.		1 2 3 4 ⑤
17. Turn off water; do not contaminate the hands; allow water to drip from elbows into sink.		1 2 3 4 ⑤

PERFORMANCE CRITERIA	Performance Rank	Performance Rating
18. Proceed to OR with hands elevated, held between waist and chest level and away from the body.		1 2 3 4 ⑤
19. Open the OR door without contaminating hands and arms; proceed to Mayo stand.		1 2 3 4 ⑤
20. Perform waterless hand scrub per manufacturer's directions (perform as a separate skill, then repeat steps 18 and 19).		1 2 3 4 ⑤

ADDITIONAL COMMENTS _____

PERFORMANCE EVALUATIONS AND RECOMMENDATIONS

☑ PASS: Satisfactory Performance
    ☑ Demonstrates professionalism
    ☑ Exhibits critical thinking
    ☑ Demonstrates proficient clinical performance appropriate for time in the program

❏ FAIL: Unsatisfactory Performance
    ❏ Critical criteria not met (see Performance Rank or Rating above)
    ❏ Professionalism not demonstrated.
    ❏ Critical thinking skills not demonstrated.
    ❏ Skill performance unsafe or underdeveloped.

❏ REMEDIATION:
    ❏ Schedule lab practice. Date: _____
    ❏ Reevaluate by instructor. Date: _____

❏ DISMISS from lab or clinicals today.
❏ Program director notified. Date: _____

100/100

SIGNATURES

Date _9-3-13_   Evaluator _____   Student _____

ACTIVITIES AND DISCUSSION QUESTIONS

Activities

1. View the Complete Perioperative Process and Focus on Skills video, Skill #5 (video can be found at www.myhealthprofessionskit.com).
2. Observe the instructor perform the skill.
3. Practice the skill in the lab, with your lab partner or in small groups.
4. Select one skill, teach a classmate, and observe and critique the performance.
5. Select two contamination errors, demonstrate them to your lab partner, and ask your partner to identify the errors. Discuss methods to prevent and correct the errors.
6. Refer to your ST textbook and this lab manual to answer the Discussion Questions (see next column).
7. Review the video and the information in this lab manual when you prepare for your certification examination.

Discussion Questions

1. What is the rationale for performing the surgical hand scrub?
2. Which U.S. agency evaluates the efficacy of hand scrub solutions in their bactericidal or bacteristatic properties?
3. List the first two steps in performing the surgical hand scrub skill.
4. During the traditional scrub, what is the rationale for scrubbing the fingernails with 30 brush strokes but only using 10 strokes on the other surfaces of the hand and arm?
5. During the traditional surgical hand scrub, you touch the faucet. What should you do next?
6. You have completed the surgical hand scrub on your first hand and arm. Now, you remember that you did not don your eye goggles. What should you do next?
7. You have completed the waterless hand scrub, and you did not don a face mask; what should you do?
8. You are performing a traditional scrub at a three-bay sink. The person standing next to you states that they saw you touch the sink with your arm while rinsing off. What should you do next? What should you not do?
9. Review the information provided in this chapter. Imagine that you are now an employee. What will you tell a new ST student about the surgical hand scrub? About the waterless hand scrub?
10. Note here any questions that you need your instructor to clarify.

Gown and Glove Self— Closed-Gloving Method

6

INTRODUCTION

The fluid-resistant sterile gown and two pairs of sterile gloves provide barriers which protect the patient and the health care worker from blood-borne pathogens during invasive surgical procedures. In this chapter you will practice donning the gown and gloves that you set up in Chapter 4.

- Before performing the following skill, your lab instructor will discuss some of the principles for practice and objectives involved in this chapter as well as the importance of following the skill sequence and instructions.
- Use the closed-gloving method to don your gloves, and practice this skill frequently until your perfect it. Work with your lab partner. Encourage and critique each other. Your instructor will offer strategies for success. Appendix E highlights the value of teaching others as a component of active learning strategies. Refer to Appendix C for an overview of the chapter.
- The lab instructor will advise you of any additional criteria to be evaluated. At a designated time, demonstration of these skills will be evaluated and graded by your lab instructor using the competency assessment tool.
- When in the clinical setting, your instructor may once again assess your performance using the same tool. Refer to Appendix A for clinical evaluation and documentation.

Team Member	Type of Role		Timing		
	Nonsterile	Sterile	Preop	Intraop	Postop
Surgical Technologist		X	X		
Assistant Circulator					
Operating Room Team		X	X		

OBJECTIVES

The learner will demonstrate this skill with 100 percent accuracy each time entering the operating room:

1. Maintain aseptic technique when relating to the sterile field and supplies on the Mayo stand.
2. Dry hands and arms thoroughly by using the sterile towel upon completion of the traditional, water-surgical scrub.
3. Allow hands and arms to air-dry upon completion of the waterless scrub.
4. Don a sterile surgical gown.
5. Double glove using the closed-gloving method.

Principles for Practice

The foundation and rationale for our practice, in the perioperative environment, stem from evidence provided by professionals, organizations, and governmental agencies. Refer to the Bibliography, Glossary of Terms, and the following documents or developmental agencies:

- Manufacturers' product guidelines
- Operating room policies

- American College of Surgeons (ACS)
- American Association of Orthopedic Surgeons (AAOS)
- Occupational Safety and Health Administration (OSHA)
- Centers for Disease Control and Prevention (CDC)
- Association of Surgical Technologists (AST)
- Association of periOperative Registered Nurses (AORN)

SKILL SEQUENCE AND INSTRUCTIONS

1. Enter the OR suite.

   - Maintain the position of your scrubbed hands and arms between your waist and midchest level.
   - Keep hands and arms in front of you, with elbows bent and away from your face mask. Refer to Chapter 5.
   - Do not touch nonsterile surfaces.
   - Monitor the movement of other team members and avoid them (see Figure 6.1).

2. Approach the front of your Mayo stand.

   - Reach into your sterile field on the Mayo stand, and pinch up the drying towel by an exposed corner or central area only.
   - Do not drip water onto your gown or gloves, and do not touch them with your hand.
   - Move into an open area nearby, but away from the Mayo stand (see Figure 6.2).

3. Unfold the towel, and dry your hands and arms while keeping both hands elevated.

   - Hold the towel by the superior edge, and dry your opposite hand and arm.
   - Move the towel with a blotting motion as you proceed from your fingertips to your elbow.
   - Bend forward at the waist to increase the distance between your OR attire and the towel.
   - Do not touch the towel onto your top or pants.
   - Switch to the lower half of the towel, and dry your opposite hand and arm.
   - Drop the drying towel into a receptacle. Keep your hands elevated (see Figure 6.3).

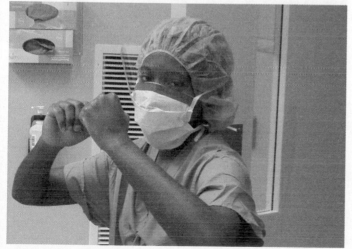

FIGURE 6.1   Enter OR.

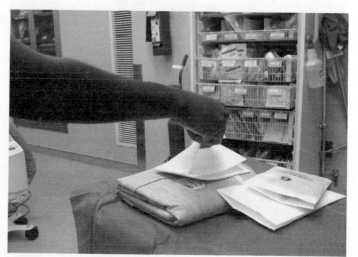

FIGURE 6.2   Lift towel in the center.

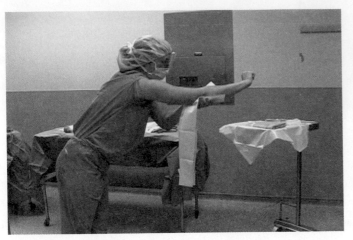

FIGURE 6.3   Blot dry.

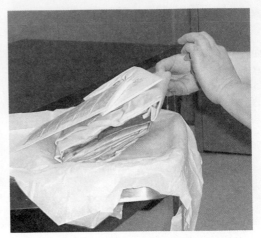

FIGURE 6.4   Grasp gown at neckline.

4. Return to the Mayo stand. Grasp the sterile gown at the neckline.

   - Step away from the field. Monitor your proximity to nonsterile surfaces and personnel traffic.
   - Do not touch nonsterile surfaces or personnel as you begin to don your gown.
   - If you drop the gown on the floor, ask your circulator for a new gown. Do not bend down to retrieve it (see Figure 6.4).

5. Slip each hand and arm into the sleeves of the gown.
   - Keep your hands and arms between your waist and the midchest area. Allow the gown to unfold.
   - Push your arms into the gown.
   - Do not allow your hands to protrude through the cuffed edges at this time (see Figures 6.5 through 6.7).

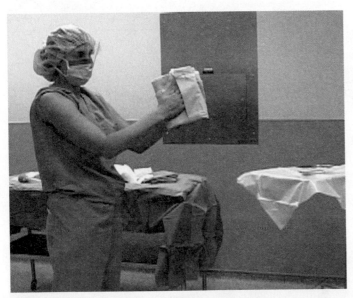

FIGURE 6.5   Slip hands into pockets.

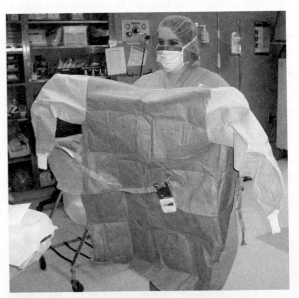

FIGURE 6.6   Unfold gown.

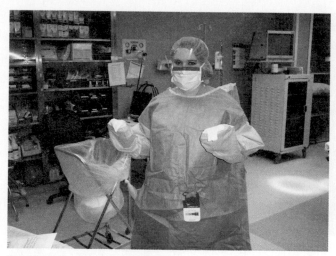

FIGURE 6.7 Slip into the gown.

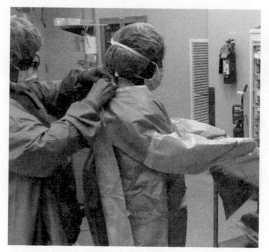

FIGURE 6.8 Circulator secures the back of your gown.

6. Perform closed-gloving.

- Return immediately to the Mayo stand, and begin to don your first pair of gloves.
- Simultaneously, the circulator or another nonsterile team member can begin to fasten the neck closure and ties in the back of the gown.
- Monitor your sterile boundaries (see Figure 6.8).

7. Open the wrapper on your first pair of gloves.

- Your hands will remain inside the gown sleeve and will be near the sleeve cuff.
- With your left hand, lift and position the right glove onto the palm of your right hand.
- For correct positioning, you can remember "palm to palm, thumb to thumb, and fingers facing you" while you are placing the glove into your outstretched hand, still under the gown sleeve (see Figures 6.9 through 6.12).

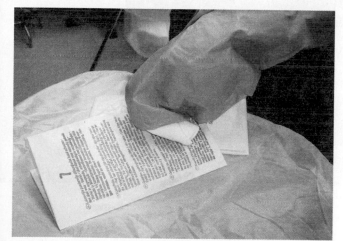

FIGURE 6.9 Open first glove package.

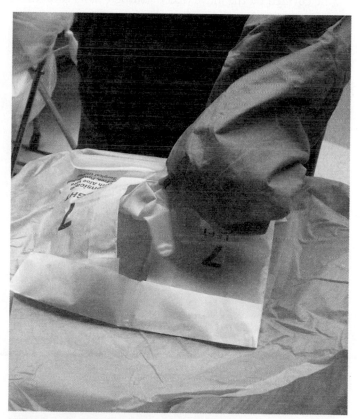

FIGURE 6.10 Grasp right glove with left "hand."

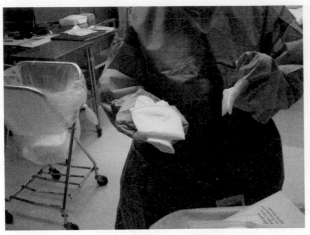

FIGURE 6.11 Position right glove with "palm to palm" and "fingers facing" yourself

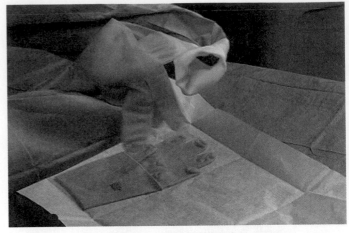

FIGURE 6.12 Grasp and stretch the right glove.

8. Stabilize the right glove.
   - Stretch and pull the glove over your sleeve cuff and hand. Push your right hand so that it emerges through the sleeve cuff into the sterile glove (see Figures 6.13 and 6.14).

9. Adjust the fit of the glove once it is in place on your right hand. The stockinet cuff on your gown must be covered by the glove. Keep your left hand covered under the sleeve and cuff at this time (see Figure 6.15).

10. Grasp the left glove with your gloved right hand, and remove it from the package on your Mayo stand.
    - Orient it as you did for the right glove.
    - Don your left glove and adjust.
    - Do not touch the stockinet cuff with the outer surface of your sterile gloves once your hands have emerged through the cuffs.
    - Pinch the sterile gloves at your wrist area if you need to adjust the fit over the sleeve cuffs (see Figures 6.16 through 6.19).

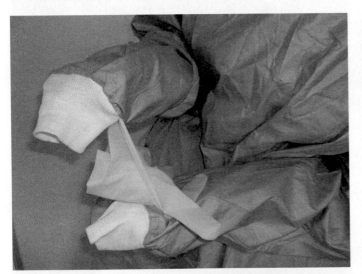

FIGURE 6.13 Secure and stretch the cuff edges of the glove.

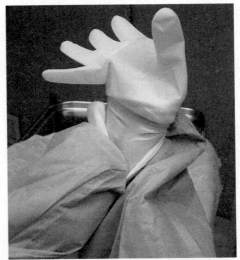

FIGURE 6.14 Stretch and pull on the glove.

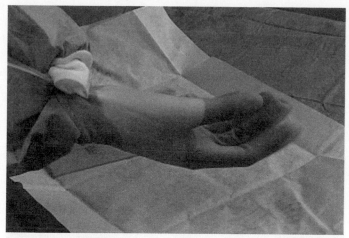

FIGURE 6.15   Adjust.

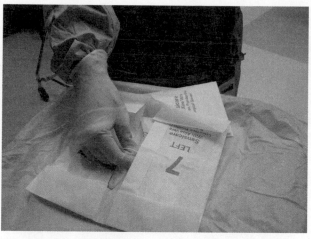

FIGURE 6.16   Grasp left glove.

11. Don the second, smaller pair of gloves, over the first. Team members may prefer the fit of two same-sized gloves.
   • Double gloving is recommended by professional organizations such as ACS, AAOS, AST, and AORN (see Figures 6.20 through 6.22).

12. Secure the gown tie around your waist.
   • Hold the proximal end of the waist tag in your right hand.
   • Pull the left end of the tie out of the tag, and hold it in your left hand.
   • Extend the distal end of the tag for a nonsterile team member to grasp (see Figures 6.23 and 6.24).

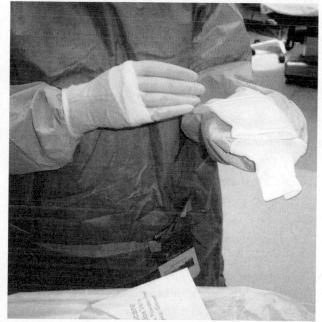

FIGURE 6.17   Position left.

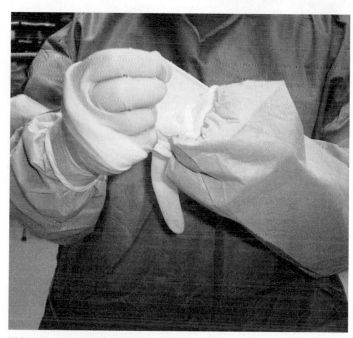

FIGURE 6.18   Pinch and stretch.

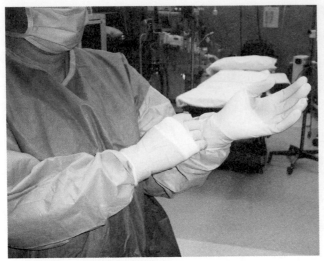

FIGURE 6.19 Sterile touches sterile.

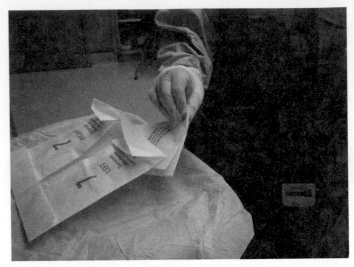

FIGURE 6.20 Grasp second pair.

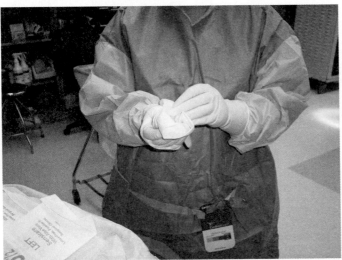

FIGURE 6.21 Don right.

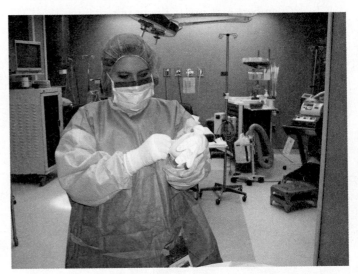

FIGURE 6.22 Don left.

13. The nonsterile team member will grasp the tagged tie and will walk around your back to your left side.

- Grasp the middle of the tie (now on your left side).
- Hold both ties as the team member pulls off the tag. The nonsterile team member will discard the tag.
- If you drop a tie, the nonsterile team member can tie them in the back of the gown for you, but must not touch the sterile areas on your gown.

14. Secure the two waist ties on your left. The process of turning and tying is called turning, or "dancing" (see Figure 6.25).

15. Maintain movement within the sterile boundaries, or zone, of your gown and work space. The sterile zone includes:

- The front of your gown from the waist to midchest (or tabletop height to midchest).
- Your sleeves up to two inches above your elbows.
- You may not touch your face mask, anywhere below your waist, the back of your gown, or any nonsterile surfaces (see Figures 6.26 through 6.28).

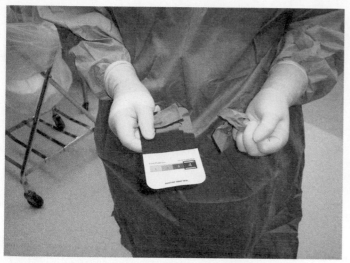

FIGURE 6.23 Hold tag in right hand, tie in left.

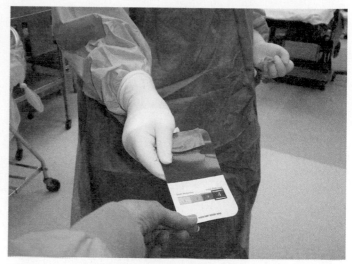

FIGURE 6.24 Tag divides sterile and nonsterile.

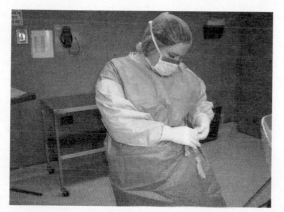

FIGURE 6.25 Secure tie.

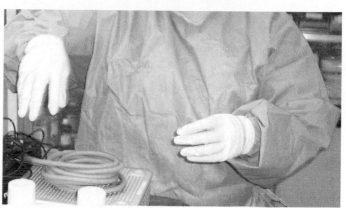

FIGURE 6.26 Sterile zone.

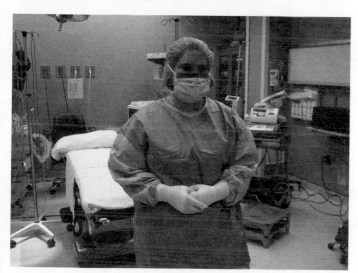

FIGURE 6.27 Sample acceptable hand position.

16. Removal of the gown wrapper on your Mayo stand will be performed by the circulator, or a nonscrubbed team member.
    • You are now gowned and gloved in sterile attire and may touch the sterile items on the back table. Your next task will be to cover the Mayo stand with a sterile drape found in your sterile, back table supplies (see Figure 6.29).

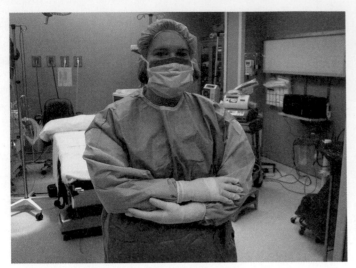

FIGURE 6.28   Hands held above waist.

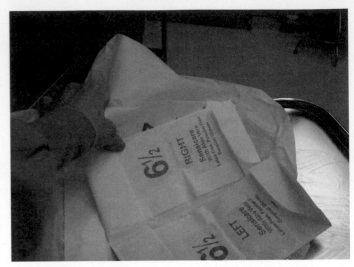

FIGURE 6.29   Nonsterile team member clears Mayo stand.

COMPETENCY ASSESSMENT

STUDENT'S NAME: _____

CHAPTER 6 GOWN AND GLOVE SELF— CLOSED-GLOVING METHOD

PERFORMANCE RANK:

S or √ = Satisfactory: Competent—safe, accurate, sequential, and timely
U = Unsatisfactory: Unsafe—inaccurate and unprepared

PERFORMANCE RATING:

5   Independent: Expert—safe, confident, seamless performance; mentors others
4   Minimally monitored: Intermediate—safe, self-corrects few errors
3   Competent: Novice—safe, revises with evaluator cues, few errors
2   Remedial: Unsafe—critical errors, unable to implement evaluator cues consistently
1   Dependent: Unsafe—unacceptable, requires multiple evaluator interventions

PERFORMANCE CRITERIA	Performance Rank	Performance Rating
1. Perform Mutual Professional and Scholastic Criteria as appropriate (see Preface or Appendix A).		1 2 3 4 ⑤
2. Approach the Mayo stand and retrieve drying towel; bend over at waist.		1 2 3 4 ⑤
3. Unfold towel held by superior edge.		1 2 3 4 ⑤
4. Dry first hand, arm, and elbow with blotting motion. *excellent drying technique*		1 2 3 4 ⑤
5. Switch towel to inferior edge and dry second side.		1 2 3 4 ⑤
6. Dispose of towel.		1 2 3 4 ⑤
7. Retrieve gown at neckline, orient it, allow it to unfold, and insert arms; keep hands inside sleeves.		1 2 3 4 ⑤
8. Retrieve right glove with your left hand; position and don it. *} handled glove a little much!*		1 2 ③ 4 5
9. Retrieve left glove with your right hand; position and don it.		1 2 ③ 4 5
10. Retrieve and don second pair of sterile gloves; adjust fit. *-- adjust much too much*		1 2 ③ 4 5
11. Prepare waist tag and tie; turn and tie with circulator.		1 2 3 ④ 5
12. Hold hands in sterile zone.		1 2 3 4 ⑤

ADDITIONAL COMMENTS <u>Be aware of how close unsterile things are</u>

PERFORMANCE EVALUATIONS AND RECOMMENDATIONS

❏ PASS: Satisfactory Performance
     ☑ Demonstrates professionalism
     ☑ Exhibits critical thinking
     ☑ Demonstrates proficient clinical performance appropriate for time in the program
❏ FAIL: Unsatisfactory Performance
     ❏ Critical criteria not met (see Performance Rank or Rating Above)
     ❏ Professionalism not demonstrated.
     ❏ Critical thinking skills not demonstrated.
     ❏ Skill performance unsafe or underdeveloped.

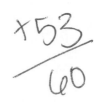

$\times 53$
$\overline{60}$

❑ REMEDIATION:
    ❑ Schedule lab practice. _____
    ❑ Reevaluate by instructor. Date: _____
❑ DISMISS from lab or clinicals today.
❑ Program director notified. Date: _____

SIGNATURES

Date _10/7/13_   Evaluator _E Bodnar_ /Student _____

ACTIVITIES AND DISCUSSION QUESTIONS

Activities

1. View the Complete Perioperative Process and Focus on Skills video, Skill #6 (video can be found at www.myhealthprofessionskit.com).
2. Observe the instructor perform the skill.
3. Practice the skill in the lab, with your lab partner or in small groups.
4. Select one skill, teach a classmate, and observe and critique the performance.
5. Select two or three possible contamination errors, demonstrate them to your lab partner, and ask your partner to identify the errors. Discuss methods to prevent and correct the errors.
6. Refer to your ST textbook and this lab manual to answer the Discussion Questions (see next column).
7. Review the video and the information in this lab manual when you prepare for your certification examination.

Discussion Questions

1. List the critical steps in performing this skill.
2. Define closed-gloving.
3. Compare closed-gloving with open-gloving. (You will need to look ahead in the lab manual to Chapter 15.)
4. What do you do to prevent contamination of the sterile drying towel? Name at least two tasks.
5. List two ways you can contaminate your gown when you are putting it on.
6. If you drop the waist ties below your waist level, how can they be tied?
7. What is the purpose of the fluid-resistant gown?
8. Why should someone else remove the wrappers (sterile field) from your Mayo stand?
9. Note here any questions that you need your instructor to clarify.

Drape Mayo Stand and Prepare Back Table

7

INTRODUCTION

Applying the concepts of aseptic technique continues in this chapter as you set up a back or instrument table and drape a Mayo stand.

- Before performing the following skill, your lab instructor will discuss some of the principles for practice and objectives involved in this chapter as well as the importance of following the skill sequence and instructions.
- Use one set-up sequence, and repeat it until you are confident and efficient. Work with your lab partner. Encourage and critique each other. Analyze any aseptic technique errors and correct them.
- Use a timer and streamline your performance. Your instructor will offer strategies for success.

Appendix E highlights the value of teaching others as a component of active learning strategies. Refer to Appendix C for an overview of the chapter.
- The lab instructor will advise you of any additional criteria to be evaluated, including a predetermined amount of time allotted to performing the skills in this chapter. At a designated time, demonstration of these skills will be evaluated and graded by your lab instructor using the competency assessment tool.
- When in the clinical setting, your instructor may once again assess your performance using the same tool. Refer to Appendix A for clinical evaluation and documentation.

Team Member	Type of Role		Timing		
	Nonsterile	Sterile	Preop	Intraop	Postop
Surgical Technologist		X	X		
Assistant Circulator					
Operating Room Team					

OBJECTIVES

The learner will demonstrate the following skills with 100 percent accuracy each time when entering the operating room:

1. Maintain aseptic technique.
2. Demonstrate movement in the sterile role.
3. Drape the Mayo stand.

4. Arrange supplies on the back table using economy of time and motion.
5. Verify and accept instruments onto the back table.
6. Organize items, and call for the count within a specified time frame.
7. Assemble a Balfour self-retaining retractor.

Principles for Practice

The foundation and rationale for our practice, in the peri-operative environment, stem from evidence provided by professionals, organizations, and governmental agencies. Refer to the Bibliography, Glossary of Terms, and the following documents or developmental agencies:

- Manufacturers' product instructions
- Operating room policies

- Surgeon's preference card
- Occupational Safety and Health Administration (OSHA)
- Centers for Disease Control and Prevention (CDC)
- Association of Surgical Technologists (AST)
- Association of periOperative Registered Nurses (AORN)

SKILL SEQUENCE AND INSTRUCTIONS

1. Demonstrate the principles of aseptic technique while draping your Mayo stand, setting up your back table, and when you navigate within the environment.

   - Respect sterile boundaries.
   - Correct all doubts of sterility at once.
   - Move furniture by only touching the top, horizontal surface with sterile gloves.

- Sterile gloved-hands may not go below the table level.
- Pass another sterile team member front to front or back to back. Sterile to sterile or nonsterile to nonsterile are the guiding principles.
- Do not turn your back and accidently touch the sterile field with the nonsterile back of your gown (see Figures 7.1 and 7.2).

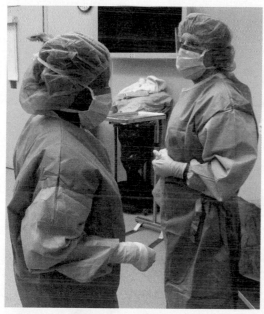

FIGURE 7.1 Pass front to front.

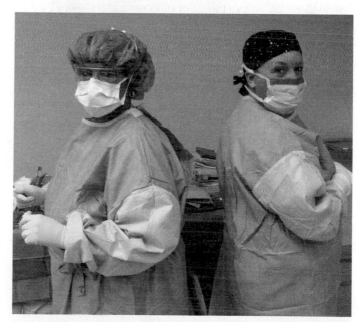

FIGURE 7.2 Pass back to back.

2. Identify and grasp the Mayo stand cover.
   - Hold it over the back table, and follow varying pre-printed instructions on the cover.
   - Prepare it for placement on your stand. Cuff your gloved hands within the drape to protect them from contamination (see Figures 7.3 and 7.4).

3. Maneuver the drape onto the stand.
   - Walk to the stand and steady the stand.
   - Protect your sterile gloves and gown from the nonsterile Mayo stand as you are draping it.
   - Feed or push the Mayo cover onto the stand.
   - Do not allow the unfolded drape to fall below table level.
   - Do not allow your gloved hands to drop below the surface of the stand (see Figures 7.5 through 7.7).

4. Prepare Mayo stand tray for use.
   - Tuck the excess Mayo cover under the side of the tray according to your OR's policy.
   - Place sterile towels over the Mayo stand to reinforce the drape (see Figures 7.8 and 7.9).

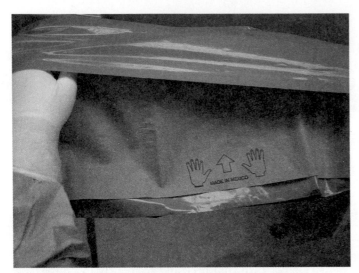

FIGURE 7.3 Follow printed illustrations on the Mayo drape.

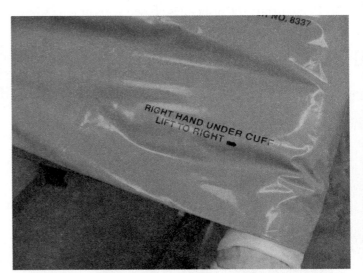

FIGURE 7.4 Follow printed instructions on the Mayo drape.

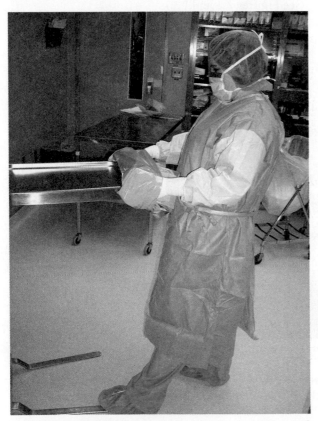

FIGURE 7.5 Steady the legs of the Mayo stand with your foot.

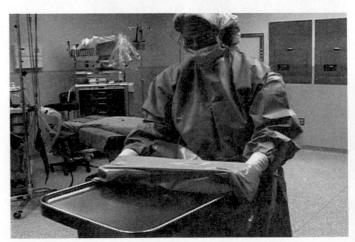

FIGURE 7.6 Feed on the drape.

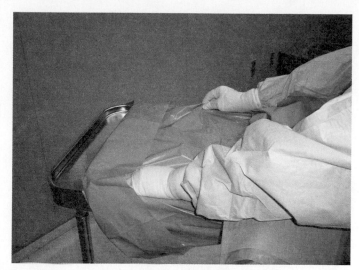

FIGURE 7.7 Sterile gloves touch sterile drape.

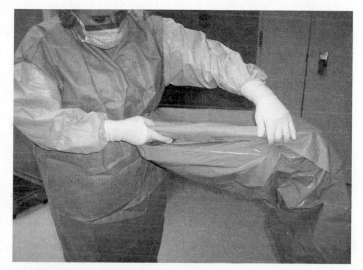

FIGURE 7.8 Fit excess drape, optional.

5. Demonstrate proficiency in moving the stand and controlling the height. A lack of proficiency may cause harm to the patient during the procedure.

6. Prepare the back, or instrument, table for use. Use economy of time and motion by arranging items only once.

- Reinforce the back table cover, and arrange supplies into work areas or stations according to the laterality of the invasive procedure—right-sided or left-sided—and the surgeon's preferences.
- Plan to stand on the opposite side from the surgeon at the surgical field, unless otherwise indicated.
- Reinforce the back table drape with opened OR towels or with a three-fouths drape, according to your OR's practices.
- Prepare four OR towels, or "4-square" for draping the abdomen in preparation for a laparotomy procedure, for example.
  - Anticipate the surgeon's order of use: prepare three with the folds facing upward and the fourth facing downward. The three layered towels on the bottom will be presented to the surgeon first.
- Arrange the abdominal drape under the "4-square" towels; anticipate order of use (top layer is used first).
- Plan a location for your tray containing the instruments.
- Layer the surgeon's drying towel, gown, and gloves in order of use.
  - Place them in a predetermined location—back table or ring stand (see 7.10 through 7.13).

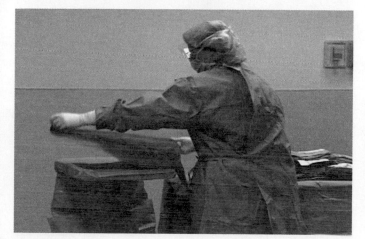

FIGURE 7.9 Reinforce top of Mayo stand drape.

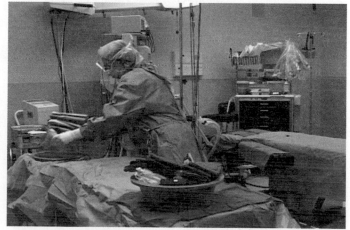

FIGURE 7.10 Arrange sterile supplies on the back table and in the ring stand basin.

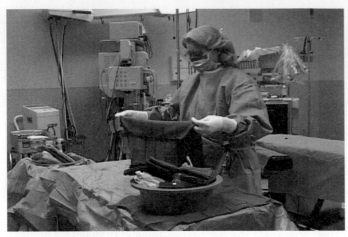

FIGURE 7.11 Prepare four towels.

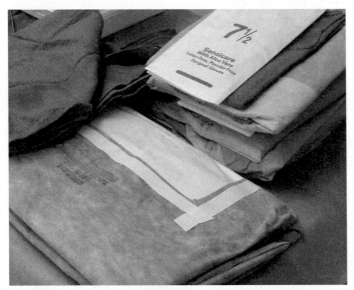

FIGURE 7.12 Layer in order of use.

7. Assess, prepare, and arrange additional surgical supplies into functional and safe areas. Follow a standardized set-up plan or develop a personal plan.

- Construct a rolled towel into a firm support for the stringed instruments.
- Prepare and arrange the suction tubing, electrocautery (Bovie) and storage holster (box), scratch pad, and light handle covers.
- Place countable items together such as: laparotomy sponges (in a pack of 5) and Ray-Tec sponges (in a pack of 10); rolled-gauze (Kitners) in a blue-pack of 5, red-needle mat, hypos, Bovie tips, and scalpel blades.
- Attach the paper trash bag. AST recommends placement on the Mayo stand edge.
- Arrange all other items: marking pen, basins, bulb syringe, medication syringes, and other requirements.
- Place basins and medication cups near the edge of the field for ease in transfer of solutions onto the field by the circulator (see Figures 7.14 through 7.17).

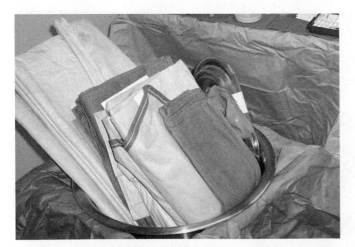

FIGURE 7.13 Arrange in ring stand.

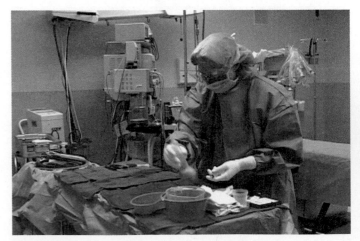

FIGURE 7.14 Implement your set-up strategy.

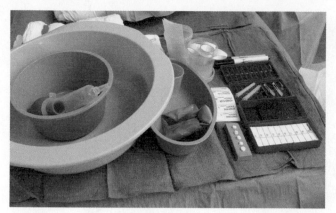

FIGURE 7.15 Arrange smaller items.

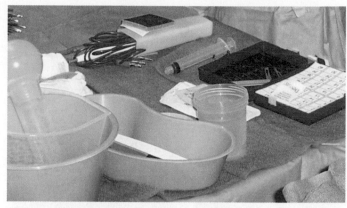

FIGURE 7.16 Group for counting.

8. Obtain instrument tray.

- Work in tandem with the circulator, who will verify the pan filters before you place the instruments onto your back table.
- Grasp the handles of the inner basket so that the outer tray is not touched with your gloved hands or the sleeves of your sterile gown.
- Lift the basket straight up and out of the outer pan.
- Hold the tray while the circulator verifies the filters.
- Do not use the instrument tray if moisture is found in the pan or holes in the filter. Obtain a new tray and change into new sterile gloves.
- Once verified, place your instrument tray onto the back table.
- Follow your OR's preferred method to verify the tray filters (see Figures 7.18 through 7.20).

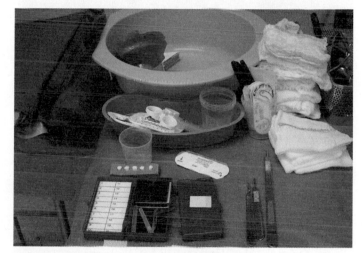

FIGURE 7.17 Groupings vary among STs.

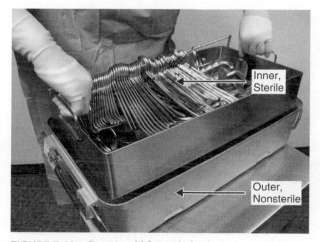

FIGURE 7.18 Grasp and lift inside basket.

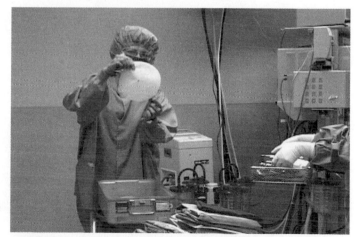

FIGURE 7.19 Assess the filter for moisture or tears. Performed by the circulator.

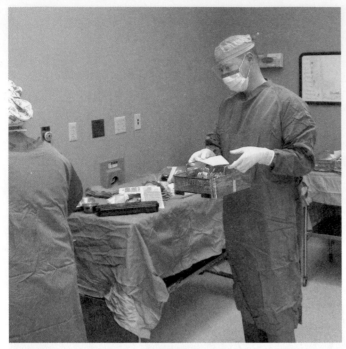
FIGURE 7.20 Place instrument tray on the sterile back table only after circulator confirms sterile processing.

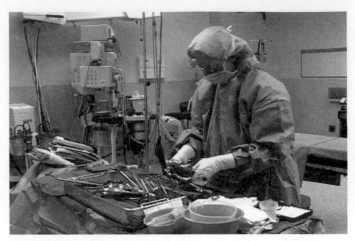
FIGURE 7.21 Group ring-handled instruments.

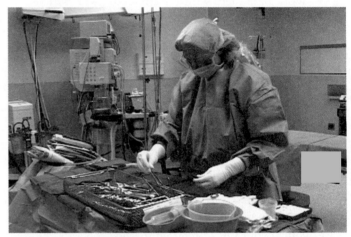
FIGURE 7.22 Arrange forceps.

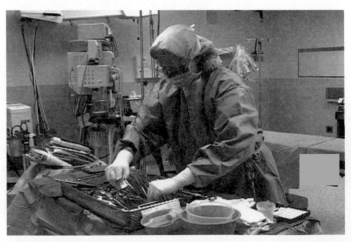
FIGURE 7.23 Group retractors.

9. Prepare instruments and supplies according to your OR's preferences. Arrange items in a functional and efficient fashion so you can access instruments quickly during the operative procedure. Promote patient safety.

- Verify any sterile processing indicators on the inside of the tray.
- Assess for cleanliness when handling the instruments. Do not use instruments containing dried debris.
- Assess instruments for proper function and parts. Tag for repair if not functional.
- Receive items from the circulator; for example, suture or larger items. Refer to Chapter 4.
- Assemble instruments with parts (disassembled for sterilization).
- Assemble a Balfour self-retaining abdominal retractor. The parts vary by manufacturer: the frame, center bladder blade, arm blades, screws, and a wing nut. Include parts in the instrument count, according to your OR's policy. Refer to Chapter 19.
- Sort and arrange instruments for the procedure.
- Protect instruments from damage.
- Arrange items to support an orderly initial count of sharps, sponges, and instruments with the circulator (see Figures 7.21 through 7.26).

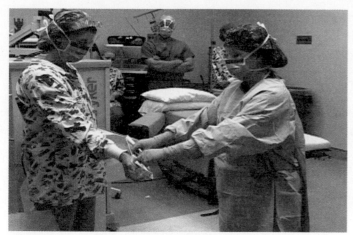

FIGURE 7.24 Receive items from the circulator.

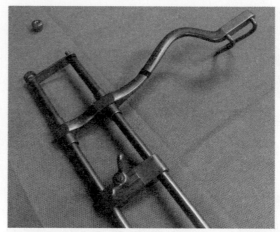

FIGURE 7.25 Assemble self-retaining Balfour retractor.

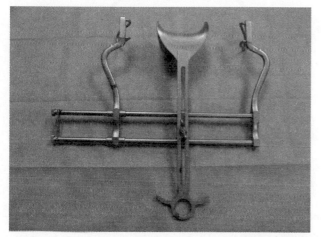

FIGURE 7.26 Balfour retractor.

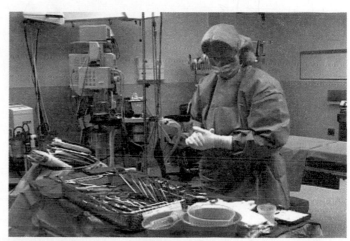

FIGURE 7.27 Evaluate for completeness.

10. Determine readiness of the setup, and call for the count with the circulator. Refer to Chapter 8 (also see Figures 7.27 through 7.30).

11. Indicate your preferences for a back table and ring stand setup. Refer to Chapter 10 to customize the Mayo stand setup (see Diagrams 7.1 and 7.2).

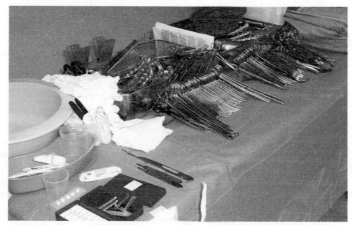

FIGURE 7.28 Back table preparation.

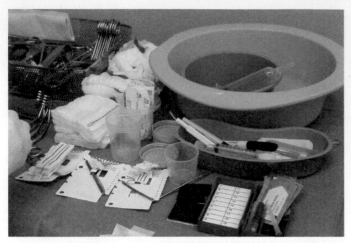

FIGURE 7.29 Locate countable items together.

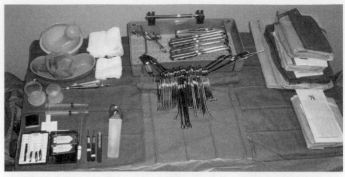

FIGURE 7.30 Evaluate arrangement of sterile supplies on the back table.

Diagram 7.1 Draw or list the sterile items in your ring stand basin.

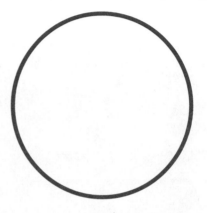

Diagram 7.2 Draw or list the sterile instruments and supplies on your back table.

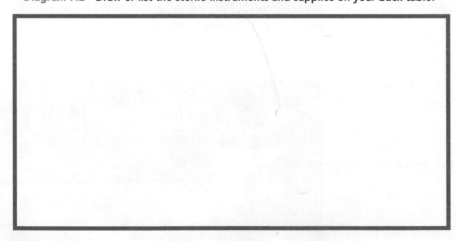

COMPETENCY ASSESSMENT

STUDENT'S NAME: _____

CHAPTER 7 DRAPE MAYO STAND AND PREPARE BACK TABLE

PERFORMANCE RANK:

    S or √ = Satisfactory: Competent—safe, accurate, sequential, and timely
    U = Unsatisfactory: Unsafe—inaccurate and unprepared

PERFORMANCE RATING:

5	Independent: Expert—safe, confident, seamless performance; mentors others
4	Minimally monitored: Intermediate—safe, self-corrects few errors
3	Competent: Novice—safe, revises with evaluator cues, few errors
2	Remedial: Unsafe—critical errors, unable to implement evaluator cues consistently
1	Dependent: Unsafe—unacceptable, requires multiple evaluator interventions

(handwritten: 89)

PERFORMANCE CRITERIA	Performance Rank	Performance Rating
1. Perform Mutual Professional and Scholastic Criteria as appropriate (see Preface or Appendix A).		1 2 3 4 (5)
2. Start time: _(handwritten)_ Laparotomy example; grasp and orient Mayo stand drape.		1 2 3 4 (5)
3. Steady Mayo stand, and cover it with the sterile drape.		1 2 3 4 (5)
4. Reinforce Mayo stand, and drape it with OR towels.		1 2 3 4 (5)
5. Move the Mayo stand, and adjust its height.		1 2 3 4 (5)
6. Reinforce back table cover. _(handwritten: Do this first prior to hanging rest)_		1 (2) 3 4 5
7. Prepare abdominal drapes, and place on sterile table/ring stand in order of use. _(handwritten: move aside for room; tray)_		1 (2) 3 4 5
8. Layer surgeon's drying towel, gown, and gloves in order of use. _(handwritten: prepare prior to surgeon)_		1 (2) 3 4 5
9. Construct rolled towel for instruments. _(handwritten: why?; work on roll)_		1 2 (3) 4 5
10. Arrange smaller items into stations.		1 2 (3) 4 5
11. Arrange sharp items for the count. _(handwritten: establish sharp zone atop)_		1 (2) 3 4 5
12. Arrange sponges for the count. _(handwritten: begin & roytex → practice)_		1 2 (3) 4 5
13. Place basins and medicine cups at table edge.		1 2 (3) 4 5
14. Lift instrument basket out of the tray; pause to allow verification of filters in tray bottom. (Verification performed by nonsterile team member.)		1 2 3 4 (5)
15. Place instrument tray onto back table, once verified. _(handwritten: center; reinforce)_		1 (2) 3 4 5
16. Verify additional chemical indicators in tray. _(handwritten: prepare for counts)_		1 2 3 4 (5)
17. Arrange instruments for the count. _(handwritten: practice)_		1 (2) 3 4 5
18. Assemble a Balfour retractor. _(handwritten: N/a)_		1 2 3 4 (5)
19. Receive sterile items from the circulator.		1 2 3 4 (5)
20. Call for the count. _(handwritten: initiate)_		1 2 (3) 4 5
21. End time: _(handwritten)_		1 (2) 3 4 5
22. Demonstrate movement in the sterile role. _(handwritten: Nice)_		1 2 3 4 (5)
23. Pass another sterile team member.		1 2 3 4 (5)
24. Pass a nonsterile team member.		1 2 3 4 (5)

(handwritten at bottom: -5 towel bth → shd fnd)

ADDITIONAL COMMENTS _____

PERFORMANCE EVALUATIONS AND RECOMMENDATIONS

☑ PASS: Satisfactory Performance
  - ❏ Demonstrates professionalism
  - ❏ Exhibits critical thinking
  - ❏ Demonstrates proficient clinical performance appropriate for time in the program

❏ FAIL: Unsatisfactory Performance
  - ❏ Critical criteria not met (See Performance Rank or Rating Above)
  - ❏ Professionalism not demonstrated.
  - ❏ Critical thinking skills not demonstrated.
  - ❏ Skill performance unsafe or underdeveloped.

❏ REMEDIATION:
  - ❏ Schedule lab practice. Date: _____
  - ❏ Reevaluate by instructor. Date: _____

❏ DISMISS from lab or clinicals today.

❏ Program director notified. Date: _____

SIGNATURES

Date ___ 10/20/13 ___   Evaluator _____   Student _____

ACTIVITIES AND DISCUSSION QUESTIONS

Activities

1. View the Complete Perioperative Process and Focus on Skills video, Skill #7 (video can be found at www.myhealthprofessionskit.com).
2. Observe the instructor perform the skill.
3. Practice the skill in the lab, with your lab partner or in small groups.
4. Select one skill, such as draping the Mayo stand, teach a classmate, observe, and critique the performance.
5. Select two or three possible performance errors, demonstrate them to your lab partner, and ask your partner to identify the errors. Discuss methods to prevent and correct the errors.
6. Refer to your ST textbook and this lab manual to answer the Discussion Questions (see next column).
7. Review the video and the information in this lab manual when you prepare for your certification examination.

Discussion Questions

1. What is the first step in draping the Mayo stand?
2. How do you protect your sterile gloved hands from touching the bare metal stand?
3. How do you correct a contamination error if you touch the Mayo stand with your sterile gloves? (Refer to Chapter 21, Maintain Sterile Technique).
4. If you are missing the needle mat from the sterile pack, what do you do?
5. Why do you cover the back table drape with OR towels or a three-fourths drape?
6. Can you imagine how you will anticipate the glove size of the surgeon? Give one example.
7. How do you stack items on the back table or in the ring stand?
8. What do you do if your room does not have a ring stand?
9. Why do you wait for the Circulator to assess the filters in the instrument pan?
10. What are your sterile boundaries on the drape covering the tabletop?
11. Where will you notice bioburden or dried debris?
12. Note here any questions that you need your instructor to clarify.

Perform Counts: Prevent Retained Surgical Items

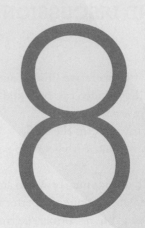

INTRODUCTION

The focal points in this chapter are: counting sponges, sharps, and instruments, and recognizing accountability of the entire operating room team for preventing unintended retention of foreign objects, or surgical items in the patient.

- Before performing the following skill, your lab instructor will discuss some of the principles for practice and objectives involved in this chapter as well as the importance of following the skill sequence and instructions.
- Role-play with your lab partner as you practice counting sponges, sharps, and instruments. Maintain aseptic technique. Attention to details and a concentrated focus are required to perform this

skill flawlessly. There is no room for error. Your instructor will offer strategies for success. Appendix E highlights the value of teaching others as a component of active learning strategies. Refer to Appendix C for an overview of the chapter.

- The lab instructor will advise you of any additional criteria to be evaluated. At a designated time, demonstration of these skills will be evaluated and graded by your lab instructor using the competency assessment tool.
- When in the clinical setting, your instructor may once again assess your performance using the same tool. Refer to Appendix A for clinical evaluation and documentation.

Team Member	Role		Timing		
	Nonsterile	Sterile	Preop	Intraop	Postop
Surgical Technologist		X	X	X	X
Assistant Circulator	X		X	X	X
Operating Room Team					

OBJECTIVES

The learner will perform this skill with 100 percent accuracy each time it is performed in the operative setting.

1. State the rationale for performing sponge, sharps, and instrument counts.

2. State the perioperative timing of the counts.
3. Demonstrate the precise method and sequence in performing the count along with the circulator.

Principles for Practice

The foundation and rationale for our practice, in the perioperative environment, stem from evidence provided by professionals, organizations, and governmental agencies. Refer to the Bibliography, Glossary of Terms, and the following documents or developmental agencies:

- OR policy
- State laws
- The Joint Commission
- Association of Surgical Technologists (AST)
- Association of periOperative Registered Nurses (AORN)

SKILL SEQUENCE AND INSTRUCTIONS

Counting Method

1. Count sponges, sharps, and instruments according to your OR policy.

   - Recognize the accountability of all team members in this patient safety mandate.
   - Count concurrently with the circulator.
   - Focus on the counting process.
   - Count items contained on the back table for the initial count.
   - Organize items for the intraoperative and postoperative counts.
   - Use the same order for each intraoperative count.
     ○ Surgical field
     ○ Mayo stand
     ○ Back table
     ○ Off the sterile field
   - Say the name of the item to be counted out loud, separate or point to each sterile item, and allow the circulator to view each item.
   - Tabulate each count. Visual aids used by the circulator may include a white board on the OR wall and an instrument count sheet initiated during instrument assembly in the sterile processing department (see Figures 8.1 through 8.3).

Count Timing

2. Perform counts for any procedure where an item could be retained unintentionally.

   - Initially, as a baseline before the skin incision
   - At the start of the closure of an organ (cavity within a cavity)
   - At the start of the closure of a body cavity
   - At the start of subcutaneous or skin closure
   - With the addition of a countable item to the sterile field
   - With the change of personnel-ST or circulator
   - Any time there is a question concerning the count

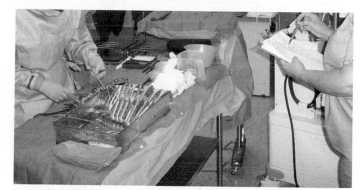

FIGURE 8.1 The ST and circulator count concurrently.

3. Perform sponge counts according to your OR policy.

   - Sponges are made of textile materials and are available in various sizes.
   - They are used during invasive surgical procedures to absorb blood and body fluids, and to aid the surgeon's view.
   - When sponges absorb blood, they take on the appearance or contour of surrounding body tissue and can be overlooked.
   - They are manufactured with an x-ray-detectable mark or stripe. Examples include 4- by 8-inch laparotomy sponges (packs of 5), Kittners (containers of 5), and 4- by 4-inch RAY-TEC sponges (packs of 10).

     ○ Remove the paper-band on the sponges, name the item, separate each sponge, and count out loud.
     ○ The circulator validates concurrently.
     ○ Sponges are the most frequently retained item (see Figure 8.4).

DESCRIPTION	CATALOG	QTY	CNT1	CNT2	CNT3
STEAM CHEMICAL INDICATOR		1	1		
Subtotal		**1**	1		
A) Stringer					
SPONGE FORCEPS	V Mueller GL650	4	4 +1 (5)		
MIXTER RIGHT ANGLE 9 1/2"	V Mueller SU10533	2	2		
KOCHER CLAMPS LONG STRAIGHT	V Mueller SU2804	2	2		
MAYO NEEDLE HOLDER 7"	V Mueller SU16061	2	2		
CRILEWOOD NEEDLE HOLDER	V Mueller SU16005	2	2		
BABCOCK FORCEP	V Mueller SU5002	2	2		
BABCOCK FORCEP 6-1/2'	V Mueller SU5000	2	2		
ALLIS CLAMP 6-1/2"	V Mueller SU4055 / SU4054	6	6		
CURVED KELLY FORCEPS	V Mueller SU2760	12	12		
CRILE FORCEP - STRAIGHT 5-1/2"	V Mueller SU2730	6	6		
CRILE FORCEP - CURVED 5-1/2"	V Mueller SU2735	12	12		
CURVED METZ SCISSORS 7"	V Mueller MO1601	1	1		
STRAIGHT MAYO SCISSOR	V Mueller SU1801	1	1		
CURVED MAYO SCISSORS 6-3/4"	V Mueller SU1826	1	1		
Subtotal for A) Stringer		**55**	55		
B)In The Tray					
RICHARDSON RETRACTOR - LARGE 2-1/2" W X 3" L	Codman 50-4117	2	2		
RICHARDSON RETRACTOR - MED/LG. 2" W X 2-1/2" L	Codman 50-4116	2	2		
RICHARDSON RETRACTOR - MED. 1-1/2" W X 2" L	Codman 50-4115	2	2		
RICHARDSON RETRACTOR - SMALL 1" W X 1-1/4" L	Codman 50-4124	2	2		
RICHARDSON RET. - APPENDECTOMY 3/4" W X 2" L	Codman 50-4131	2	2		
POOLE SUCTION TIP 30FR	V Mueller SU13000	1	1	1	
ARMY NAVY RETRACTORS	V Mueller SU3660	2	2		
RAKE RETRACTORS 4 PRONG BLUNT 8 3/4"	V Mueller SU3552-01	2	2		
CUSHING VEIN RETRACTORS	V Mueller NL1003	2	2		
WEITLANER RETRACTOR BLUNT 6 1/2"	V Mueller SU3112-001	1	1		
LARGE TOWEL CLIPS	V Mueller SU2905	6	6	6	
UNIVERSAL BANDAGE SCISSORS- BLACK HANDLES	V Mueller SU2014-001	1	1		
ZIMM CLIP	Zimmer 57-02	2	2	2	
Subtotal for B)In The Tray		**27**	27		
C)Peel Pouch					
DEBAKEY FORCEP 9 1/2"	V Mueller CH5904	2	2	(11)	
DEBAKEY FORCEP 6-1/4"	V Mueller CH5900	2	2		
SINGLEY INTESTINAL FORCEP 9 3/4"	V Mueller SU5075	1	1		+3

FIGURE 8.2 Paper count sheet.

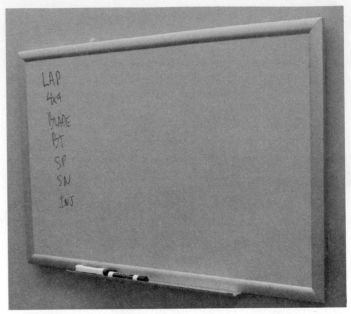

FIGURE 8.3 White wallboard used for tracking and tallying countable items.

4. Perform sharp and small item counts according to your OR policy. Examples include: scalpel blades, hypodermic needles, suture needles, electrocautery tips, tip scratch pads, vessel loops, and broken parts.

- Identify each sharp item individually, say the name of the item out loud, and count out loud (see Figure 8.5).

5. Perform instrument counts according to your OR policy. Included in this category are metal or plastic instruments designed to be extensions or aides for the surgeon's hand. Examples include scissors, forceps, Yankauer suction tube, knife handles, and retractors.

- Identify, name, separate, and count out loud. Use an unarmed knife handle to assist with locating and separating instruments.
- Count removable parts separately (see Figures 8.6 through 8.8).

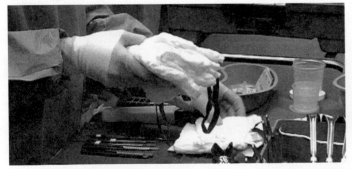

FIGURE 8.4 Separate sponges.

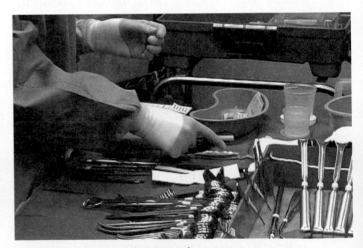

FIGURE 8.5 Count each separately.

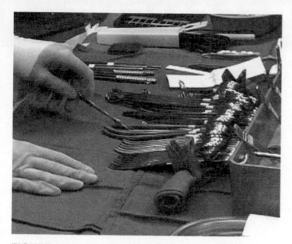

FIGURE 8.6 Separate and identify instruments.

6. The surgeon is notified of a "correct" or "incorrect" count by the circulator.
7. Perform the count again, if the count is incorrect. Manual, visual, technology enhanced, and x-ray verification may occur to rectify the error.
   - Inspect the surgical site, sterile drapes, and sterile surfaces on the Mayo stand or back table. Inspection of sterile surfaces is performed by the ST and sterile team members.
   - Inspect the floor and trash receptacles. Nonsterile team members will search under the OR bed, on low-hanging drapes, under OR furniture, and in the paper trash receptacles.
   - Adjunct technologies, such as bar coding, electronic surveillance, and radio-frequency identification, supplement the traditional counting process.
   - If an item is still missing, an X-ray may be taken to determine if the item has been retained in the patient.
8. Postpone counts in an extreme emergency, according to OR policy. At the conclusion of the case, an x-ray may be taken, or adjunct technologies will be used to confirm nonretention.
9. Corral all broken instrument or needle parts in a designated area, such as the needle mat. Count all parts.
10. Document according to the counting policy in the patient's chart, electronic or paper. The circulator will record correct counts and discrepancies along with actions taken to rectify the error.

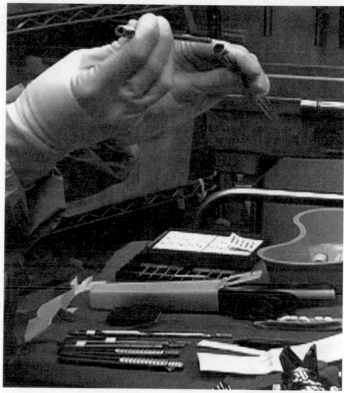

FIGURE 8.7 Count the two Poole suction parts. Say "Poole suction, one and two."

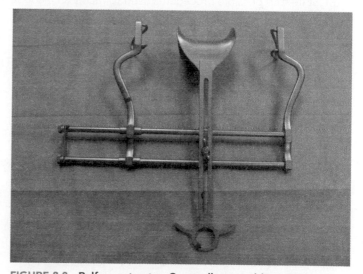

FIGURE 8.8 Balfour retractor. Count all removable parts.

STUDENT'S NAME: _____

CHAPTER 8 PERFORM COUNTS: PREVENT RETAINED SURGICAL ITEMS

(16)

PERFORMANCE RANK:

S or √ = Satisfactory: Competent—safe, accurate, sequential, and timely

U = Unsatisfactory: Unsafe—inaccurate and unprepared

PERFORMANCE RATING:

5   Independent: Expert—safe, confident, seamless performance; mentors others

4   Minimally monitored: Intermediate—safe, self-corrects few errors

3   Competent: Novice—safe, revises with evaluator cues, few errors

2   Remedial: Unsafe—critical errors, unable to implement evaluator cues consistently

1   Dependent: Unsafe—unacceptable, requires multiple evaluator interventions

PERFORMANCE CRITERIA	Performance Rank	Performance Rating
1. Perform Mutual Professional and Scholastic Criteria as appropriate (see Preface or Appendix A).		1 2 3 4 (5)
2. Perform preoperative initial counts with circulator, concurrently and audibly, and separate for clear visibility; count sponges, sharps, and instruments.		1 (2) 3 4 5
3. Organize and perform intraoperative counts with the circulator, concurrently and audibly, and separate for clear visibility; perform in the same order each time: Field, Mayo stand, back table, and off the field.		1 (2) 3 4 5
4. Perform postoperative final counts with the circulator, concurrently and audibly, and separate for clear visibility.		1 (2) 3 4 5
5. State four possible procedures used to rectify an incorrect count.		1 2 3 4 (5)

ADDITIONAL COMMENTS _____

PERFORMANCE EVALUATIONS AND RECOMMENDATIONS

❑ PASS: Satisfactory Performance
    ❑ Demonstrates professionalism
    ❑ Exhibits critical thinking
    ❑ Demonstrates proficient clinical performance, appropriate for time in the program

❑ FAIL: Unsatisfactory Performance
    ❑ Critical criteria not met (See Performance Rank or Rating Above)
    ❑ Professionalism not demonstrated.
    ❑ Critical thinking skills not demonstrated.
    ❑ Skill performance unsafe or underdeveloped.

☑ REMEDIATION:
    ☑ Schedule lab practice. Date: _10_/_30_/_13_
    ❑ Reevaluate by instructor. Date: _____

❑ DISMISS from lab or clinicals today.

❑ Program director notified. Date: _____

SIGNATURES

Date _10_/_30_/_13_   Evaluator _____   Student _____

ACTIVITIES AND DISCUSSION QUESTIONS

Activities

1. View the Complete Perioperative Process and Focus on Skills video, Skill #8 (video can be found at www.myhealthprofessionskit.com).
2. Observe the instructor perform the skill.
3. Practice the skill in the lab, with your lab partner or in small groups.
4. Teach this skill to a classmate, and observe and critique the performance.
5. Select two or three possible performance errors, demonstrate them to your lab partner, and ask your partner to identify the errors. Focus on accuracy. Discuss methods to prevent and correct the errors.
6. Refer to your ST textbook and this lab manual to answer the Discussion Questions (see next column).
7. Review the video and the information in this lab manual when you prepare for your certification examination.

Discussion Questions

1. State the rationale for performing counts.
2. State when counts are performed for sharps.
3. State when counts are performed for sponges.
4. State when counts are performed for instruments.
5. How is the initial, baseline count different than any subsequent counts?
6. Once the case is in progress, what is the method for counting the retainable items?
7. Which characteristics of surgical sponges make them the most frequently retained items in the abdomen or pelvis?
8. If a suture needle breaks during the case, what should you do with the parts?
9. Note here any questions that you need your instructor to clarify.

Prepare Medications and Solutions

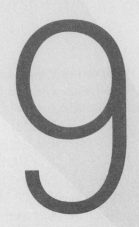

INTRODUCTION

The surgical technologist has a vital role in receiving, preparing, and passing medications and solutions on the sterile field. The ST and the circulator visibly, audibly, and concurrently verify all medications and solutions. The ST passes only validated medications to the surgeon. Meticulous attention to detail paired with dedicated practice are required for safe, seamless performance.

- Your lab instructor will discuss some of the principles for practice and objectives involved in this chapter as well as the importance of following the skill sequence and instructions.
- Role-play with your lab partner as you practice the sequential process. Encourage and critique each other. Your instructor will offer strategies for success. Appendix E highlights the value of teaching others as a component of active learning strategies. Refer to Appendix C for an overview of the chapter.
- The lab instructor will advise you of any additional criteria to be evaluated. At a designated time, demonstration of these skills will be evaluated and graded by your lab instructor using the competency assessment tool.
- When in the clinical setting, your instructor may once again assess your performance using the same tool. Refer to Appendix A for clinical evaluation and documentation.

Team Member	Type of Role		Timing		
	Nonsterile	Sterile	Preop	Intraop	Postop
Surgical Technologist		X	X	X	
Assistant Circulator	X		X	X	
Operating Room Team					

OBJECTIVES

The learner will perform this skill with 100 percent accuracy each time it is performed in the operative setting:

1. State rationale for verifying all medications and solutions managed on the sterile field.
2. Demonstrate a precise method and sequence for verifying, labeling, receiving, preparing, and passing medications.
3. Demonstrate a precise sequence for verifying, labeling, receiving, preparing, and passing solutions.
4. Read the amount of fluid or medication contained in differently sized and calibrated syringes.
5. Anticipate and request replenishment of supplies, medications, and solutions.
6. Calculate and report the amount of medications and solutions used by the surgeon.

Principles for Practice

The foundation and rationale for our practice, in the perioperative environment, stem from evidence provided by professionals, organizations, and governmental agencies. Refer to the Bibliography, Glossary of Terms, and the following documents or developmental agencies:

- Operating room policies
- State laws
- The Joint Commission
- Occupational Safety and Health Administration (OSHA)
- Centers for Disease Control and Prevention (CDC)
- Association of Surgical Technologists (AST)
- Association of periOperative Registered Nurses (AORN)

SKILL SEQUENCE AND INSTRUCTIONS

1. Verify and obtain the correct medication or solution for the patient (circulator role).

   - Verify preoperatively the medications and solutions listed on the preference card with the surgeon and verify the patient's allergies before obtaining medications from the storage system or solutions from the warming cabinet.
   - Read the medication label, and any package instructions (see Figures 9.33 and 9.34).
     - Validate the generic and brand names, concentration or dosage, amount or volume, and expiration date.
     - Validate any specific instructions such as methods of dilution or reconstitution.
   - Verify the "six rights" for medication preparation:
     Right patient
     Right medication   *Right documentation*
     Right dose
     Right route
     Right time
     Right label

   - Contact the pharmacist, or use an electronic or printed drug reference resource, if you do not recognize the medication or know why you are using it.
   - Read the preprinted label twice to verify it with the preference card or order. Do not assume the stock has been correctly sorted.
   - Assess a vial of medication for integrity and medication color. As an example, assess a vial of local anesthetic. Do not use if the seal is broken, the vial is cracked, the medication is discolored, or the date on the label has expired.
   - Local anesthetic medications, for subcutaneous injection by the surgeon, are available in various strengths or concentrations and with or without additives, such a epinephrine.
     - Bupivacaine "plain" is illustrated in two of its concentrations 0.5% or 5 mg/1 mL and 0.25% or 2.5 mg/1 mL (see Figure 9.1).
     - Bupivacaine "with epi." 0.5% with 1:200,000 epinephrine is shown with a red label alerting OR personnel to the addition of epinephrine, a potent vasoconstrictor (see Figure 9.2).

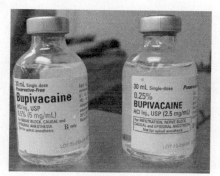

FIGURE 9.1   Bupivacaine "plain."

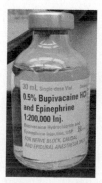

FIGURE 9.2   Bupivacaine with "epi."

2. Verify the medication—concurrently and audibly.

- The circulator reads out loud the name of the medication, the strength, and the expiration date while the ST simultaneously views the label.
- The ST reads and repeats out loud the name, strength, and expiration date of the medication printed on the label (see Figure 9.3).

3. Label the sterile container that will receive the medication.

- Label the containers after verifying and before receiving the medication onto the sterile field.
- Use a preprinted label or write with a sterile pen.
- Place the label on the side of the container or syringe that is free of measurement marks (see Figure 9.4).

4. Receive the medication via transfer from the circulator.

- Follow your OR policy when selecting a method to transfer and receive medication.
  - Use handheld medication basins or those located at the corner or edge of the back table or Mayo stand.
  - Use a sterile syringe or a sterile transfer device.
- The circulator may transfer the medication via a sterile transfer decanter into a sterile basin, recommended by AORN.
- The circulator may remove the stopper from the vial and pour the medication into a sterile basin, not recommended by AORN or AST.
- The circulator may hold the vial as the ST withdraws the medication from the vial with a sterile syringe attached to a large bore needle, 18 gauge, for example (see Figures 9.5 and 9.6).

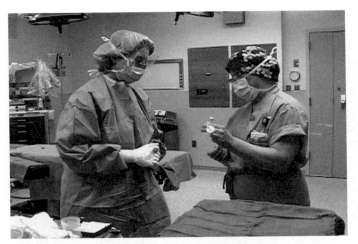

FIGURE 9.3   Verify.

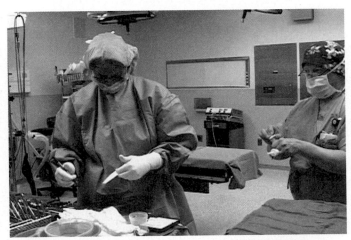

FIGURE 9.4   Label.

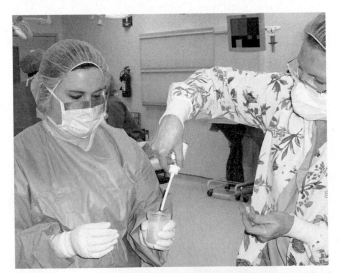

FIGURE 9.5   Use a sterile transfer decanter. Preferred method.

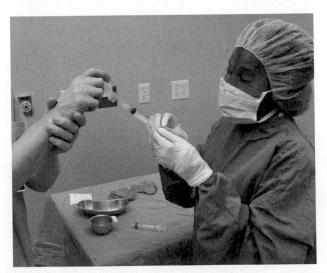

FIGURE 9.6   Use a sterile syringe. Not preferred.

5. Prepare the medication for injection by the surgeon.
   - Fill a 10 mL Leur-lock tip syringe from the basin containing the medication.
   - Remove any air bubbles from the syringe. Point the syringe tip upwards and gently push on the plunger to remove the excess bubbles.
   - Secure a new, capped-hypo (needle) onto the Leur-lock tip of the syringe; use a clockwise, twisting motion to seat the hypo. Select a small bore needle (25 gauge) if the patient will be conscious during the injection of a local anesthetic.
   - Remove the cap, and push a small amount of medication slowly through the hypo to ensure that it is patent.
   - Recap the hypo, if necessary, using the one-handed scooping technique.
   - Place the syringe in a safe area on the back table until requested by the surgeon (see Figures 9.7 through 9.9).
   - Refer to Figures 9.21–9.32 for additional syringe management skills.

6. Pass the prepared syringe to the surgeon. Promote patient and OR team safety and prevent accidental needlestick injuries.
   - Remove the cap and place it near the needle mat on the back table.
   - Note: Remove a firmly attached cap with a clamping instrument. Do not use your hands. Use clamps to grasp the cap, near the needle hub, and twist the cap clockwise while lifting the cap off. Resecure the hypo.
   - Communicate or announce that a sharp is being made available or is ready to be passed.
   - State the name, strength, and amount of the medication to the surgeon prior to passing the syringe.
   - Use a no-touch neutral zone or basin to pass the syringe to the surgeon. The sharp (syringe with needle) will only be handled by one person at a time, thereby decreasing the risk of a needlestick injury (see Figures 9.10 and 9.11).
   - Pass hand-to-hand (not recommended by OSHA or CDC).
   - Communicate and focus.
   - Remove the cap. Place cap near the needle mat.
   - Hold the syringe barrel by the superior surface, with the needle facing toward you. Place the barrel of the syringe into the surgeon's hand (see Figure 9.12).

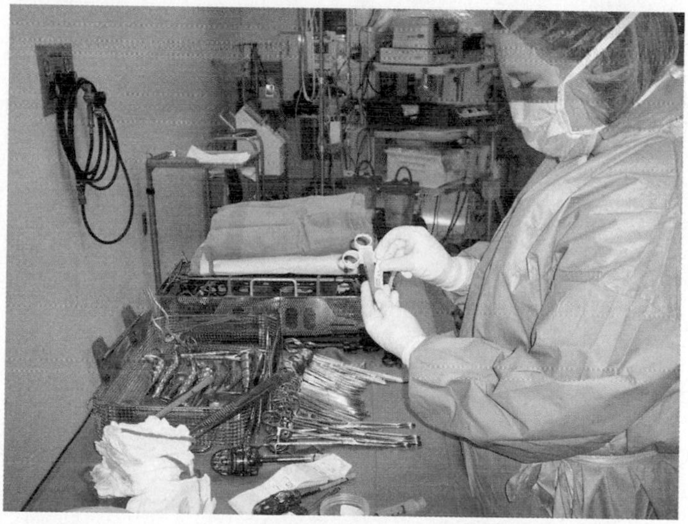

FIGURE 9.7 Place a label indicating the contents.

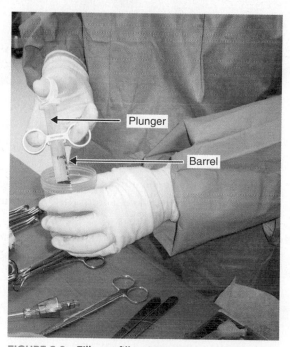

FIGURE 9.8 Fill or refill syringe. Hypo not attached.

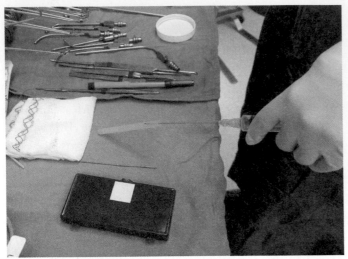

FIGURE 9.9   One-handed scoop re-capping.

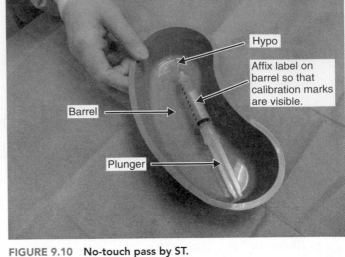

FIGURE 9.10   No-touch pass by ST.

Hypo

Affix label on barrel so that calibration marks are visible.

Barrel

Plunger

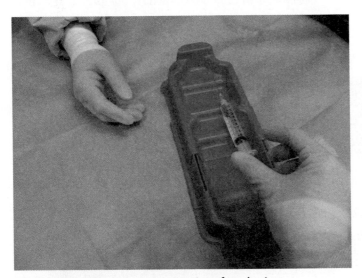

FIGURE 9.11   Surgeon retrieves syringe from basin.

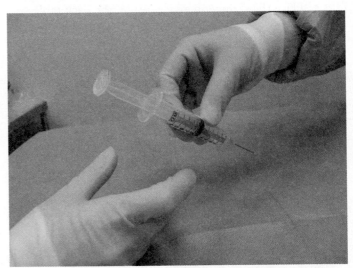

FIGURE 9.12   Hand-to-hand pass. Not recommended.

7. Remove firmly attached needles by using a forceps or clamping instrument.

 • Grasp the needle at the hub and twist the needle counterclockwise. Remove it from the syringe and place it into the needle mat.
 • Directional cues for twisting are helpful reminders of the process: "righty-tighty and left-loosey" (see Figure 9.13).

8. Tabulate the total amount of medication administered by the surgeon during the procedure.

 • Write the amount of medication used on the back table cover or a sterile piece of paper on the back table.
 • After each pass, refill the syringe in anticipation of subsequent use.
 • State the total amount of medication used at the conclusion of the procedure, or when asked to report.
 • Document the amount of medication administered to the patient (circulator and anesthesia care providers' role).

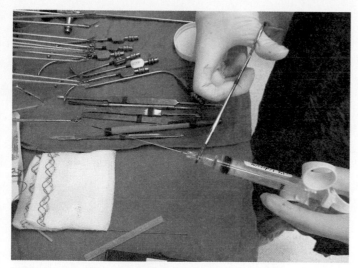

FIGURE 9.13 Remove needle with forceps; turn hub counterclockwise.

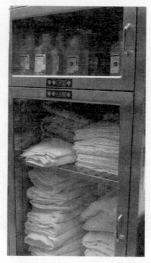

FIGURE 9.14 Warming cabinet with solutions on top.

9. Validate the solution to be used on the sterile field.

- The circulator will use a safety process to verify any solutions to be used on the sterile field such as normal saline 0.9%, irrigation solution, or sterile water used to clean instruments.
- Retrieve irrigation solutions from the warming cabinet.
- Examine the warmed-bottle for after-market labels affixed to indicate a 72-hour expiration date.
- Verify the solution with the ST in the sterile role—visually, audibly, and concurrently.
- Deliver the solution into a labeled sterile basin large enough to hold the contents of the bottle, usually 1 L.
- Do not reuse or repour any solution remaining in the bottle (see Figures 9.14 through 9.17).

10. The ST places a sterile and labeled bulb syringe, or Asepto, into the basin, and fills the bulb syringe with the solution in anticipation of use by the surgeon.

- Assess the solution's warmth. An intraoperative electronic fluid warmer may be used. This type of fluid warmer will be covered with a sterile drape during your back table set up, as performed in Chapter 7 (see Figure 9.18).
- Compress or squeeze the bulb on the 120–150 mL capacity Asepto syringe, submerge tip end into solution, release bulb, and allow syringe to fill.
- Tilt syringe tip upward, slowly depress bulb again, and resubmerge tip into solution to complete filling.
- Fill the syringe to capacity and place it in the basin.
- Pass the syringe to the surgeon so that the solution does not drip over the sterile filed. Orient the syringe tip so that it is pointed upward.

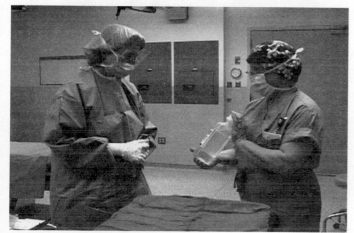

FIGURE 9.15 Verify solution.

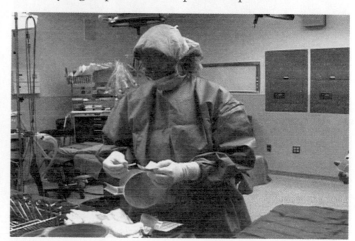

FIGURE 9.16 Label.

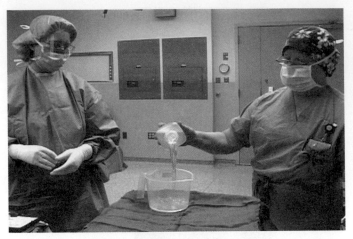

FIGURE 9.17 Sterile basin placed for delivery.

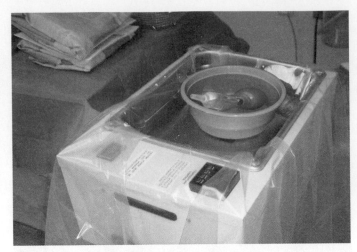

FIGURE 9.18 Electric fluid warmer.

11. Wipe off instruments during the procedure with sterile water.
   • Verify and label, as previously indicated, and place this basin in a separate location on your back table, according to your hospital policy. Do not confuse the two solutions. Sterile water is hypotonic and will cause body cells to swell and rupture.

12. Dispose of unused solutions or medications according to your OR's policy at the end of the procedure.
   • Solidify, absorb with OR towels, or use an automated collection system.
   • Dilute and dispose of any remaining narcotics on the sterile field, such as cocaine which is used for hemostasis during some nasal procedures. This disposal is witnessed by two licensed team members. The circulator will document the disposal (see Figures 9.19 and 9.20).

13. The circulator will report to the post–anesthesia care unit (PACU) nurse pertinent information concerning the patient and the procedure, including information related to the medications received, the amount, administration route, timing, and any unusual patient responses to the medication. Medications taken by the patient on a daily basis are also part of the hand-off report.

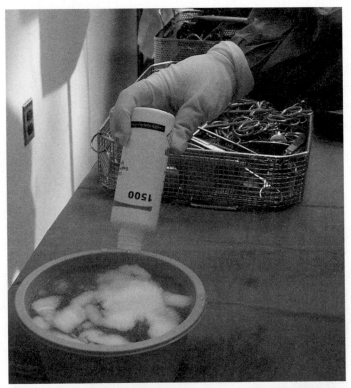

FIGURE 9.19 Solidify liquids at the conclusion of the procedure.

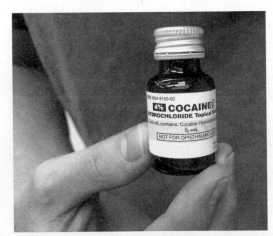

FIGURE 9.20 Nasal hemostatic agent, cocaine, is diluted for disposal at procedure end.

14. Practice syringe management skills.
   - Identify differently sized and calibrated syringes (see Figures 9.21 through 9.28).
     - Syringes are available in various sizes, typically holding 1 through 60 milliliters (mL). Selection is based on the intended use during invasive procedures.
     - Each syringe is calibrated so that a single mark on the barrel represents either one-hundredth, one-tenth, two-tenths, one, or more of volume in milliliters.
   - Read the amount of fluid or medication contained in prepared syringes (see Figures 9.29 through 9.32).

15. Identify pertinent information on various medication labels. The medications may be supplied by the manufacturer or mixed by a pharmacist.
   - Locate and interpret the brand and generic names, concentration or strength, total volume, expiration date, and any instructions for preparation and administration.
   - Refer to steps 1 and 2 and also to Figures 9.33 and 9.34.

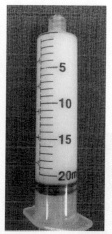

FIGURE 9.21 20 mL syringe with 1 mL marks on barrel.

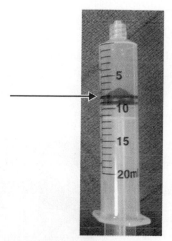

FIGURE 9.22 Read superior plunger ridge at 8 mL.

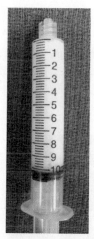

FIGURE 9.23 10 mL syringe with 0.2 mL marks.

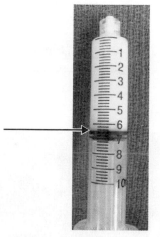

FIGURE 9.24 Read superior plunger ridge at 6.4 mL

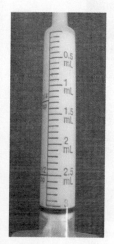

FIGURE 9.25 3 mL syringe with 0.1 mL marks.

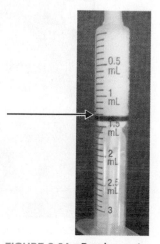

FIGURE 9.26 Read superior plunger ridge at 1.3 mL.

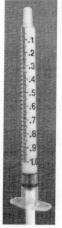

FIGURE 9.27 1mL syringe with 0.01 marks.

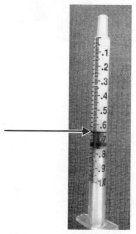

FIGURE 9.28 Read superior plunger ridge at 0.65 mL.

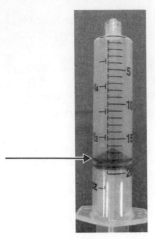

FIGURE 9.29 20 mL syringe. Read _____ mL.

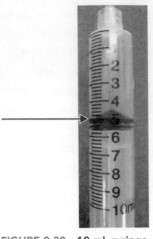

FIGURE 9.30 10 mL syringe. Read _____ mL.

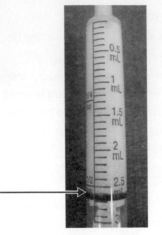

FIGURE 9.31 3 mL syringe. Read _____ mL.

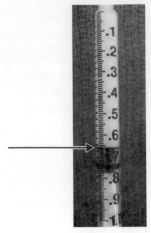

FIGURE 9.32 1 mL syringe. Read _____ mL.

Answer key

Figure 9.29: 18mL; Figure 9.30: 5 mL; Figure 9.31: 2.6 mL; Figure 9.32: 0.66 mL

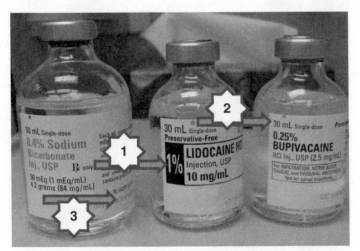

FIGURE 9.33 Irrigation solution name and strength (1), total amount (2), and expiration date (3).

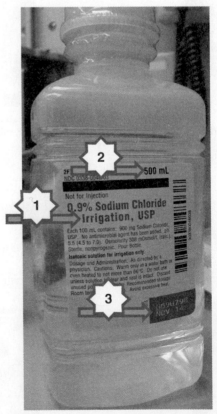

FIGURE 9.34 Medication name and strength (1), total amount (2), and expiration date (3).

COMPETENCY ASSESSMENT

STUDENT'S NAME: _____

CHAPTER 9 PREPARE MEDICATIONS AND SOLUTIONS

PERFORMANCE RANK:

S or √ = Satisfactory: Competent—safe, accurate, sequential, and timely
U = Unsatisfactory: Unsafe—inaccurate and unprepared

PERFORMANCE RATING:

5   Independent: Expert—safe, confident, seamless performance; mentors others
4   Minimally monitored: Intermediate—safe, self-corrects few errors
3   Competent: Novice—safe, revises with evaluator cues, few errors
2   Remedial: Unsafe—critical errors, unable to implement evaluator cues consistently
1   Dependent: Unsafe—unacceptable, requires multiple evaluator interventions

PERFORMANCE CRITERIA	Performance Rank	Performance Rating
1. Perform Mutual Professional and Scholastic Criteria as appropriate (see the Preface or Appendix A).		1 2 3 4 (5)
2. Read a medication label—generic and brand names, total volume, strength and concentration, expiration date, and any manufacturer's instructions.	*verbalize under*	1 2 (3) 4 5
3. State at least two resources for medication information.		1 2 3 4 (5)
4. State the "6 rights" of medication preparation.		1 2 3 4 (5)
5. Demonstrate the ST role using a local anesthetic vial: verify medication with the circulator, label syringe/basin, and receive.		1 2 3 4 (5)
6. Prepare a 10 mL syringe for use by the surgeon.		1 2 3 4 (5)
7. Pass the syringe to the surgeon; state the name, strength, and amount. Use delivery method of choice.		1 2 3 4 (5)
8. Recap hypo/needle with a one-handed scoop technique. *Nice*		1 2 3 4 (5)
9. Remove hypo/needle from the syringe with a forceps. *Practice technique*		1 2 (3) 4 5
10. Express solution from the syringe and refill to the 10 mL mark.		1 2 3 4 (5)
11. Tabulate total medication used.		1 2 3 4 (5)
12. Demonstrate the ST role with normal saline (NS); for the irrigation solution: verify the solution with the circulator, label the basin, and receive solution. *repeat*		1 2 3 4 (5)
13. Prepare the bulb syringe. Pass the filled syringe to the surgeon while stating the name of the solution. Refill the syringe.		1 2 3 4 (5)
14. Tabulate the total solution used.		1 2 3 4 (5)
15. Read the volume of fluid contained in differently sized and calibrated syringes. Instructor will provide at least 2 samples.		1 2 3 4 (5)

ADDITIONAL COMMENTS _____

PERFORMANCE EVALUATIONS AND RECOMMENDATIONS

☑ PASS: Satisfactory Performance

    ❏ Demonstrates professionalism

    ❏ Exhibits critical thinking

    ❏ Demonstrates proficient clinical performance, appropriate for time in the program

❏ FAIL: Unsatisfactory Performance

    ❏ Critical criteria not met (see Performance Rank or Rating Above)

    ❏ Professionalism not demonstrated.

    ❏ Critical thinking skills not demonstrated.

    ❏ Skill performance unsafe or underdeveloped.

❏ REMEDIATION:

    ❏ Schedule lab practice. Date: _____

    ❏ Reevaluate by instructor. Date: _____

❏ DISMISS from lab or clinicals today.

❏ Program director notified. Date: _____

SIGNATURES

Date _____   Evaluator _____   Student _____

ACTIVITIES AND DISCUSSION QUESTIONS

Activities

1. View the Complete Perioperative Process and Focus on Skills video, Skill #9 (video can be found at www.myhealthprofessionskit.com).

2. Observe the instructor perform the skill.

3. Practice reading the amount of fluid in differently sized and calibrated syringes. Work with your lab partner, and quiz each other. Refer to Figures 9. 21 through 9.32.

4. Practice performing the sterile and nonsterile roles with your lab partner.

5. Teach this skill to a classmate, and then observe and critique the performance.

6. Select two or three possible performance errors, demonstrate them to your lab partner, and ask your partner to identify the errors. Focus on sharps safety and accuracy. Discuss methods to prevent and correct the errors.

7. Refer to your ST textbook and this lab manual to answer the Discussion Questions (see next column).

8. Review the video and the information in this lab manual when you prepare for your certification examination.

Discussion Questions

1. Why are national organizations (such as the Joint Commission, AORN, and AST) recommending that all medications and fluids be labeled on the sterile field?

2. What are the essential steps in placing medications on the sterile field, such as the back table or Mayo stand?

3. List the essential steps in receiving sterile solutions onto the back table or Mayo stand.

4. What do you say to the surgeon when you are passing a syringe filled with medication?

5. Why do you inform the surgeon in the previous question? Aren't you afraid that you may break his or her concentration?

6. How can an electronic medication record help to prevent medication errors?

7. What can happen if the ST does not securely fasten the hypo onto the Leuer-lock end of the syringe?

8. Develop a plan to calculate the amount of medication used from a syringe that is refilled multiple times.

9. If you do not know the generic and brand name of a drug, how will you find out? Why do you need to know both names?

10. You are relieving a co-worker for lunch and you notice that the syringe with medication in it is not labeled. What should you do?

11. Note here any questions that you need your instructor to clarify.

Select Mayo Stand Instruments

10

INTRODUCTION

Instruments are selected for the Mayo stand according to the sequence of the procedure and the surgeon's preferences. Thoughtful planning permits the surgical technologist to set up this contained workspace safely and efficiently.

- Before performing this skill, your lab instructor will discuss some of the principles for practice and objectives involved in this chapter as well as the importance of following the skill sequence and instructions.
- Set up a Mayo stand with the instruments needed to begin a laparotomy procedure. Handle all sharps safely, and state the rationale for your selections. Practice with your lab partner, and encourage

and critique each other. Your instructor will offer strategies for success. Appendix E highlights the value of teaching others as a component of active learning strategies. Refer to Appendix C for an overview of the chapter.
- The lab instructor will advise you of any additional criteria to be evaluated. At a designated time, demonstration of these skills will be evaluated and graded by your lab instructor using the competency assessment tool.
- When in the clinical setting, your instructor may once again assess your performance using the same tool. Refer to Appendix A for clinical evaluation and documentation.

Team Member	Type of Role		Timing		
	Nonsterile	Sterile	Preop	Intraop	Postop
Surgical Technologist		X	X	X	
Assistant Circulator					
Operating Room Team					

OBJECTIVES

The learner will demonstrate this skill with 100 percent accuracy each time it is performed in the operative setting:

1. Maintain aseptic technique.
2. Demonstrate preparation of the Mayo stand with appropriate instruments and equipment for a selected surgery procedure.

3. Use critical thinking and economy of time and motion in the selection and preparation of instrumentation.
4. Load a blade onto a knife handle using a needle holder.
5. Unload the blade using a needle holder.
6. Assemble a sponge on a sponge forceps.
7. Load a Kitner sponge on a curved forceps.

Principles for Practice

The foundation and rationale for our practice, in the perioperative environment, stem from evidence provided by professionals, organizations, and governmental agencies. Refer to the Bibliography, Glossary of Terms, and the following documents or developmental agencies:

- OR guidelines
- Surgeon's preference card
- ST's preferences
- Association of Surgical Technologists (AST)
- Association of periOperative Registered Nurses (AORN)

SKILL SEQUENCE AND INSTRUCTIONS

1. Prepare a stable base for the ringed instruments on the Mayo stand.
   - Make a rolled towel, and place it on the Mayo stand. It will support your ringed instruments (see Figure 10.1).

2. Select instruments from the back table to be used initially according to the procedure and the surgeon's preferences.
   - Place your selection on your Mayo stand.
   - Construct your own arrangement plan, or use a standardized one specific to your OR.
   - Plan to change the inventory of instruments on the stand as the procedure progresses. Refer to Chapters 19, 20, and 22 for additional information.
   - Select ring-handled forceps, squeeze closed the ratchets to the first tooth, and place in pairs on your Mayo stand the following: Criles, Kellys, Curved Kellys, Kochers, Allises, and Babcocks.
   - Select and place scissors, straight and curved. Straight Mayo scissors may be called "suture scissors" and are used to cut suture. Curved Mayo scissors may be used to cut tissue. Metzenbaum scissors may be used to cut delicate tissue.
   - Select and place forceps, with or without teeth.
   - Select and place retractor pairs according to the depth of the procedure in the body (see Figures 10.2 through 10.5).

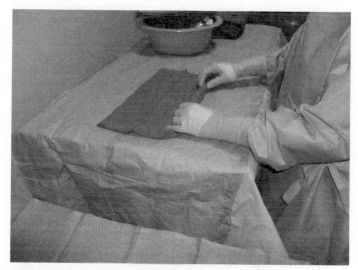

FIGURE 10.1   Make a rolled towel.

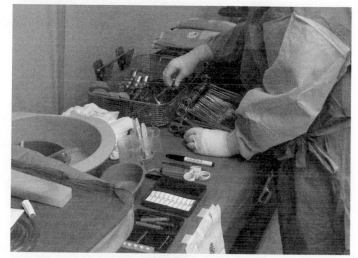

FIGURE 10.2   Select from the back table.

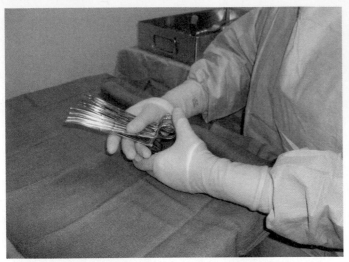

FIGURE 10.3 Close ringed instruments to the first tooth.

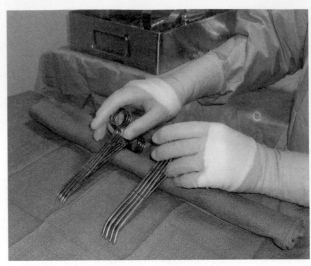

FIGURE 10.4 Place ringed instruments on the rolled towel.

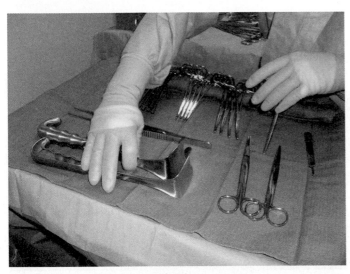

FIGURE 10.5 Arrange two Richardson retractors.

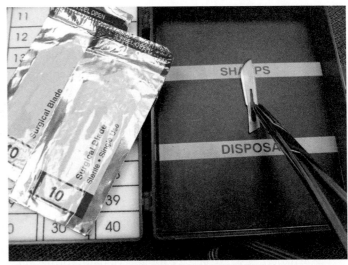

FIGURE 10.6 Grasp blade with a needle holder.

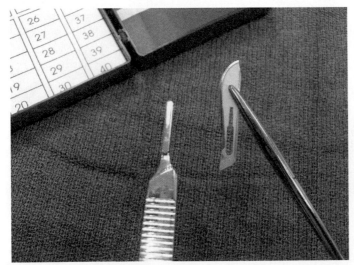

FIGURE 10.7 Align angles and slots.

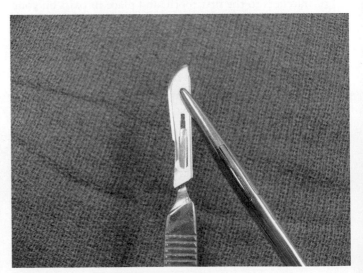

FIGURE 10.8 Slide blade onto handle.

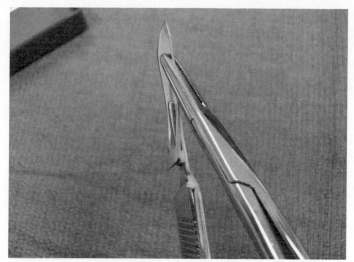

FIGURE 10.9 Side view of seating the blade.

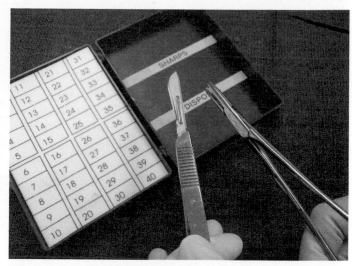

FIGURE 10.10 Loaded knife handle.

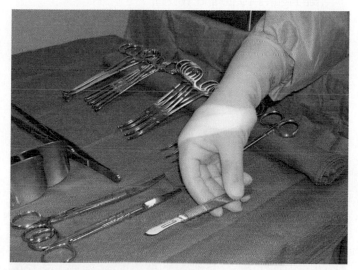

FIGURE 10.11 Position scalpel onto the Mayo stand.

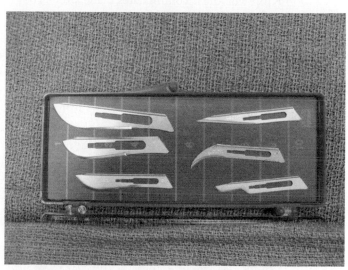

FIGURE 10.12 View various blade sizes.

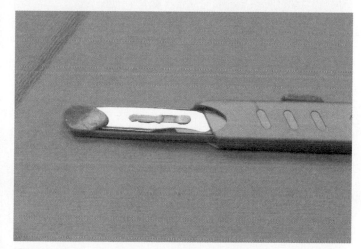

FIGURE 10.13 View preloaded safety knife handle with sheath.

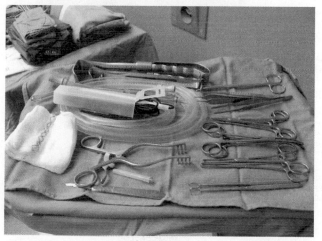

FIGURE 10.14 Move this knife handle to a safer location.

3. Load or arm the knife handle.
   - Identify and open the #10 blade packet. Place the blade into the needle counter.
   - Grasp the blade with a needle holder (needle driver).
   - Align the blade with the slots on the #3 knife handle; align the angle of the blade with the angle on the knife handle.
   - Slide, or seat, the blade into place on the handle.
   - Do not rush or force the blade.
   - Place the knife blade on the Mayo stand in a safe location, or in a no-touch basin. Do not place it where it cannot be seen.
   - Place two Ray-Tec sponges on the Mayo stand for use by the surgeon during the incision.
   - Knife handle and blades:
     # 3 Knife Handle accommodates blade sizes #10, #11, #12, and #15.
     # 4 Knife Handle accommodates blade sizes #20, and #21.
     # 7 Knife Handle accommodates blade sizes #10, #11, #12, and #15 (see Figures 10.6 through 10.14)

4. Unload the blade from the handle.
   - Grasp the end of the blade with a needle holder, point the blade downward and facing the needle mat, lift the blade, and slide it off of the handle.
   - Place the blade into the needle mat.
   - Perform this skill at the end of the surgical procedure (see Figure 10.15).

5. Assemble a Ray-Tec sponge on a sponge forceps (sponge stick); use an x-ray detectable sponge. Follow the surgeon's preference for construction. (see Figures 10.16 through 10.19).

6. Load an x-ray detectable-Kitner sponge on a curved forceps; it will be used as an extension of the surgeon's finger during blunt dissection, or for blood absorption. A Kitner may also be known as a peanut or pusher. (see Figures 10.20 and 10.21).

7. Mayo stand setups will vary depending on the facility, preceptor, procedure, and preferences. Some procedures do not use a Mayo stand, and the ST works directly from the back table. Mayo stands will be used for various sterile items, other than instruments (see Figures 10.22 through 10.24).

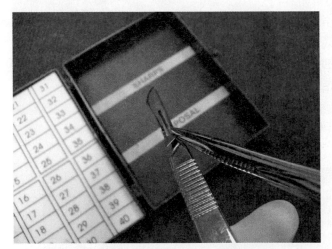

FIGURE 10.15   Point toward needle mat, and lift off blade.

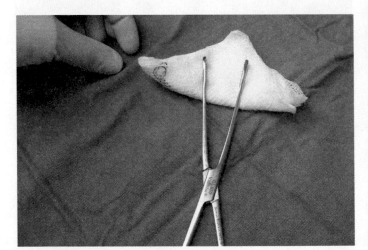

FIGURE 10.16   Fold sponge.

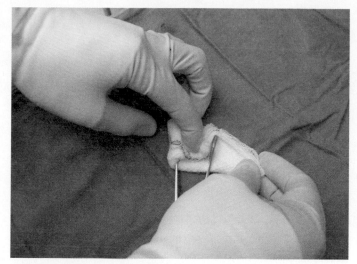

FIGURE 10.17 Enclose forceps.

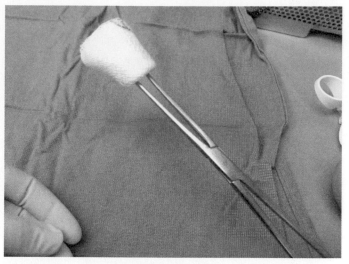

FIGURE 10.18 One type of sponge stick.

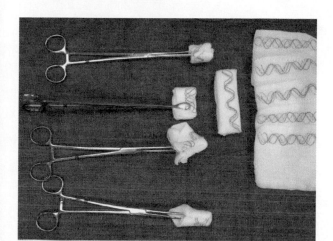

FIGURE 10.19 Sponge stick variations.

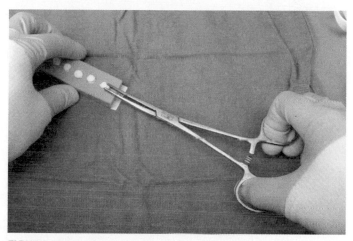

FIGURE 10.20 Grasp Kitner sponge with curved forceps.

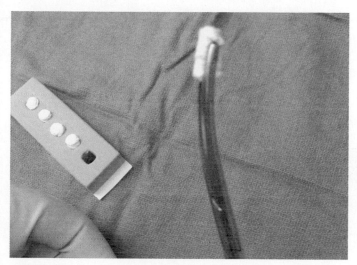

FIGURE 10.21 Kitner loaded on a curved forceps or passer.

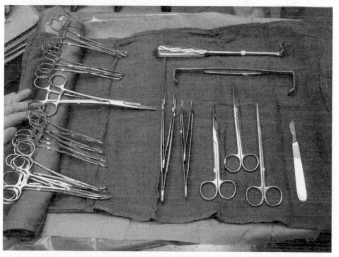

FIGURE 10.22 General surgery setup.

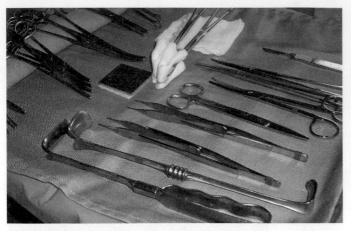

FIGURE 10.23   Lab setting Mayo stand.

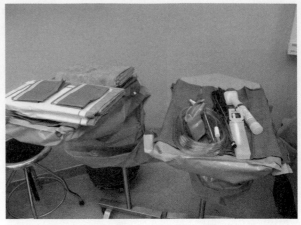

FIGURE 10.24   Mayo stands can hold sterile supplies.

Indicate your preferences for a Mayo stand setup in
Diagram 10.1.

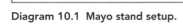

Diagram 10.1 Mayo stand setup.

COMPETENCY ASSESSMENT

STUDENT'S NAME: _____

CHAPTER 10 SELECT MAYO STAND INSTRUMENTS

PERFORMANCE RANK:

S or √ = Satisfactory: Competent—safe, accurate, sequential, and timely
U = Unsatisfactory: Unsafe—inaccurate and unprepared

PERFORMANCE RATING:

5   Independent: Expert—safe, confident, seamless performance; mentors others
4   Minimally monitored: Intermediate—safe, self-corrects few errors
3   Competent: Novice—safe, revises with evaluator cues, few errors
2   Remedial: Unsafe—critical errors, unable to implement evaluator cues consistently
1   Dependent: Unsafe—unacceptable, requires multiple evaluator interventions

PERFORMANCE CRITERIA	Performance Rank	Performance Rating
1. Perform Mutual Professional and Scholastic Criteria as appropriate (see the Preface or Appendix A).		1 2 3 4 5
2. Prepare a stable base, such as a rolled towel, and place on the Mayo stand.		1 2 3 4 5
3. Select and place ringed forceps; close the ratchets.		1 2 3 4 5
4. Select and place scissors.		1 2 3 4 5
5. Select and place forceps, with and without teeth.		1 2 3 4 5
6. Select and place retractors.		1 2 3 4 5
7. Pair appropriately sized knife handles and blades.		1 2 3 4 5
8. Load and place a knife handle.		1 2 3 4 5
9. Remove the blade; place it into a needle mat (state timing in the procedure when the blade is routinely removed).		1 2 3 4 5
10. Place two x-ray detectable sponges for the surgeon.		1 2 3 4 5
11. Construct a sponge stick using an x-ray detectable sponge.		1 2 3 4 5
12. Load a Kitner sponge onto a curved forceps.		1 2 3 4 5

ADDITIONAL COMMENTS _____

PERFORMANCE EVALUATIONS AND RECOMMENDATIONS

❑ PASS: Satisfactory Performance
    ❑ Demonstrates professionalism
    ❑ Exhibits critical thinking
    ❑ Demonstrates proficient clinical performance appropriate for time in the program
❑ FAIL: Unsatisfactory Performance
    ❑ Critical criteria not met (See Performance Rank or Rating Above)
    ❑ Professionalism not demonstrated.
    ❑ Critical thinking skills not demonstrated.
    ❑ Skill performance unsafe or underdeveloped.
❑ REMEDIATION:
    ❑ Schedule lab practice. Date: _____
    ❑ Reevaluate by instructor. Date: _____
❑ DISMISS from lab or clinicals today.
❑ Program director notified. Date: _____

SIGNATURES

Date _____   Evaluator _____   Student _____

ACTIVITIES AND DISCUSSION QUESTIONS

Activities

1. View the Complete Perioperative Process and Focus on Skills video, Skill #10 (video can be found at www.myhealthprofessionskit.com).
2. Observe the instructor perform the skill.
3. Practice the skill in the lab, with your lab partner or in small groups.
4. Direct observation by your instructor may be mandatory when loading and unloading scalpel blades.
5. Select one skill, teach it to a classmate, and then observe and critique the performance.
6. Select two possible performance errors, demonstrate them to your lab partner, and ask your partner to identify the errors. Focus on sharps safety and accuracy. Discuss methods to prevent and correct the errors.
7. Refer to your ST textbook and this lab manual to answer the Discussion Questions (see next column).
8. Review the video and the information in this lab manual when you prepare for your certification examination.

Discussion Questions

1. List the essential steps of this skill in order.
2. Discuss the different uses for the Mayo scissors and the Metzenbaum scissors.
3. Why should the scrub tech identify malfunctioning pieces of equipment?
4. Why are you taught to arm a knife handle by holding the blade with a needle holder?
5. You notice that the screw lock on the scissors is loose. What should you do?
6. During the procedure, the surgeon asks the anesthesia care provider to elevate the OR bed. What is your role? (You may refer to Chapter 7.)
7. It is the end of the case, and skin closure is imminent. What supplies do you think you will need on your Mayo stand now?
8. Note here any questions that you need your instructor to clarify.

PEARSON
myhealthprofessionskit™

Use this address to access the Companion Website created for this textbook. Simply select "Surgical Technology" from the choice of disciplines. Find this book and log in using your username and password to access interactive activities, videos, and much more.

11 Prepare the Patient for Operating Room Entry

INTRODUCTION

During preparation for the procedure in the operating room, the patient is being prepared in a separate location, the pre-operative holding area. In the nonsterile role, prepare the patient for surgery, obtain vital signs, and transfer and transport the patient to the operating room using proper body mechanics and safety.

- Before performing this skill, your lab instructor will discuss some of the principles for practice and objectives involved in this chapter as well as the importance of following the skill sequence and instructions.
- Role-play with your lab partner and prepare the patient for OR entry. Encourage and critique each other. Your instructor will offer strategies for success. Appendix E highlights the value of teaching others as a component of active learning strategies. Refer to Appendix C for an overview of the chapter.
- The lab instructor will advise you of any additional criteria to be evaluated. At a designated time, demonstration of these skills will be evaluated and graded by your lab instructor using the competency assessment tool.
- When in the clinical setting, your instructor may once again assess your performance using the same tool. Refer to Appendix A for clinical evaluation and documentation.

Team Member	Type of Role		Timing		
	Nonsterile	Sterile	Preop	Intraop	Postop
Surgical Technologist	X		X		
Assistant Circulator	X		X		
Operating Room Team	X		X		

OBJECTIVES

The learner will demonstrate the following with 100 percent accuracy each time the operative environment is entered.

1. Identify the patient using established parameters.
2. Facilitate completion of the preoperative checklist.
3. Obtain and appraise vital signs—pain, pulse, respirations, blood pressure, temperature, and pulse oximetry.
4. Prepare the OR bed for the patient.
5. Promote patient safety during transfers and transportation.
6. Promote normothermia.
7. Uphold the patient's privacy.
8. Assist OR team members with positioning and padding of bony prominences.

Principles for Practice

The foundation and rationale for our practice, in the perioperative environment, stem from evidence provided by professionals, organizations, and governmental agencies. Refer to the Bibliography, Glossary of Terms, and the following documents or developmental bodies:

- Manufacturers' product instructions
- Operating room policies

- State practice acts
- American Heart Association (AHA)
- National Institute for Occupational Safety and Health (NIOSH)
- Occupational Safety and Health Administration (OSHA)
- Association of Surgical Technologists (AST)
- Association of periOperative Registered Nurses (AORN)

SKILL SEQUENCE AND INSTRUCTIONS

Prepare the OR Bed

1. Prepare the OR Bed for the patient.

   - Position the bed with the head closest to the anesthesia care provider for a laparotomy procedure, in this example.
   - Cover the bed with clean, hospital-laundered linens.
   - Place positioning aids, including ulnar pads (elbow) and occipital pads (head).
   - Prepare the bed according to the requirements of the surgical procedure; configurations and padding will vary among surgical specialties (see Figures 11.1 through 11.4).
   - Go to the separate pre-op holding area to meet the patient scheduled in the room you prepared.

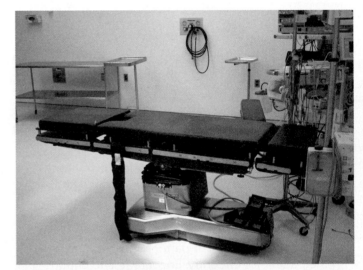

FIGURE 11.1 OR bed; headrest on right.

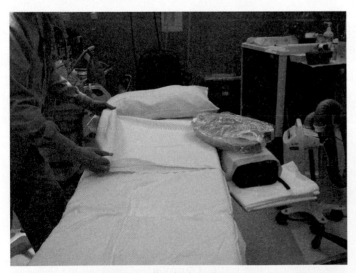

FIGURE 11.2 Make the bed with clean linens.

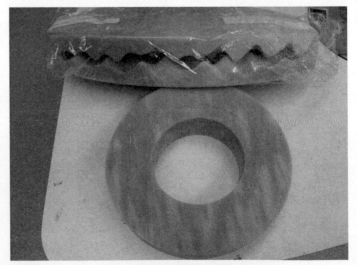

FIGURE 11.3 Gather and place disposable padding.

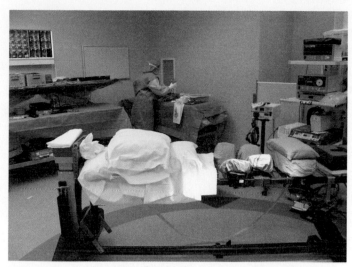

FIGURE 11.4   View example of bed variations: Neurosurgery Jackson table, Wilson frame, and padding.

Preoperative Preparation

2. Perform Preoperative Preparation of the patient and assist to complete the preoperative checklist, in the pre-op holding room.

   - Identify yourself, and explain your role to the patient.
   - Identify the patient according to your hospital policy. For example, verify by asking the patient to state their name and birth date. Compare with the patient's name band or chart.
   - Assist the patient to remove fingernail polish, face makeup, clothing, earrings, and any body jewelry.
   - Assist the patient to use the bathroom, urinal, or bedpan, as needed, before surgery; document the time and amount of the last void before surgery. Refer to Chapters 1 through 3 and Appendix D.
   - Label and store personal belongings per your OR policy. Valuables should be left at home.
   - Assist the patient to put on a hospital gown and OR cap to cover their hair.
   - Obtain coveralls, mask, and OR hat for a translator, parent, or law enforcement personnel who will accompany the patient into the OR.
   - The surgeon will identify and confer with the patient, answer questions, obtain the consent for surgery from the patient or a legal guardian, review radiology and laboratory data, and mark the incision site.

- Perform appropriate hair removal with clippers per the surgeon's order. Explain the procedure to the patient. Maintain patient privacy.
- Note: The CDC guidelines recommend not removing hair prior to an operation. If hair will interfere with the incision site then hair removal should be performed with clippers and just prior to the procedure. Shaving promotes microabrasions and SSIs.
- Physical assessments are completed by the patient's surgeon, the anesthesia care provider, and the registered nurse. Review of the chart includes evaluating orders, diagnostic tests, laboratory values, the history and physical, when the patient ate or drank fluids last, or NPO status, completion of at-home-preparation, allergy status, communication barriers, baseline data, and a signed surgical consent.
- Perform a Braden risk assessment to determine the risk of skin breakdown, and perform the risk-to-fall assessment to determine those at higher risk for injury. Plan on using additional padding or precautions, as indicated. Follow your hospital policy regarding which team member is responsible for these assessments.
- Obtain vital signs and document.

Vital Signs

3. Obtain Vital Signs and document these as the preprocedure baseline: Pain, Pulse, Respirations, Blood Pressure, Temperature, and Pulse Oximetry. (Skill sequence follows.)

   - Report readings outside of the expected parameters to the surgeon or manager.
     - Note: Any abnormal vital sign reading obtained during lab practice with fellow classmates is confidential information. Your classmate is responsible for seeking medical advice from his or her own health care practitioner.
     - Vital sign parameters are listed in Table 11.1.

TABLE 11.1 Average Vital Signs

Vital Signs Average Parameters							
Temperature		Pulse: Beats per Minute		Respirations: Breaths per Minute	Blood Pressure: mm Hg	Pain	Pulse Oximetry %
Site	Normal °F						
Axillary	97.6	Birth	130–160	30–60	60/30	0	98–100
Oral	98.6	Infant 1 yr.	110–130	20–30	80/50	0	98–100
Temporal	99.4	Child 1–11 yr.	80–110	16–26	110/60	0	98–100
Rectal	99.6	Adult 12 +	60–100	12–20	120/80	0	95–100

TABLE 11.2 Adult Number Scale

Adult Pain Scale										
0	1	2	3	4	5	6	7	8	9	10
No Pain										Worst Pain Experienced

Pain

4. Assess Pain using the age-appropriate scale: numerical, caricatures, crying, and body language or positioning.

   - For the alert adult, a number scale of 0 to 10 is used where "0" indicates no pain and "10" indicates the worst pain experienced. Refer to Table 11.2.
   - Explain the rating scale. Ask the adult patient to rate their pain on a scale of 0 to 10, and document the rating.
   - Follow hospital policy for appropriate interventions related to the rating of pain. It is customary to report pain ratings to the RN.
   - Record "0" on a scale of 0–10.
   - For the young child who is unable to use a number scale, use the facility-approved method, such as the *Wong-Baker Faces Pain Rating Scale*. Refer to Table 11.3.
     ○ Ask the child to point to the face depicting how they feel.
   - Infant pain is assessed using crying patterns and ability to be consoled.
     ○ Document and follow facility policy regarding appropriate interventions related to a pain rating.

Pulse

5. Measure and record the radial pulse rate and rhythm, and the patient's position for an adult patient, for example.

   - Locate the radial artery by feeling for the pulse. Use gentle pressure with your first two or three fingers as you count the number of beats per minute. Do not use your thumb.
   - Evaluate the pattern of the beats—regular or irregular.
   - Use a wall clock or wrist watch with a second hand as a timer.
   - Count for one full minute, and record the rate, regularity, and location.
   - Record Pulse: 60, regular, right radial. Refer to Table 11.5 (see also Figure 11.5).

TABLE 11.3   Child Faces Scale

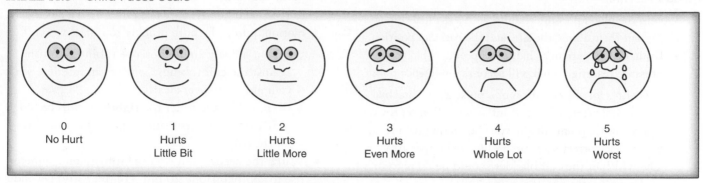

0	1	2	3	4	5
No Hurt	Hurts Little Bit	Hurts Little More	Hurts Even More	Hurts Whole Lot	Hurts Worst

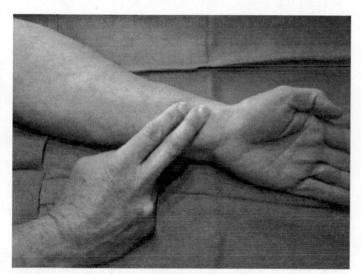

FIGURE 11.5   Count the radial pulse rate.

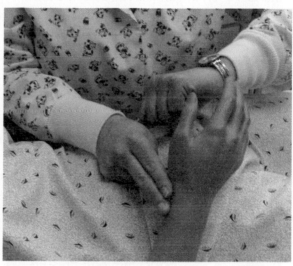

FIGURE 11.6   Monitor respirations while taking the pulse.

Respirations

6. Measure and record the respiratory rate and rhythm. Watch the chest rise with each inspiration.

- Count the number of inspirations per minute.
- Observe the rhythm.
- Do not tell the patient that you are watching them breathe, to prevent voluntary control over their inspirations.

- Monitor the respiratory rate and rhythm after counting the pulse rate, but do not change your position.
- If you cannot see the chest rise with inspirations, then gently rest your hand or forearm on the patient's chest or abdomen to feel the rise and fall of the chest, if not contraindicated.
- Record respiratory rate and rhythm: Rate 16, regular. Refer to Table 11.5 (see also Figure 11.6).

Blood Pressure

7. Obtain the blood pressure reading with a manual cuff, and document the reading, the site, and the patient's position.
   - Evaluate the patient's chart for a previous blood pressure reading which will serve as a reference point.
     - Feeling for the cessation of a pulse at the brachial or radial artery after cuff inflation will also provide a reference point for the systolic blood pressure.
   - Secure the correct size cuff around the upper arm. The width of the cuff bladder should be 40 percent of the circumference of the arm.
   - Follow the arrow on the cuff for placement over the brachial artery. Secure the cuff at least 1 inch above the antecubital space to provide room for stethoscope placement.
   - Position the patient's upper arm so it is supported at heart level, and keep the gauge in the same location.
   - Refer to Table 11.4 for erroneous errors.
   - Instruct the patient to relax the arm.
   - Palpate the brachial artery on the medial aspect of the antecubital fossa with your first two fingers.
   - Place the bell/diaphragm of the stethoscope over the artery and the earpieces into your ears. Apply continuous and gentle pressure on the diaphragm.

TABLE 11.4   Skill Performance Errors

Cuff and Position Errors	Errors in Blood Pressure Reading	
	False Low	False High
B/P Cuff Too Narrow		X
B/P Cuff Too Wide	X	
Arm Held Too High	X	
Arm Held Too Low		X

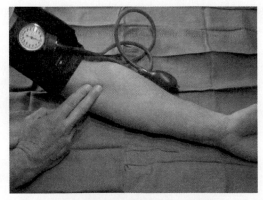

FIGURE 11.7   Palpate the brachial artery.

- With your other hand, grasp the pressure bulb on the cuff, and gently close the roller with a clockwise motion; pump the bulb quickly to inflate the cuff.
  - Do not allow your stethoscope tubing to brush against the cuff tubing. Contact can interfere with your ability to hear clearly.
  - Do not close the roller too tightly. It will be too difficult to open resulting in pain or discomfort for the patient.
- Watch the needle gauge on the sphygmomanometer rise to approximately 20 mm Hg (mercury) beyond the last blood pressure reading.
- Slowly release the roller using a counterclockwise motion as you listen for the pumping or tapping sounds in your stethoscope.
- Release at the rate of 2 to 4 mm per second. Each mark on the gauge represents 2 mm Hg.
- Listen for the first sound (tapping pulse): Karotkoff phase I, or the systolic reading, which is an indirect measure of the pressure in the large arteries during systole.
- Listen for additional sounds first louder, followed by dull and muffled.
- Listen for the sound to disappear. Karotkoff phase V, or the diastolic reading, is an indirect measure of the pressure on the arteries during diastole.
- Record the systolic and diastolic readings; remove the cuff.
- Refer to a physical assessment text for additional information.
- Alternately, the B/P may be obtained with an automated device. A stethoscope is not used. Follow the manufacturer's instructions for use.
- Record B/P via a manual cuff: 120/68, left arm, lying position.
- Refer to Table 11.5 (see also Figures 11.7 through 11.11).

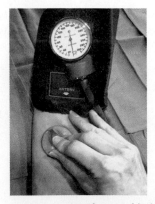

FIGURE 11.8   Place and hold the stethoscope over the artery.

TABLE 11.5 Medical or Surgical Variables related to Vital Sign Changes

Rationale for Vital Sign Changes

Readings	T	P	R	B/P	Pain	Pulse Ox
Elevated	Infection	Fever	Fever	CV disease	Trauma	Deep breathing
	Metabolic disease	Pain	Pain	Kidney disease	Surgery	Supplemental oxygen therapy
	Head injury	Hemorrhage	Hemorrhage	Fluid overload	Arthritis	Falsely elevated with CO
		Heart disease	Hypoxia	Pain	Medical diagnoses	
		Hypoxia	Hypercapnia	Anxiety	Anxiety	
		Hypercapnia	Anxiety			
		Anxiety				
		Medications				
Decreased	Hemorrhage	Heart block	Resting	Hemorrhage	Neuromuscular disease	Lung disease
	Cold environment	Metabolic disease	Head injury	Heredity	Paralysis	Hemorrhage
	Head injury	Vagus nerve stimulation	Narcotics	Physically fit	Chemical nerve blocks	Hypotension
		Physically fit				Hypothermia
		Medications				Motion
						Ambient light
						Dyes
						Falsely decreased with oxidized iron

Note: This table is not inclusive and is intended to be an example to encourage additional reading.

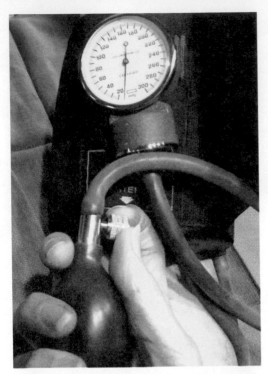

FIGURE 11.9   Regulate cuff inflation with the roller and bulb.

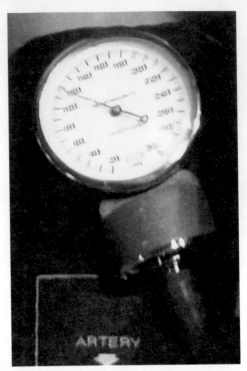

FIGURE 11.10   Record systolic reading.

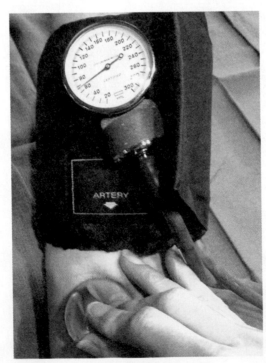

FIGURE 11.11   Record diastolic reading.

Temperature

8. Obtain and record a temperature.

- Wash your hands, gather all equipment, and explain the procedure to the patient.
- Instruct the patient not to eat or drink for 20 minutes before an oral reading.
- Wear appropriate PPE for the patient's diagnosis—gloves, mask, eye goggles, or a disposable isolation gown. Refer to Chapter 3.
- Measure and record the temperature using the preferred method: oral, axillary, tympanic, temporal, or rectal. Follow the manufacturer's instructions for use of the thermometer. Record site and reading.
- Temperature: Temporal, 99.2°F.
  Refer to Table 11.5, which lists sample rationales for deviations from the norm. (see also Figures 11.12 and 11.13).

Pulse Oximetry

9. Obtain and record a pulse oximetry reading.

- Pulse oximetry, or "Pulse ox," is a noninvasive method used to assess the saturation of hemoglobin molecules in the blood with oxygen. The probe uses light sources and a microprocessor to calculate the saturation.
  - Low readings indicate the need for respiratory care intervention and oxygen therapy.
  - Use your emergency CPR training to provide rescue breaths and chest compressions if the patient is not breathing and there is no pulse. Activate the Code (Blue) button or call the operator.
- Obtain the pulse oximeter device and explain the procedure to the patient; follow manufacturer's instructions for use.
- Turn the device on.
- Clip the sensor to one of the patient's warm fingertips or toes, if they are free of nail polish or acrylics. Do not allow movement.
  - Good perfusion to the fingertips or toes is required by the sensor. Warm toes and fingertips with brisk capillary refill indicate adequate perfusion.
  - Measure capillary refill by gently squeezing the tip of the index finger. Notice blanching or white color. Release your grip and monitor the return of color. Good perfusion is evidenced by a refill or return of color in less than 3 seconds.
  - Black, green, and blue, and, to a lesser degree, red nail polishes will result in a falsely low pulse ox reading.
  - IV dyes, especially methylene blue, also falsely lower the reading for a brief interval.
  - Refer to Table 11.5 for deviations.
- For acrylic nails, turn the probe 90 degrees and place it with the sensor reading through the skin of the fingertip.
- Use manufacturer-supplied sensors for earlobes or the bridge of the nose, or an infant's sole or palm, as needed. Remove all jewelry, including earrings. Secure the jewelry in a sealed container, and label it with the patient's name.
- Read the pulse ox on the monitor screen, and record as a percentage. Most monitors also provide a pulse rate.
  - Compare the radial pulse rate with the rate obtained by the monitor. The values should be the same.
- Survey the patient for the use of supplemental oxygen.
- Record the reading and the use of supplemental oxygen or none (room air).
- Report abnormal reading to your supervisor—your surgeon or manager.
- Document: Pulse oximetry, 98% on room air, and the pulse rate, if provided by the device (see Figure 11.14).
- Provide appropriate comfort measures for the waiting patient; these may include warm blankets and magazines (see Figure 11.15).

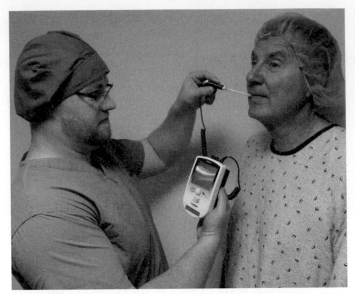

FIGURE 11.12 Obtain digital oral temperature reading.

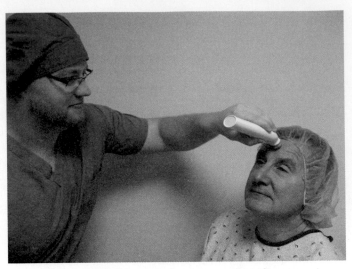

FIGURE 11.13 Obtain temporal temperature reading.

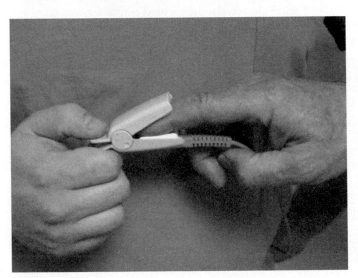

FIGURE 11.14 Attach pulse oximetry probe.

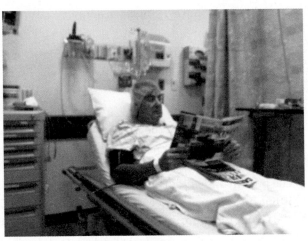

FIGURE 11.15 Comfort measures for waiting patient.

Transport and Transfer

10. Transport the patient from the preoperative holding room to the OR suite and to the OR bed.

- Obtain the necessary equipment.
- Position the stretcher next to the bed, and lock the wheels. Describe to the alert patient how they will assist with the transfer to the stretcher—lift your "bottom" as you slide onto the stretcher.
- Respect privacy; cover the patient with her or his gown or the blanket.
- Secure personal belongings, per hospital policy.
- Once the patient is transferred, elevate and secure the side rails on the stretcher.

- Cover the patient with a warm blanket for comfort.
- Unlock the wheels; move the stretcher slowly, smoothly, and feet first.
- Align the stretcher with the OR bed, equalize the heights, lock the wheels on the stretcher and on the OR bed, and describe the transfer process to the patient.
- Use minimal assistance to transfer the alert patient.
- Use at least four team members to assist with the transfer of a nonalert patient.
- Demonstrate the principles of ergonomics: push rather than pull heavy items; lift with your legs, not with your lower back; bend at your knees, not with your back; do not twist at your waist (see Figure 11.16).

11. Prepare the patient on the OR bed.

- To prepare the patient on the OR bed, introduce the patient to the team members in the room.
- Apply a safety strap around the patient's legs, approximately two inches above the knees. Adjust the fit so that you can place one hand between the strap and the patient.
- Place pillows under the patient's knees for comfort.
- Uncross the patient's feet at the ankles.
- Do not leave the patient unattended.
- Attach padded arm boards to the bed frame to prevent ulnar nerve damage. Position each arm board at an angle less than 90° to prevent stretching of the patient's brachial plexus.
- Position the patient's arm on the arm board with their palms facing the ceiling and the fingers extended, not flexed.
- Apply sequential compression devices to the lower extremities, per your OR policy, to prevent deep vein thrombosis.

- Provide emotional support and therapeutic communication.
- Assist the anesthesia care provider with placement of the automatic blood pressure cuff, EKG leads, and pulse oximeter, according to your OR policy.

Additional Practice:

- Position the patient in a prone position (on their stomach) or in a lateral (side-lying) position, as indicated by the operative site.
- Obtain additional padding and positioning devices (see Figures 11.17 through 11.19).

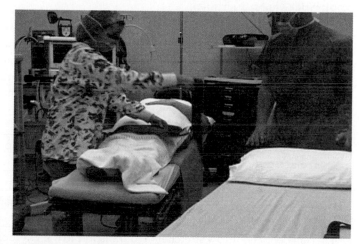

FIGURE 11.17   Apply the safety strap.

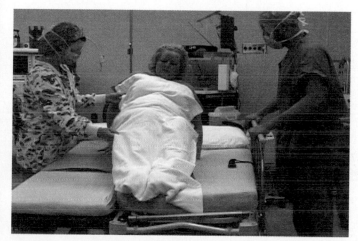

FIGURE 11.16   Transfer safely from the stretcher to OR bed.

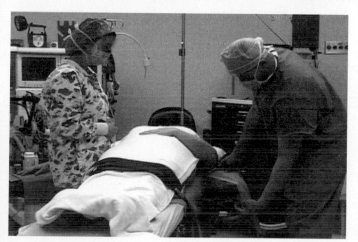

FIGURE 11.18   Position the padded arm board.

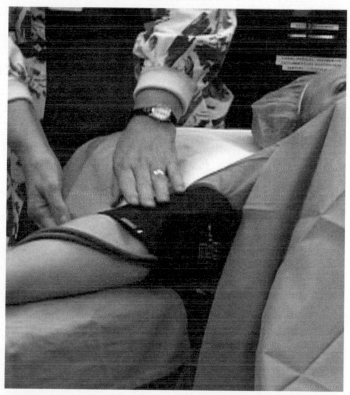

FIGURE 11.19   Apply automatic blood pressure cuff.

COMPETENCY ASSESSMENT

STUDENT'S NAME: _____

CHAPTER 11 PREPARE THE PATIENT FOR OPERATING ROOM ENTRY

PERFORMANCE RANK:

S or √ = Satisfactory: Competent—safe, accurate, sequential, and timely
U = Unsatisfactory: Unsafe—inaccurate and unprepared

PERFORMANCE RATING:

5   Independent: Expert—safe, confident, seamless performance; mentors others
4   Minimally monitored: Intermediate—safe, self-corrects few errors
3   Competent: Novice—safe, revises with evaluator cues, few errors
2   Remedial: Unsafe—critical errors, unable to implement evaluator cues consistently
1   Dependent: Unsafe—unacceptable, requires multiple evaluator interventions

PERFORMANCE CRITERIA	Performance Rank	Performance Rating
1. Perform Mutual Professional and Scholastic Criteria as appropriate (see the Preface or Appendix A).		1 2 3 4 5
2. Appraise the preoperative checklist for completeness.		1 2 3 4 5
3. Obtain vital signs and document; use a student actor or simulation manikin in the laboratory setting: T, P, R, B/P, Pain, Pulse Oximetry.		1 2 3 4 5
4. Transfer patient to a stretcher, and transport to the OR room; use safety precautions and proper body mechanics.		1 2 3 4 5
5. Transfer patient to an OR bed; use safety precautions and proper body mechanics.		1 2 3 4 5
6. Introduce patient to the OR team members present in the room.		1 2 3 4 5
7. Prepare the patient on the OR bed; position in the supine position.		1 2 3 4 5
8. Demonstrate alternate positions; lateral and prone.		1 2 3 4 5

ADDITIONAL COMMENTS _____

PERFORMANCE EVALUATIONS AND RECOMMENDATIONS

❏ PASS: Satisfactory Performance
    ❏ Demonstrates professionalism
    ❏ Exhibits critical thinking
    ❏ Demonstrates proficient clinical performance appropriate for time in the program
❏ FAIL: Unsatisfactory Performance
    ❏ Critical criteria not met (see Performance Rank or Rating Above)
    ❏ Professionalism not demonstrated.
    ❏ Critical thinking skills not demonstrated.
    ❏ Skill performance unsafe or underdeveloped.
❏ REMEDIATION:
    ❏ Schedule lab practice. Date: _____
    ❏ Reevaluate by instructor. Date: _____
❏ DISMISS from lab or clinicals today.
❏ Program director notified. Date: _____

SIGNATURES

Date _____   Evaluator _____   Student _____

ACTIVITIES AND DISCUSSION QUESTIONS

Activities

1. View the Complete Perioperative Process and Focus on Skills video, Skill #11, Transport and Transfer the Patient (video can be found at www.myhealthprofessionskit.com).
2. Observe the instructor perform the skill.
3. Practice the skill in the lab, with your lab partner or in small groups.
4. Observe any variations in the blood pressure and pulse ox readings when obtained in different positions: lying, standing, and sitting. Observe changes to respirations and pulse after running or lying quietly. Apply black, green, or blue nail polish to one fingernail and observe corresponding changes in the pulse ox readings.
5. Select one skill, teach a classmate, and observe and critique the performance.
6. Refer to your ST textbook and this lab manual to answer the Discussion Questions (see next column).
7. Review the video and the information in this lab manual when you prepare for your certification examination.

Discussion Questions

1. List the essential steps in transferring and transporting the patient from pre-op holding to the OR in logical order.
2. What are two essential themes in the steps you listed in #1?
3. Measure your patient's vital signs. The temporal thermometer registers the temperature as 95.9°F. What is your next action?
4. Your patient's chart lists the last B/P as 130/85, height and weight are 5' 2", and 250 lbs. You obtain a reading of 180/100. Your patient is awake, talkative, denies pain, and states the usual B/P is about 130/80. What is your next action?
5. Why do we pad the bony prominences, such as the olecranon process or the occiput?
6. If the patient is uncooperative and does not want to slide onto the OR bed, what should you do?
7. Note here any questions that you need your instructor to clarify.

Participate in Preanesthesia Skills

12

INTRODUCTION

Operating room team members pause before invasive procedures and validate, as a group through verbal communication and with a checklist, that all key factors are accounted for. Soon thereafter, the anesthesia care provider begins to administer anesthesia to the patient. The surgical technologist (ST) may be called to assist with cricoid pressure, during intubation. In an emergency, the ST may work with other team members by performing cardio-pulmonary resuscitation (CPR).

- Before performing these skills, your lab instructor will discuss some of the principles for practice and objectives involved in this chapter as well as the importance of following the skill sequence and instructions.

- Use a manikin, and practice the chapter skills with your lab partner. Encourage and critique each other. Your instructor will offer strategies for success. Appendix E highlights the value of teaching others as a component of active learning strategies. Refer to Appendix C for an overview of the chapter.
- The lab instructor will advise you of any additional criteria to be evaluated. At a designated time, demonstration of these skills will be evaluated and graded by your lab instructor using the competency assessment tool.
- When in the clinical setting, your instructor may once again assess your performance using the same tool. Refer to Appendix A for clinical evaluation and documentation.

Team Member	Type of Role		Timing		
	Nonsterile	Sterile	Preop	Intraop	Postop
Surgical Technologist	X	X	X		
Assistant Circulator	X		X		
Operating Room Team	X	X	X		

OBJECTIVES

The learner will demonstrate the following with 100 percent accuracy each time the operative environment is entered.

1. Demonstrate collaboration with team members when verifying key components on a safe surgery checklist.
2. Evaluate the significance of using a checklist prior to complex processes.

3. Describe the timing of the safe surgery checklist in relationship to the administration of anesthesia.
4. Demonstrate hand placement for cricoid pressure.
5. Demonstrate cardiopulmonary resuscitation techniques—face mask, Ambu bag, and hand placement for chest compressions in the operating room.
6. Demonstrate positioning of oxygen therapy devices—nasal cannula.

Principles for Practice

The foundation and rationale for our practice, in the perioperative environment, stem from evidence provided by professionals, organizations, and governmental agencies. Refer to the Bibliography, Glossary of Terms, and the following documents or developmental agencies:

- Operating room policies
- The Joint Commission
- World Health Organization (WHO)
- Association of Surgical Technologists (AST)
- Association of periOperative Registered Nurses (AORN)
- Emergency Care Research Institute (ECRI)
- American Heart Association (AHA)
- American Society of Anesthesiologists (ASA)

SKILL SEQUENCE AND INSTRUCTIONS

Preprocedure Validation

1. Collaborate with OR team members, and concur with validation of key components of a preprocedure, safe surgery checklist. This process may also be known as the intraoperative pause.

   - Recognize the importance of actively participating in prevention strategies.
     - The Joint Commission estimates that approximately 40 wrong site surgeries occur each week in hospitals and clinics in the US. Although reporting errors is confidential and voluntary in about half of the states, only a portion of the errors are reported to the commission.
   - Appraise information pertinent to the surgical procedure preoperatively, before induction into anesthesia: name of patient, medical record number, date of birth, surgeon, procedure, laterality, site markings, positioning, equipment, supply or implant needs, allergy status, antibiotics, diagnostic images or pathology reports, blood product requirements, plan for specimens, signed operative consent, special safety precautions, sterilization indicators, and fire risk score. Refer to Chapters 10 and 13.
   - Introduce yourself to the patient, along with the other OR team members.
   - Maintain awareness of the unique components of the checklist for each patient.
   - Do not become complacent.
   - Be attentive to the announcement, by the circulator or surgeon, of the pause for the safe surgery checklist.

   - Focus on the process of validation before induction into anesthesia or the skin incision. Give your attention to the announcement of the key facts.
   - Respond verbally to affirm the correctness of the key parameters, as a member of the OR team, according to your hospital's policy.
   - Document agreement in the patient's chart, which is the circulator's role (see Figure 12.1).

2. Compare your OR policy to those designed by the World Health Organization (WHO) and the Association of periOperative Registered Nurses (AORN) (see Figures 12.2 and 12.3).

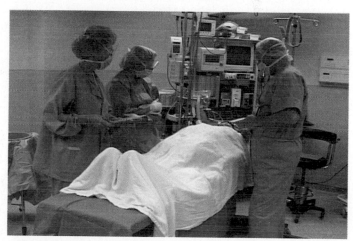

FIGURE 12.1   Pause for patient safety.

TABLE 12.1   Perioperative Safe Surgery Checklist

Stakeholders	Components	
Patient	Personal identity	History and Physical
	Surgical site	Medications
	Allergies	Risk factors
	Anesthesia	Discharge instructions
Surgeon	Consent	Blood loss
	Images	Specimens
	Special equipment	Timing
	Surgical site	New orders
		Discharge instructions
Anesthesia provider	Airway	Antibiotics
	IV site	Medications
	Blood products	Postanesthesia care
	VS & Normothermia	Discharge instructions
Nursing Team	Assessment	Sterile parameters
	Preop-checklist	Postanestheisa care
	Prevention of risk factors	Medications
		Discharge instructions

Cricoid Pressure

3. Assist the anesthesia care provider (ACP) during the patient's emergency induction into anesthesia (see Figures 12.2 through 12.4).

- Following verification of key components, general anesthesia is administered by the ACP as appropriate for the procedure.
- Vital signs—temperature, pulse, respirations, blood pressure, pulse oximetry, and EKG—are monitored by the ACP.
- Be attentive to assist the ACP during placement of an endotracheal tube for use with general anesthesia.
- Move to the head of the bed and assist as instructed.
- Use a Yankauer suction catheter to remove oral secretions.

- Perform cricoid pressure as instructed by the ACP.
  - Locate the patient's prominent thyroid cartilage along the anterior neck.
  - Press your thumb and forefinger into the area inferior to the prominence. This area, or round cricoid cartilage, is displaced backwards against the body of the sixth cervical vertebrae, thereby occluding the esophagus. The goal is to prevent a chemical pneumonitis due to aspiration of vomited stomach contents.
  - Maintain backward, occluding pressure, until the ACP verifies placement of the endotracheal tube and gives permission to release your hand position.
  - Regown and reglove to perform in the sterile role or return to the assistant circulator role.

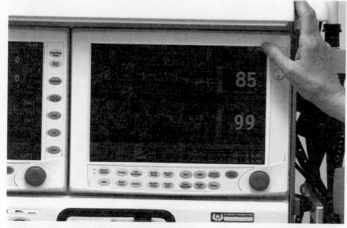
FIGURE 12.2 Monitoring of vital signs.

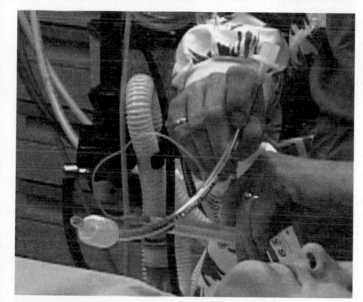
FIGURE 12.4 Simulated endotracheal intubation.

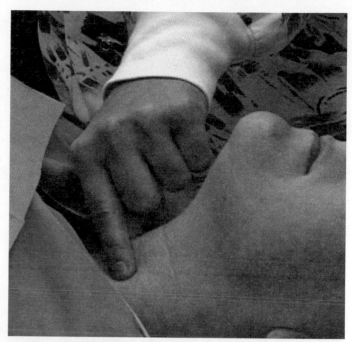
FIGURE 12.3 Cricoid pressure.

Cardiopulmonary Resuscitation

4. Assist the OR team during cardio-pulmonary resuscitation. The anesthesiologist will alert you to an emergency.

- Obtain CPR certification. Refer to your training manual for additional instructions. The American Heart Association teaches rescuers this sequence: "CAB"—compressions-airway-breathing.
- Demonstrate hand placement for chest compressions on an adult manikin.

  ○ Use step stools or kneel on the OR bed, so you can position your shoulders and arms directly over the sternum of the manikin. The OR team will place a firm back board under the patient, if needed.
  ○ Use the heels of both hands placed over the lower half of the manikin's sternum and compress hard and fast, at least two inches, and at a rate of at least 100/min. Compress 30 times then give 2 ventilations with the Ambu bag.
  ○ Two team members will coordinate compressions and ventilations.

- Demonstrate placement and use of a one-way valve face mask with Ambu bag for rescue breaths. Stand at the head of the bed.

  ○ Perform a head-tilt, chin lift maneuver and secure the mask over the patient with your fingers in the E–C configuration.
  ○ Squeeze the bag; watch the manikin's chest rise and fall. Give 10–12 breaths per minute for the adult or 1 breath every 5–6 seconds. Coordinate breaths with the chest compressions. (see Figures 12.5 and 12.6).

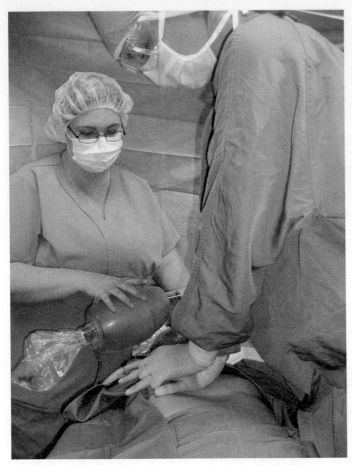

FIGURE 12.5 Hand placement over the lower half of the sternum.

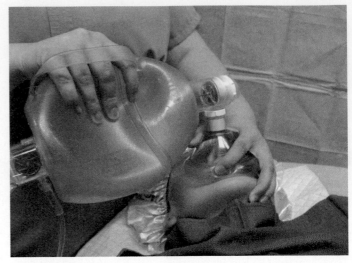

FIGURE 12.6 E-C hand grip on face mask with Ambu bag.

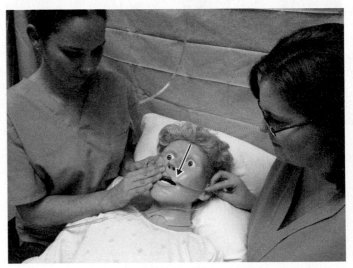

FIGURE 12.7 Reposition displaced prongs and oxygen tubing.

Oxygen Therapy

5. Assist with the management of oxygen therapy, in the nonsterile ST role. Oxygen therapy is ordered by the anesthesiologist; it is similar to a medication.

- Know your hospital's policy. The ST may obtain vital signs, including pulse oximetry readings. The ST may not initiate oxygen therapy or perform a physical assessment. Refer to Chapter 11.
- Ensure attachment of oxygen tubing to the green (oxygen) flow meter on the wall or to a portable oxygen tank during transportation of the patient.
- Reposition nasal cannula prongs in the patient's nose, for example, if they become dislodged. The prongs should follow the natural curve of the nasal passage. Secure the tubing around the patient's ears. (see Figure 12.7).

STUDENT'S NAME: _____

CHAPTER 12 PARTICIPATE IN PREANESTHESIA SKILLS

PERFORMANCE RANK:

S or √ = Satisfactory: Competent—safe, accurate, sequential, and timely
U = Unsatisfactory: Unsafe—inaccurate and unprepared

PERFORMANCE RATING:

5   Independent: Expert—safe, confident, seamless performance; mentors others
4   Minimally monitored: Intermediate—safe, self-corrects few errors
3   Competent: Novice—safe, revises with evaluator cues, few errors
2   Remedial: Unsafe—critical errors, unable to implement evaluator cues consistently
1   Dependent: Unsafe—unacceptable, requires multiple evaluator interventions

PERFORMANCE CRITERIA	Performance Rank	Performance Rating
1. Perform Mutual Professional and Scholastic Criteria as appropriate (see the Preface or Appendix A).		1 2 3 4 5
2. State the rationale for a safe surgery checklist.		1 2 3 4 5
3. Name a minimum of five criteria or key components validated before anesthesia is given.		1 2 3 4 5
4. State the rationale for performing cricoid pressure.		1 2 3 4 5
5. Demonstrate cricoid pressure (Sellick's maneuver) on a simulation manikin.		1 2 3 4 5
6. Demonstrate chest compressions, and rescue breaths with an Ambu bag, on a manikin.		1 2 3 4 5
7. Demonstrate placement of nasal cannula tubing for oxygen therapy.		1 2 3 4 5

ADDITIONAL COMMENTS _____

PERFORMANCE EVALUATIONS AND RECOMMENDATIONS

❑ PASS: Satisfactory Performance
    ❑ Demonstrates professionalism
    ❑ Exhibits critical thinking
    ❑ Demonstrates proficient clinical performance appropriate for time in the program
❑ FAIL: Unsatisfactory Performance
    ❑ Critical criteria not met (see Performance Rank or Rating Above)
    ❑ Professionalism not demonstrated.
    ❑ Critical thinking skills not demonstrated.
    ❑ Skill performance is unsafe or underdeveloped.
❑ REMEDIATION:
    ❑ Schedule lab practice. Date: _____
    ❑ Reevaluate by instructor. Date: _____
❑ DISMISS from lab or clinicals today.
❑ Program director notified. Date: _____

SIGNATURES

Date _____   Evaluator _____   Student _____

ACTIVITIES AND DISCUSSION QUESTIONS

Activities

1. View the Complete Perioperative Process, Introduction to Anesthesia, and Focus on Skills video, Skill #12. (video can be found at www.myhealthprofessionskit.com).
2. Observe the instructor perform the skill.
3. Practice CPR skills and use of an Ambu bag for artificial ventilations on a manikin.
4. Practice performing cricoid pressure on a manikin in the lab setting.
5. Select one skill, teach a classmate, then observe and critique the performance.
6. Refer to your ST textbook and this lab manual to answer the Discussion Questions (see next column).
7. Review the video and the information in this lab manual when you prepare for your certification examination.

Discussion Questions

1. List the essential steps to verify a safe surgery checklist.
2. Why does the OR need a safe surgery checklist?
3. Why do some ORs ask the ST to pass the scalpel to the surgeon after the safe surgery checklist has been validated?
4. While you are in preop holding with the patient, she says that she is having her right toe amputated but the consent form indicates a left-sided procedure. What do you do next?
5. What information will be documented about the time-out process in your facility?
6. Who performs cricoid pressure and when?
7. Note here any questions that you need your instructor to clarify.

13

Facilitate Electrosurgery, Demonstrate Surgical Fire Awareness

INTRODUCTION

Electrocautery is a modality used to assist the surgeon to alter, cut, dissect, and coagulate tissue with high-frequency electrical current. To prevent unintentional damage to the patient, any electrical device is grounded. If the three components of the fire triangle merge, oxygen, fuel, and an ignition source (such as the electrocautery), then accidental fires in the operating room can begin. In this chapter you will learn how to work safely with electrocautery and how to perform emergency fire suppression skills.

- Before performing these skills, your lab instructor will discuss some of the principles for practice and objectives involved in this chapter as well as the importance of following the skill sequence and instructions.

- Practice the skills in this chapter with your lab partner. Encourage and critique each other. Your instructor will offer strategies for success. Appendix E highlights the value of teaching others as a component of active learning strategies. Refer to Appendix C for an overview of the chapter.
- The lab instructor will advise you of any additional criteria to be evaluated. At a designated time, demonstration of these skills will be evaluated and graded by your lab instructor using the competency assessment tool.
- When in the clinical setting, your instructor may once again assess your performance using the same tool. Refer to Appendix A for clinical evaluation and documentation.

Team Member	Type of Role		Timing		
	Nonsterile	Sterile	Preop	Intraop	Postop
Surgical Technologist	X	X	X	X	X
Assistant Circulator	X	X	X	X	X
Operating Room Team	X	X	X	X	X

OBJECTIVES

The learner will demonstrate the following with 100 percent accuracy each time the perioperative environment is entered.

1. Apply the principles of electrical safety.
2. Select the proper grounding pad and position it to minimize the risk of patient burns.
3. Remove eschar from an active electrode tip during the procedure.
4. State the policy for reporting and impounding malfunctioning equipment.
5. Perform a fire risk assessment related to the fire triangle.
6. Practice fire suppression techniques.
7. Practice evacuation techniques.

Principles for Practice

The foundation and rationale for our practice, in the peri-operative environment, stem from evidence provided by professionals, organizations, and governmental agencies. Refer to the Bibliography, Glossary of Terms, and the following documents or developmental agencies:

- Manufacturers' product instructions
- Operating room policies
- Emergency Care Research Institute (ERCI)
- National Fire Protection Agency (NFPA)
- The American Society of Anesthesiologists (ASA)
- The Association of Surgical Technologists (AST)
- The Association of periOperative Registered Nurses (AORN)

SKILL SEQUENCE AND INSTRUCTIONS

Facilitate Electrosurgery

1. Gather and position the electrosurgery supplies and equipment.

- Nonsterile role:
- Position the generator unit to facilitate connection with the return electrode (grounding pad) used with monopolar electrosurgery.
- Position the foot-pedal control unit on the floor for use by the surgeon. Use your OR's equipment which may supply the surgeon with a hand-activated electrode instead of a foot control.
- Obtain the return electrode (grounding pad). Verify the expiration date on the package.
- Position the patient for the operative procedure: supine, prone, or lateral.
- Place the grounding pad, adhesive side down, on the patient's intact skin and over a large muscle near the operative site. Note, excess hair will be clipped preferably in the preoperative holding area.
- Ensure adhesion of the pad. Do not cut the pad.
- Do not place the pad over bony prominences, scar tissue, hairy surfaces, excess fatty tissue, a tattoo (because of metallic dyes), an implanted metal prosthesis, pacemaker, electrical implants, or internal cardioverter-defibrillator (ICD).

- Follow OR policy regarding the removal of body jewelry. A body jewelry removal tool kit is routinely available. Secure and tag along with other belongings of the patient.
- Special precautions are used if the patient has a pacemaker or ICD. The surgeon may order bipolar electrosurgery instead of using monopolar. A pacemaker programmer unit or magnet will be available in the OR. The ICD may be deactivated. A defibrillator is available in the event of a cardiac emergency.
- Attach the cord from the pad to the generator unit, and set the parameters for the cut and coagulation modes per the surgeon's order.
- Maintain the volume of the audible safety alarms on the generator unit.
- Open, onto the sterile back table cover, the electrosurgical pencil (active electrode), holster, and scratch pad, if they are not in the back table pack. Variations include a hand-activated pencil and those with an integral smoke evacuator (see Figures 13.1 through 13.7).

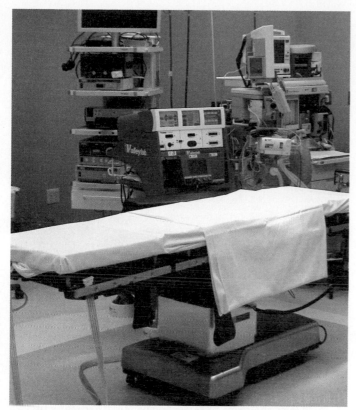

FIGURE 13.1 Generator positioned adjacent to the OR bed.

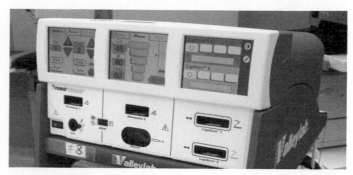

FIGURE 13.2 Generator unit.

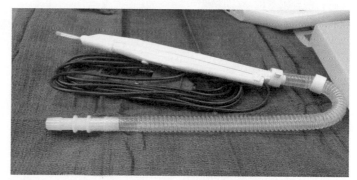

FIGURE 13.4 Hand-activated "pencil" with smoke evacuator tubing.

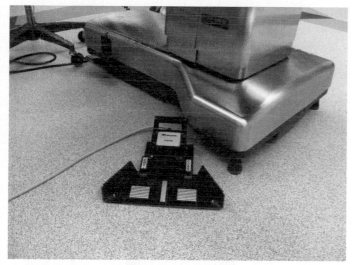

FIGURE 13.3 Foot-activated control.

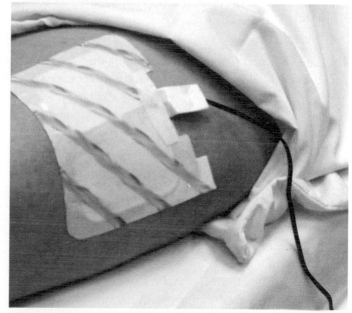

FIGURE 13.5 Anterior thigh placement; patient supine.

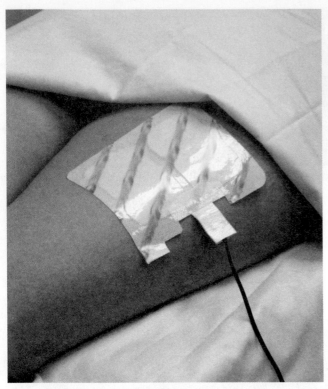

FIGURE 13.6 Posterior thigh placement; patient prone.

2. Prevent OR fires when electrosurgery is used. According to the Emergency Care Research Institute (ERCI), 70 percent of OR fires involve the hot electrosurgery pencil tip.

- The OR is an oxygen-enriched environment where all three of the basic components required for combustion exist together. These elements are known as the fire triangle.
  - Oxidizers: oxygen and nitrous oxide.
  - Fuels: alcohol in skin preps and suture packs, flatus, smoke gases, eschar, dry sponges, drapes, ointments, tinctures, bedding, hair grooming products, and hair.
  - Ignition sources: electrosurgery devices, high speed drills, LASERS, and fiberoptic lights.
- Collaborate during the fire risk assessment, performed by the circulator. The National Fire Protection Agency, in Standard NFPA 99, recommends a time out while flammable skin prep solutions dry.
- Assist the OR team to follow manufacturer's guidelines for drying times of flammable skin prep solutions. Refer to Chapter 16.

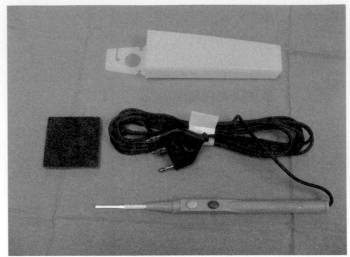

FIGURE 13.7 Hand-activated electrocautery pencil, holster, and scratch pad.

- Apply the instructions for use (IFU) when using flammable prepping solutions. Allow a minimum of 3 minutes of drying time on a hairless body part and up to 1 hour for a surface with hair. Wet hair is flammable.
- Assist the team to separate the three elements of combustion.
  - Refer to professional organizations, such as AORN, for fire risk assessment tools.
- Preoperatively, the patient is instructed to wash hair and to remove petroleum products and hair spray.
- Protect the patient's eyebrows with a nonpetroleum product, such as KY Jelly.
- Prepare dull, anodized instruments for use during LASER procedures.
- The entire OR team is vigilant (see Figure 13.8).

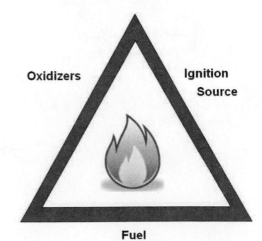

FIGURE 13.8 Three components support fire.

3. Prepare and maintain the electrosurgery equipment and supplies for the surgical procedure.

• Sterile role:
• Position the pencil, holster, and scratch pad near the surgeon and the operative site, after the surgical drapes have been placed over the patient. Use nonpenetrating clamps or Velcro tabs on the drape. Refer to Chapter 18.
• Do not wrap the cords around a metal instrument; this may cause a fire or burn.
• Pass the distal end of the pencil cord to the circulator for attachment into the generator unit with audible alarms "on."
• Prepare and store moist towels on the back table for use during a fire.
• Wipe clean the tip of the pencil by using the scratch pad during the surgical procedure. Eschar, a fuel source for a fire, builds up on the tip after use. The surgeon and the ST can use the scratch pad.
• Exchange the tips, according to the depth of the surgical plane.
• Store the pencil in the plastic holster. The tip of the pencil can reach 1100°F; if accidently activated, the drapes will burn.
• Disconnect the foot pedal when not in use, as appropriate for the equipment (circulator role).
• Place fiberoptic cables (endoscopy procedures) in the standby mode when not in use (circulator role).
• Alert the circulator to place light sources on standby-mode when not in use.
• Do not place hot cable ends on the drapes (ST role; see Figures 13.9 through 13.13).

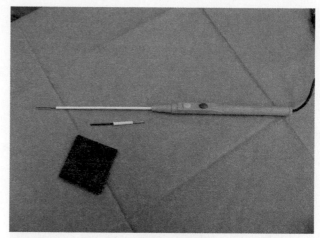

FIGURE 13.9   Long electrocautery tip.

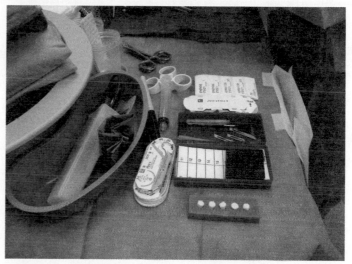

FIGURE 13.10   Group pencil, holster, and scratch with countable items during your setup.

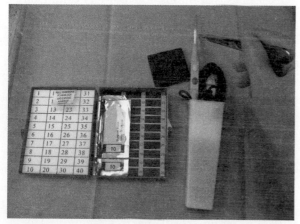

FIGURE 13.11   Identify and count sharp tip.

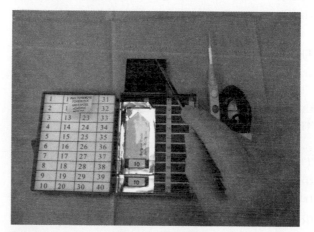

FIGURE 13.12   Count the scratch pad.

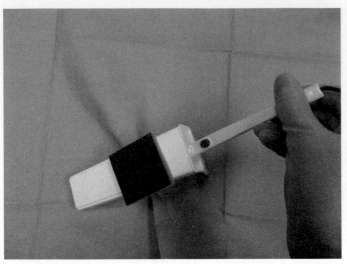

FIGURE 13.13 Place pencil into the holster when not in use.

4. Dispose of all electrosugery or Bovie tips into the sharps container at the conclusion of the procedure. The circulator will remove the grounding pad from the patient.
   - Slowly pull the pad off of the skin, use a rolling motion.
   - Discard it in the proper receptacle.
   - Assess the skin for intactness, tears, or burns. Document the skin integrity before and after the procedure and the use of safety precautions.

SURGICAL FIRE AWARENESS: EMERGENCY PREPAREDNESS

1. Participate in fire safety drills.
   - Know hospital policy and locate the evacuation routes.
   - Keep the hallways clear for a potential evacuation with the patient on the OR bed.
   - Locate carbon dioxide fire extinguishers.
   - Locate gas turn-off valves for each OR room.
2. Separate the three fire triangle components during a procedure. Awareness and prevention are paramount in fire safety.
3. In the event of a patient fire, many actions occur simultaneously.
   - The anesthesia care provider turns off the oxygen and manages the airway.
   - The surgeon controls bleeding and helps suppress the fire.
   - The circulator assists to suppress the fire and contacts the hospital operator, as needed.
   - The surgical technologist smothers the flames with a towel or douses the flames with water from the back table.
4. Perform the following fire suppression techniques as recommended by ERCI educators.

- Call out "Fire, shut off the gasses," when you see a flame or smell smoke. This notice will alert all team members to act quickly.
- Team members perform tasks simultaneously: Pull off the drapes; douse the fire with water; cover the fire; and sweep the fire out and away from the patient's head. Pat or tuck to extinguish flames on an extremity.
- Protect the patient and protect yourself from unnecessary injury.
- If needed, use a carbon dioxide fire extinguisher; it releases CO_2 at minus 400°F—very cold. Don't get it on your hands.
  - Pull, aim, squeeze, and sweep—PASS.
- Protect your face when smothering the fire with a towel.
- Place a towel on the patient's chest, rest your upper arm on the upper edge the towel, and hold it there to block the fire from moving toward the patient's head (see Figures 13.14 and 13.15).
- Drop the lower edge of the towel over the flame, and smooth (sweep) your hand towards the patient's feet to suppress the fire (see Figures 13.16 through 13.18).
- Pour water into the flames (see Figure 13.19)

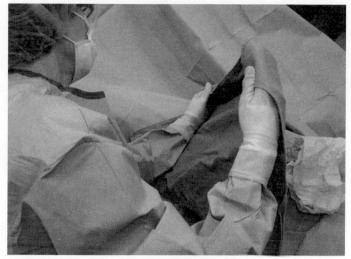
FIGURE 13.14 Block fire to patient's head.

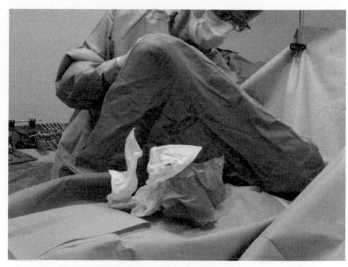
FIGURE 13.15 Protect your face.

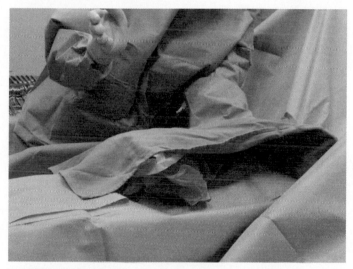
FIGURE 13.16 Cover.

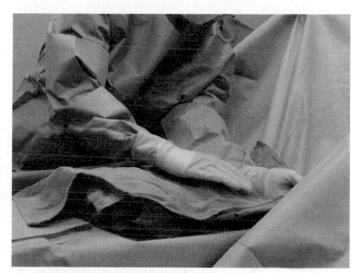
FIGURE 13.17 Smooth.

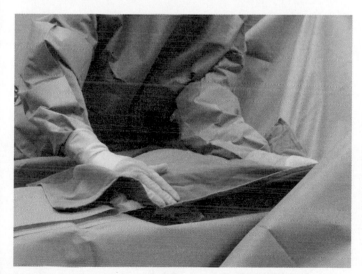
FIGURE 13.18 Direct or sweep towards patient's feet.

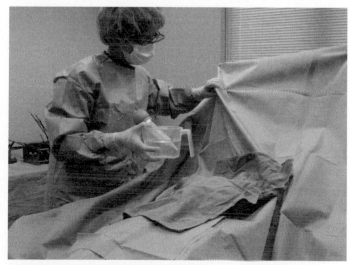
FIGURE 13.19 Pour water into flames.

Emergency Evacuation

5. In the event of an emergency evacuation due to a large fire or smoke in the room, facility policy is followed. An example evacuation is listed here.

   - Alert the manager and operator of the "Code Red" fire.
   - Pass moist laps to the surgeon; the surgeon will pack the wound with the moistened sponges.
   - Gather the required instruments in a basin or towel that will be transported with the patient.
   - The anesthesia care provider manages the airway, and brings along extra IV fluids and medications.

- The circulator notifies the operator, assists to clear the pathway, and secures the patient.
- All team members push the patient out of the room.
- The last person to leave the OR closes the door.
- Do not call a "Code Blue" (cardiac arrest) because hospital staff will rush to the area and they could be harmed by the fire (see Figures 13.20, 13.21, 13.22, and 13.23).

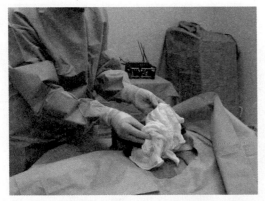

FIGURE 13.20   Place moist lap sponges into the wound.

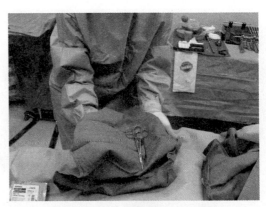

FIGURE 13.21   Gather instruments needed by the surgeon.

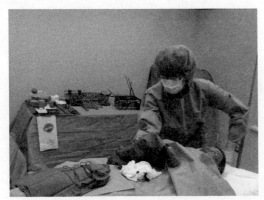

FIGURE 13.22   Evacuate the patient.

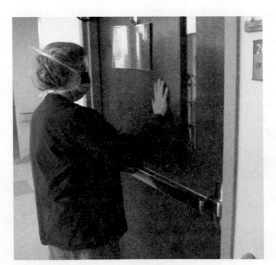

FIGURE 13.23   Close the OR door.

Facilitate Investigation

6. Follow hospital policy if an unplanned burn, or sentinel event, occurs to the patient or staff.

   • Assist to provide emergency treatment.

   • Keep all parts and packaging from the malfunctioning device so they may be included in the reporting process.

   • Document the generator number, and tag it for evaluation. Remove the unit to the bioengineering department.

STUDENT'S NAME: _____

CHAPTER 13 FACILITATE ELECTROSURGERY AND DEMONSTRATE SURGICAL FIRE AWARENESS

PERFORMANCE RANK:

S or √ = Satisfactory: Competent—safe, accurate, sequential, and timely
U = Unsatisfactory: Unsafe—inaccurate and unprepared

PERFORMANCE RATING:

5   Independent: Expert—safe, confident, seamless performance; mentors others
4   Minimally monitored: Intermediate—safe, self-corrects few errors
3   Competent: Novice—safe, revises with evaluator cues, few errors
2   Remedial: Unsafe—critical errors, unable to implement evaluator cues consistently
1   Dependent: Unsafe—unacceptable, requires multiple evaluator interventions

PERFORMANCE CRITERIA	Performance Rank	Performance Rating
1. Perform Mutual Professional and Scholastic Criteria as appropriate (see the Preface or Appendix A).		1 2 3 4 5
2. Facilitate electrosurgery; perform in the nonsterile role: position the equipment in the room, ensure function; maintain safety alarms.		1 2 3 4 5
3. Place grounding pad on the patient; connect the cord to the generator.		1 2 3 4 5
4. Open ESU-required sterile supplies onto the sterile back table (refer to Chapter 4).		1 2 3 4 5
5. Assess the environment for the fire triangle components.		1 2 3 4 5
6. Demonstrate smothering a patient "fire" with an OR towel in the scrubbed ST or circulator role.		1 2 3 4 5
7. Simulate dousing a patient "fire" with water in the ST or circulator role.		1 2 3 4 5
8. Simulate evacuating a patient from the OR with additional team members.		1 2 3 4 5

ADDITIONAL COMMENTS _____

PERFORMANCE EVALUATIONS AND RECOMMENDATIONS

❏ PASS: Satisfactory Performance
    ❏ Demonstrates professionalism
    ❏ Exhibits critical thinking
    ❏ Demonstrates proficient clinical performance, appropriate for time in the program
❏ FAIL: Unsatisfactory Performance
    ❏ Critical criteria not met (see Performance Rank or Rating above)
    ❏ Professionalism not demonstrated.
    ❏ Critical thinking skills not demonstrated.
    ❏ Skill performance unsafe or underdeveloped.
❏ REMEDIATION:
    ❏ Schedule lab practice. Date: _____
    ❏ Reevaluate by instructor. Date: _____
❏ DISMISS from lab or clinicals today.
❏ Program director notified. Date: _____

SIGNATURES

Date _____   Evaluator _____   Student _____

ACTIVITIES AND DISCUSSION QUESTIONS

Activities

1. View the Complete Perioperative Process and Focus on Skills video, Skill #13. (video can be found at www.myhealthprofessionskit.com).
2. Observe the instructor perform the skill.
3. Practice applying a grounding pad to a manikin or a patient actor in the supine and prone positions in the lab with your lab partner.
4. Simulate flames with red, orange, or yellow paper, and practice fire suppression techniques on a manikin in the lab setting, along with your lab partner.
5. Select one skill, teach a classmate, then observe and critique the performance.
6. Refer to your ST textbook and this lab manual to answer the Discussion Questions (see next column).
7. Review the video and the information in this lab manual when you prepare for your certification examination.

Discussion Questions

1. List the essential steps of this skill in order for the sterile and nonsterile team members.
2. Which team members are responsible for counting the ESU pencil tip and scratch pad?
3. You are preparing for an incision and drainage of a skin lesion on the posterior calf. Predict the placement of the dispersive electrode (grounding pad).
4. The surgeon places the active electrode, or pencil, onto the drapes after he finishes using it. Which strategy would you use to keep the patient safe from injury?
5. A RN student nurse enters the suite to observe the case and stumbles over the electrical cord that extends from the generator to the wall plug. No one is injured. After the case is over, you and your team members discuss how to prevent this situation again. Formulate two strategies of prevention.
6. Associate the fire triangle with potential surgical fire risks related to a procedure.
7. Note here any questions that you need your instructor to clarify.

Gown and Glove Another Team Member

14

INTRODUCTION

The surgical technologist anticipates and prepares the appropriate size gown and gloves needed by the surgeon and sterile team members. While maintaining aseptic technique, the ST in the sterile role gowns and gloves the surgeon and any other assistants.

- Before performing the following skill, your lab instructor will discuss some of the principles for practice and objectives involved in this chapter as well as the importance of following the skill sequence and instructions.
- Role-play with your lab partner and practice until you perform this skill smoothly and with confidence. Encourage and critique each other. Your instructor

will offer strategies for success. Appendix E highlights the value of teaching others as a component of active learning strategies. Refer to Appendix C for an overview of the chapter.

- The lab instructor will advise you of any additional criteria to be evaluated. At a designated time, demonstration of these skills will be evaluated and graded by your lab instructor using the competency assessment tool.
- When in the clinical setting, your instructor may once again assess your performance using the same tool. Refer to Appendix A for clinical evaluation and documentation.

Team Member	Type of Role		Timing		
	Nonsterile	Sterile	Preop	Intraop	Postop
Surgical Technologist		X	X	X	
Assistant Circulator					
Operating Room Team					

OBJECTIVES

The learner will demonstrate this skill with 100 percent accuracy each time the perioperative environment is entered.

1. Anticipate and prepare the correct size gown and gloves for the surgeon and team members.
2. Maintain aseptic technique.

3. Introduce self using professional etiquette.
4. Present drying towel to the team member after they perform a traditional, surgical scrub.
5. Gown and glove the surgeon and other team members.

Principles for Practice

The foundation and rationale for our practice, in the perioperative environment, stem from evidence provided by professionals, organizations, and governmental agencies. Refer to the Bibliography, Glossary of Terms, and the following documents or developmental agencies:

- Operating room policies
- Occupational Safety and Health Administration (OSHA)
- Centers for Disease Control and Prevention (CDC)
- Association of Surgical Technologists (AST)
- Association of periOperative Registered Nurses (AORN)

SKILL SEQUENCE AND INSTRUCTIONS

1. Prepare the sterile supplies in the order of use.
   - Place the drying towel, or the first item to be used, on the top of the stack. Refer to Chapter 7.
   - Layer the surgeon's gown over the appropriate size gloves (see Figure 14.1).

2. Introduce yourself to the surgeon.
   - The surgeon will approach the sterile back table upon entering the room with hands elevated, after performing the surgical scrub.
   - Introduce yourself to the surgeon and state your role. Engage in appropriate conversation—follow the surgeon's lead.

3. Present the drying towel to the surgeon.
   - Offer the drying towel only if the surgeon's hands are wet. The towel is not used following a surgical scrub with a waterless scrub product.
   - Open the towel horizontally, cuff your sterile gloved hands under the corners, and drop the towel into the surgeon's open hand (see Figure 14.2).
   - The ST will not watch the surgeon dry his hands, but will turn towards the back table and begin to prepare the surgeon's gown.
   - The surgeon will dry both hands and arms and will drop the towel into a receptacle in a manner that promotes aseptic technique (or may hand the towel to the circulator.)
   - Prevent contamination of your back table which can occur if the surgeon or assistants retrieve the towel or gown themselves.

4. Open and present the sterile gown.
   - Secure the sterile gown in both hands and move away from the back table to allow the gown to unfold.
   - Lift the gown at the shoulders and present it so that the surgeon can push both arms into the sleeves of the gown.
   - Tuck or cuff your sterile gloves under the gown to protect them from touching the skin or scrub suit of the surgeon to prevent contamination.
   - The circulator or another nonsterile team member will secure the neck closure and waist ties in the back of the gown (see Figures 14.3 and 14.4).

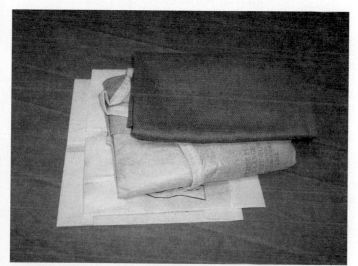

FIGURE 14.1   Prepare in order of use.

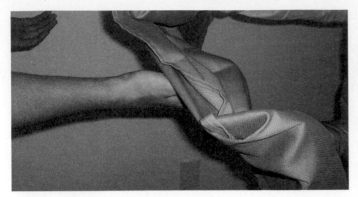

FIGURE 14.2 Present sterile towel.

5. Prepare and present the sterile gloves.

- Grasp the right glove. Milk or stretch the glove to release the elasticity.
- Orient the right glove so that the thumb or palm surface faces the surgeon. This orientation will match the presentation of the surgeon's hand into the glove. Think "thumb to thumb and fingers facing down."
- Insert your thumbs inside the glove. Turn the edges over to make a wide cuff.
- Protect your sterile gloves under the cuff of the surgeon's glove.
- Spread the right glove opening into the shape of an oval or circle.
- Offer the glove to the surgeon's right hand. Pull up on the glove as the surgeon inserts his hand.
- Release the cuff, and pull your hands away (see Figures 14.5 through 14.7).

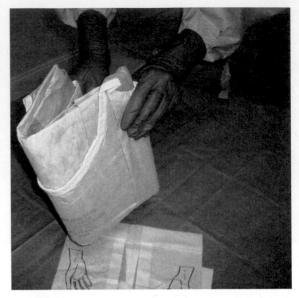

FIGURE 14.3 Grasp surgeon's gown.

6. Prepare the left glove in the same manner. The surgeon will assist with donning the left hand by using their sterile-gloved right hand.

- Present the left glove so that the surgeon can reach it with the gloved right hand. The surgeon will assist to stretch open the left glove.
- Simultaneously pull open the left glove.
- Pull up the left glove as the surgeon pushes their left hand into the glove.
- Release your grip as the glove slides over the gown sleeve.
- Focus on only touching the surgeon's sterile gown or gloves with your sterile gloves (see Figure 14.8).

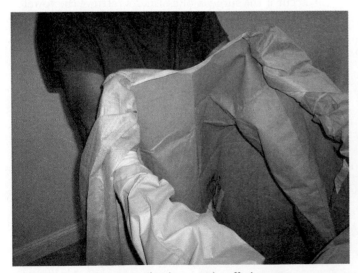

FIGURE 14.4 Protect sterile gloves with cuffed gown.

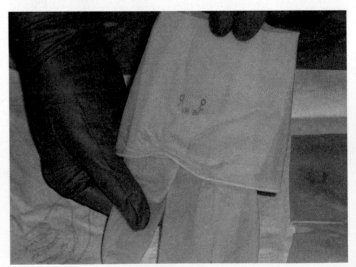

FIGURE 14.5 Prepare gloves.

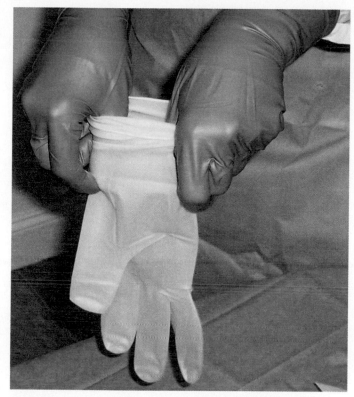

FIGURE 14.6 Prepare to make a protective cuff.

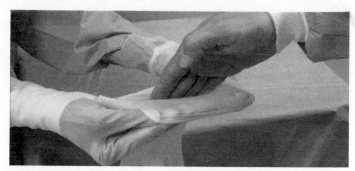

FIGURE 14.7 Stretch the opening wide.

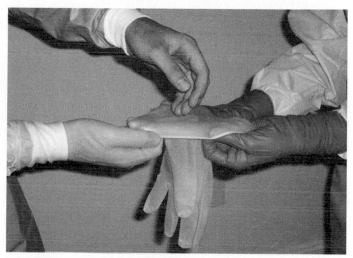

FIGURE 14.8 Assist to glove left.

7. Prepare and present the second pair of gloves.

   - Use the assisted-gloving technique.
   - The surgeon can assist with his gloved hands and will adjust the fit (see Figures 14.9 and 14.10).

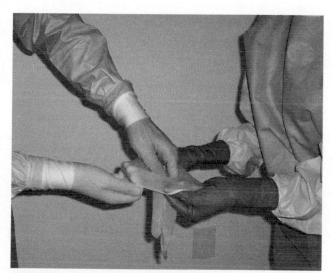

FIGURE 14.9 Assist with second pair.

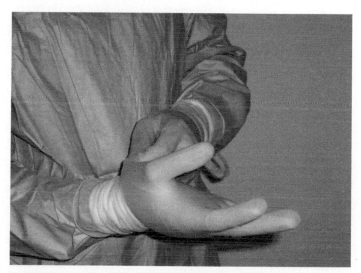

FIGURE 14.10 Surgeon makes adjustments.

8. Assist the surgeon to turn and tie their sterile gown. One possible method is described here.

   • The surgeon holds the left tie in their hand as he or she passes the tag and right tie to the ST. The surgeon turns counterclockwise so that the right tie wraps around the back of the gown.

   • Pull the right tie out of the tag, and present the tie to the surgeon. The surgeon secures both ties on the left.

   • Discard the paper tag (see Figure 14.11).

9. Perform assisted gloving if the surgeon requests a new pair of gloves during the procedure.

   • Obtain a pair of sterile gloves from the circulator as needed. Refer to steps 5 and 6 above.

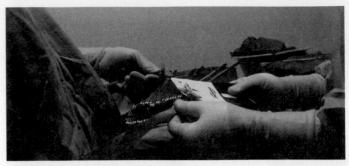

FIGURE 14.11   Assist to turn and tie.

STUDENT'S NAME: _Manjula_

CHAPTER 14 GOWN AND GLOVE A[...] TEAM MEMBER

PERFORMANCE RANK:

S or √ = Satisfactory: Competent—safe, accurate, sequential, and timely

U = Unsatisfactory: Unsafe—inaccurate and unprepared

PERFORMANCE RATING:

5   Independent: Expert—safe, confident, seamless performance; mentors others

4   Minimally monitored: Intermediate—safe, self-corrects few errors

3   Competent: Novice—safe, revises with evaluator cues, few errors

2   Remedial: Unsafe—critical errors, unable to implement evaluator cues consistently

1   Dependent: Unsafe—unacceptable, requires multiple evaluator interventions

PERFORMANCE CRITERIA	Performance Rank	Performance Rating
1. Perform Mutual Professional and Scholastic Criteria as appropriate (see the Preface or Appendix A).		1 2 3 4 (5)
2. Prepare sterile supplies in order of use (refer to Chapter 4).		1 2 (3) 4 5
3. Introduce self to the surgeon.		(1) 2 3 4 5
4. Prepare and present drying towel (water-based scrub only). *not properly*		1 (2) 3 4 5
5. Prepare and present sterile gown. *saw hands*		(1) 2 3 4 5
6. Prepare and present right glove. *contaminated*		(1) 2 3 4 5
7. Prepare and present left glove.		(1) 2 3 4 5
8. Prepare and present second pair of gloves: right then left.		1 2 3 4 (5)
9. Turn and tie surgeon's gown.		1 2 3 4 (5)

ADDITIONAL COMMENTS _____

PERFORMANCE EVALUATIONS AND RECOMMENDATIONS

❏ PASS: Satisfactory Performance

     ❏ Demonstrates professionalism

     ❏ Exhibits critical thinking

     ❏ Demonstrates proficient clinical performance appropriate for time in the program

❏ FAIL: Unsatisfactory Performance

     ❏ Critical criteria not met (see Performance Rank or Rating Above)

     ❏ Professionalism not demonstrated.

     ❏ Critical thinking skills not demonstrated.

     ❏ Skill performance is unsafe or underdeveloped.

❏ REMEDIATION:

     ☑ Schedule lab practice. Date: _____

     ☑ Reevaluate by instructor. Date: _____

❏ DISMISS from lab or clinicals today.

❏ Program director notified. Date: _____

SIGNATURES

Date ___11/4/13___   Evaluator _____   Student _____

Discussion Questions

...e Complete Perioperative Process and
...s on Skills video, Skill #14. (video can be
...und at www.myhealthprofessionskit.com).

... Observe the instructor perform the skill.

3. Practice this skill with your lab partner. Use clear communication and introduce yourself to your "surgeon" lab partner.

4. Teach this skill to your lab partner, then observe and critique the performance.

5. Refer to your ST textbook and this lab manual to answer the Discussion Questions (see next column).

6. Review the video and the information in this lab manual when you prepare for your certification examination.

1. In your own words, recall the essential steps in this skill.

2. What will you do if the surgeon's glove size is not listed on the preference card?

3. You are prepared to gown and glove the surgical team. A medical student enters the room, walks to the back table, and grasps the drying towel. Water drips onto your back table. What should you do next?

4. You are preparing the right sterile glove for the surgeon. As you stretch the cuff open, the edge rips. What should you do now?

5. The surgeon prefers not to double glove. What should you do with the second pair of gloves?

6. Note here any questions that you need your instructor to clarify.

PEARSON
myhealthprofessionskit™

Use this address to access the Companion Website created for this textbook. Simply select "Surgical Technology" from the choice of disciplines. Find this book and log in using your username and password to access interactive activities, videos, and much more.

15 Perform Open-Gloving Technique

INTRODUCTION

Open gloving is a skill routinely performed when in the nonsterile role in preparation for completing a sterile skill, including urinary catheterization or skin preparation. Under special circumstances, a sterile team member may don sterile gloves with the open-gloving technique. Refer to Chapter 21.

- Before performing this skill, your lab instructor will discuss some of the principles for practice and objectives involved in this chapter as well as the importance of following the skill sequence and instructions.
- Don sterile gloves while your lab partner observes for breaks in aseptic technique. Encourage and critique each other. Your instructor will discuss strategies for success. Appendix E highlights the value of teaching others as a component of active learning strategies. Refer to Appendix C for an overview of the chapter.
- The lab instructor will advise you of any additional criteria to be evaluated. At a designated time, demonstration of these skills will be evaluated and graded by your lab instructor using the competency assessment tool.
- When in the clinical setting, your instructor may once again assess your performance using the same tool. Refer to Appendix A for clinical evaluation and documentation.

Team Member	Type of Role		Timing		
	Nonsterile	Sterile	Preop	Intraop	Postop
Surgical Technologist	X		X	X	
Assistant Circulator	X		X	X	
Operating Room Team	X		X	X	

OBJECTIVES

The learner will demonstrate the following with 100 percent accuracy each time the skill is used:

1. Apply the principles of aseptic technique.
2. State the rationale for using open gloving.
3. Select and prepare the appropriate gloves.
4. Don sterile gloves while in nonsterile attire.
5. Remove, doff, sterile gloves.

Principles for Practice

The foundation and rationale for our practice, in the perioperative environment, stem from evidence provided by professionals, organizations, and governmental agencies. Refer to the Bibliography, Glossary of Terms, and the following documents or developmental agencies:

- Manufacturers' product instructions
- Operating room policies
- Occupational Safety and Health Administration (OSHA)
- Centers for Disease Control and Prevention (CDC)
- Association of Surgical Technologists (AST)
- Association of periOperative Registered Nurses (AORN)

SKILL SEQUENCE AND INSTRUCTIONS

1. Perform hand hygiene. Refer to Chapter 2 (see also Figure 15.1).
2. Prepare supplies and equipment.
   - Position a clean prep table or Mayo stand in a convenient location; this will be your work space.
   - Secure a sterile pack of gloves, inspect, and open the glove packet on the stand. Discard the outer peel-package.
   - Open the inner glove packet and touch only the 1-inch margin around the paper edges.
   - Secure the edges and establish a sterile field (see Figures 15.2 through 15.4).

3. Don sterile gloves with the open-gloving method. Don your dominant hand first. See right hand example.
   - Pinch the bottom edge of the right glove cuff, lift the glove up, move away from the sterile field, and slide the glove onto your right hand.
   - Do not touch the sterile glove with your nonsterile left hand (see Figures 15.5 and 15.6).

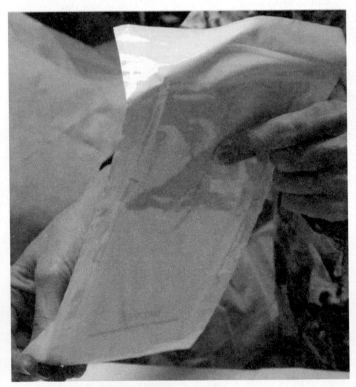

FIGURE 15.1 **Wash your hands.**

FIGURE 15.2 **Inspect the peel-package.**

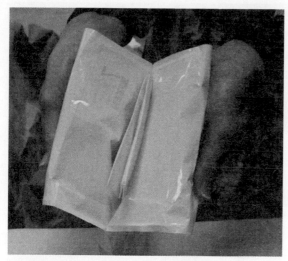

FIGURE 15.3 Open the peel wrapper.

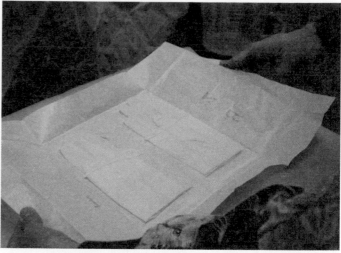

FIGURE 15.4 Prepare a sterile field.

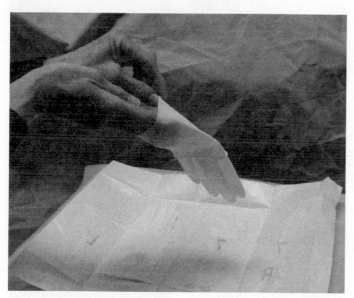

FIGURE 15.5 Don right glove.

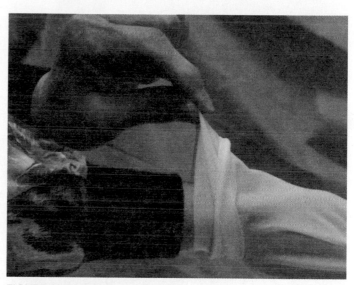

FIGURE 15.6 Adjust at cuff only.

4. Lift the left glove under the cuff with the sterile right-gloved hand.

- Slide your left hand into the left glove. Protect your gloved right hand.
- Do not touch the sterile glove with your bare left hand.
- Adjust the fit by touching sterile surfaces only (see Figures 15.7 through 15.9).

5. Perform the sterile procedure, such as a urinary catheterization or skin preparation.

6. Don sterile gloves in a sterile procedure kit.

Note: Obtain a separate pair of gloves if your hands are sized smaller or larger than the "medium" pair in the kit.

- Inspect and open the procedure kit, and establish a sterile field.
- Grasp the enclosed glove pack by pinching the top and lift it to another flat surface. Do not touch the drapes or contents of the kit with your hands.
- Don the sterile gloves. Refer to steps 2–4.
- Return to the kit and perform the sterile procedure. Refer to Chapter 16 (see also Figure 15.10).

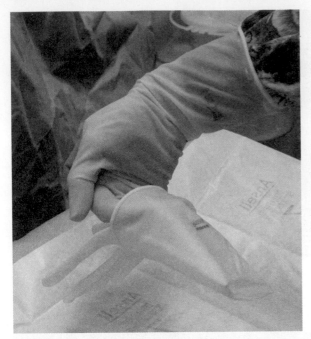

FIGURE 15.7 Touch sterile to sterile surfaces.

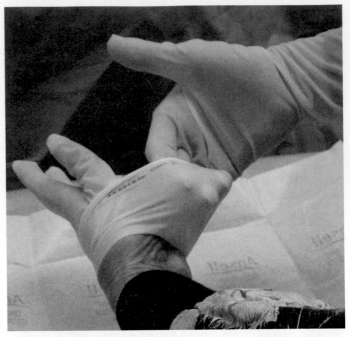

FIGURE 15.8 Pull on left glove.

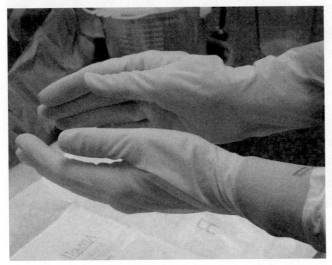

FIGURE 15.9 Only touch sterile surfaces.

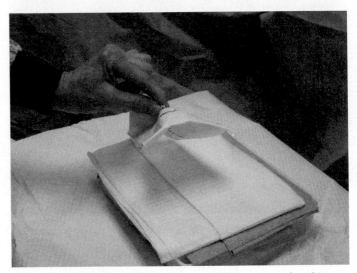

FIGURE 15.10 Don sterile gloves provided in a procedure kit.

7. When in the sterile role, use open-gloving to correct a contamination error if you cannot correct the error by other preferred methods. Refer to Chapter 21.

8. Doff or remove the gloves after use.

- Pinch palm surface of right glove with the left glove and pull off the right glove. Hold right glove in a tight ball in the left glove.
- Insert bare right index finger under the left glove (touch the palm of the left hand) and lift off the left glove.
- Think: touch "glove to glove, then "skin to skin."
- Discard gloves into a proper receptacle.
- Perform hand hygiene. Refer to Chapter 2 (see also Figure 15.11).

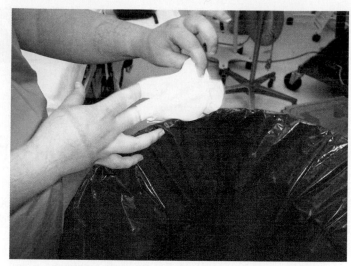

FIGURE 15.11 Remove gloves.

STUDENT'S NAME: _____

CHAPTER 15 PERFORM OPEN-GLOVING TECHNIQUE

PERFORMANCE RANK:

S or √ = Satisfactory: Competent—safe, accurate, sequential, and timely
U = Unsatisfactory: Unsafe—inaccurate and unprepared

PERFORMANCE RATING:

5	Independent: Expert—safe, confident, seamless performance; mentors others
4	Minimally monitored: Intermediate—safe, self-corrects few errors
3	Competent: Novice—safe, revises with evaluator cues, few errors
2	Remedial: Unsafe—critical errors, unable to implement evaluator cues consistently
1	Dependent: Unsafe—unacceptable, requires multiple evaluator interventions

PERFORMANCE CRITERIA	Performance Rank	Performance Rating
1. Perform Mutual Professional and Scholastic Criteria as appropriate (see the Preface or Appendix A).		1 2 3 4 5
2. Inspect and open selected glove package; discard outer dust cover.		1 2 3 4 5
3. Establish a sterile field on a nonsterile surface, prep table, or Mayo stand.		1 2 3 4 5
4. Don sterile gloves; use open gloving method.		1 2 3 4 5
5. Remove gloves; prevent self-contamination.		1 2 3 4 5
6. Perform hand hygiene.		1 2 3 4 5

ADDITIONAL COMMENTS _____

PERFORMANCE EVALUATIONS AND RECOMMENDATIONS

❑ PASS: Satisfactory Performance
    ❑ Demonstrates professionalism
    ❑ Exhibits critical thinking
    ❑ Demonstrates proficient clinical performance appropriate for time in the program
❑ FAIL: Unsatisfactory Performance
    ❑ Critical criteria not met (see Performance Rank or Rating Above)
    ❑ Professionalism not demonstrated.
    ❑ Critical thinking skills not demonstrated.
    ❑ Skill performance is unsafe or underdeveloped.
❑ REMEDIATION:
    ❑ Schedule lab practice. Date: _____
    ❑ Reevaluate by instructor. Date: _____
❑ DISMISS from lab or clinicals today.
❑ Program director notified. Date: _____

SIGNATURES

Date _____   Evaluator _____   Student _____

ACTIVITIES AND DISCUSSION QUESTIONS

Activities

1. View the Complete Perioperative Process and Focus on Skills video, Skill #15 (video can be found at www.myhealthprofessionskit.com).
2. Observe the instructor perform the skill.
3. Practice this skill with your lab partner, in the nonsterile role.
4. Teach this skill to your lab partner, then observe and critique the performance.
5. Refer to your ST textbook and this lab manual to answer the Discussion Questions (see next column).
6. Review the video and the information in this lab manual when you prepare for your certification examination.

Discussion Questions

1. List five essential steps in this skill.
2. When you assess the package integrity, you notice a tear in the inner wrapper. The outer wrapper appears to be intact. Is it acceptable to use this package? Why or why not?
3. Give two examples explaining how a glove in this skill could become contaminated.
4. How do you control package memory?
5. Formulate a plan to keep the gloves sterile, once they are on, until you need to touch sterile items in a kit.
6. Note here any questions that you need your instructor to clarify.

Perform Urinary Catheterization and Skin Preparation

16

INTRODUCTION

Urinary catheterization is a sterile procedure used to drain the bladder and to monitor kidney function. During preoperative skin preparation, an antiseptic solution is used around the proposed incision site to inhibit growth of transient and resident microorganisms thereby, decreasing the risk of a surgical site infection.

- Before performing these skills, your lab instructor will discuss some of the principles for practice and objectives involved in this chapter as well as the importance of following the skill sequence and instructions.
- Use a manikin to perform a urinary catheterization and a skin prep for a laparotomy procedure. Practice with a lab partner, and encourage and critique each other. Your instructor will offer strategies for success. Appendix E highlights the value of teaching others as a component of active learning strategies. Refer to Appendix C for an overview of the chapter.
- The lab instructor will advise you of any additional criteria to be evaluated. At a designated time, demonstration of these skills will be evaluated and graded by your lab instructor using the competency assessment tool.
- When in the clinical setting, your instructor may once again assess your performance using the same tool. Refer to Appendix A for clinical evaluation and documentation.

Team Member	Type of Role		Timing		
	Nonsterile	Sterile	Preop	Intraop	Postop
Surgical Technologist	X		X		
Assistant Circulator	X		X		
Operating Room Team	X		X		

OBJECTIVES

The learner will demonstrate the following with 100 percent accuracy each time the operative environment is entered:

1. Maintain aseptic technique.
2. State the rationale for performing a urinary catheterization.
3. Differential between a straight and an indwelling catheterization.
4. Perform a male and a female catheterization.
5. Obtain a sterile urine specimen with a straight catheter.
6. State at least two methods of preventing injury to the patient related to the surgical skin preparation.
7. State the rationale for performing the skin preparation.
8. Prep the skin for a selected procedure—such as an abdominal laparotomy.

Principles for Practice

The foundation and rationale for our practice, in the perioperative environment, stem from evidence provided by professionals, organizations, and governmental agencies. Refer to the Bibliography, Glossary of Terms, and the following documents or developmental agencies:

- Manufacturers' product instructions
- Operating room policies

- Surgeon's preference card
- The Joint Commission
- Surgical Care Improvement Project (SCIP)
- National Fire Prevention Agency (NFPA)
- Federal Drug Administration (FDA)
- Occupational Safety and Health Administration (OSHA)
- Centers for Disease Control and Prevention (CDC)
- Association of Surgical Technologists (AST)
- Association of periOperative Registered Nurses (AORN)

SKILL SEQUENCE AND INSTRUCTIONS
URINARY CATHETERIZATION

Indwelling Urinary Catheterization: Prepare Patient and Supplies

1. Wash and dry your hands. Refer to Chapter 2.
2. Complete preliminary requirements.

   - Recognize the importance of preventing catheter associated urinary tract infections (CAUTI's). Maintain aseptic technique. Only insert a sterile catheter into the urinary tract. Refer to chapters 1 through 7 and 14.
     ○ The CDC reports that a urinary tract infection is the most common type of healthcare-associated infection in the healthcare setting.
   - Verify the surgeon's preference card or orders.
   - Identify the patient.
   - Verify the patient's allergy status before proceeding. Most urinary prep kits contain a Povidone-Iodine solution. Contact the surgeon for a new order if the patient has an allergy.
   - Perform the time out. Refer to Chapter 12.
   - Explain the procedure to the alert patient.

3. Gather the supplies and equipment for a urinary catheterization.

   - Position a table or stand near the patient's thighs so that you can reach it with your dominant hand. Your dominant hand should be near the foot of the bed.
   - Position a trash receptacle within easy reach.

- Obtain an indwelling-retention catheterization kit.
- Read the package label for a retention or indwelling catheter kit; the contents are arranged in layers.

  ○ Top layer: sterile gloves, underpad, and fenestrated drape
  ○ Second layer: Povidone-Iodine swab sticks, dry swabs, 10mL syringe, filled with 10 mL sterile water, lubricating jelly
  ○ Bottom layer: 16 Fr. 5 mL catheter connected to a drainage bag, and specimen container with lid.

- Gather supplemental supplies or a different kit, as needed.

  ○ Obtain a sterile red rubber, Robinson, catheter for a straight catheterization procedure to drain urine or obtain a specimen; this catheter does not remain in the bladder and the drainage bag is not required. Refer to step 14.
  ○ Obtain your own sterile gloves if your hands are very small or very large. The kit contains medium sterile gloves.
  ○ Obtain a 3-way catheter if the surgeon orders continuous urinary irrigation.

- Place the catheterization kit on the stand.

4. Position the patient. Note variations for males and females.

   - Explain the procedure to the alert patient. Seek their assistance with positioning.
   - **MALE:** Position the anesthetized male patient in the supine position with his legs abducted approximately 30° from the midline.
   - **FEMALE:** Position the anesthetized female patient in the supine position and obtain assistance from a second nonsterile team member to flex the patient's hips and knees simultaneously. Place the soles of her feet together for support.
   - Position the lights to assist with visualization.

5. Perform perineal hygiene.

   - Don nonsterile gloves and wash the genitalia and perineal area with soap and water, as needed, and dry the area.
   - **MALE, UNCIRCUMCISED:** Retract the foreskin and perform hygiene care. Do not return the foreskin to the natural position until after the catheter has been inserted.
   - Remove your gloves. Wash your hands.

6. Inspect the catheterization kit and open the outer dust cover. Open the sterile kit on a separate table. Maintain aseptic technique. Refer to Chapter 4 (see also Figure 16.1).

7. Don your sterile gloves and prepare the sterile supplies.

   - Pinch the glove package, lift it up, and remove it to a separate area.
   - Don your sterile gloves using the open-gloving technique.
   - Prepare and arrange the supplies according to the provisions in your kit.
   - Open the swab stick packet; arrange the sticks for easy access. Squeeze lubricating jelly into the tray.
   - Note: For Bard catheter kits, the manufacturer does not recommend pretesting the balloon.
   - Remove the plastic covering as you secure the catheter in your gloved hand.
   - Perform a pretest on the balloon, as recommended by the manufacturer. Attach the prefilled syringe to the catheter port, and fill the balloon with 10 mL of sterile water. Observe for leaking or irregularities. Discard and obtain a new catheter, if found. Deflate the balloon; withdraw the water into the syringe.
   - Lubricate the catheter tip with the lubricant.
   - Coil the catheter in the sterile container on the field (see Figures 16.2 through 16.5).

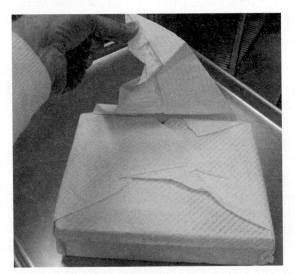

FIGURE 16.1   Open sterile kit.

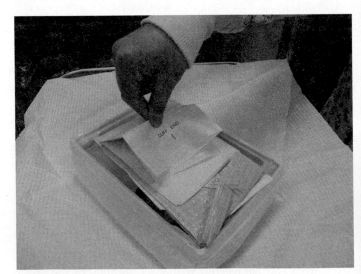

FIGURE 16.2   Grasp sterile gloves in a package.

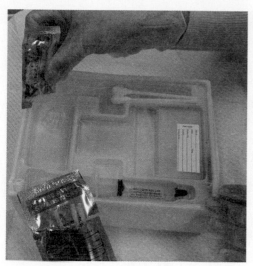

FIGURE 16.3 Prepare swabs and lubricant.

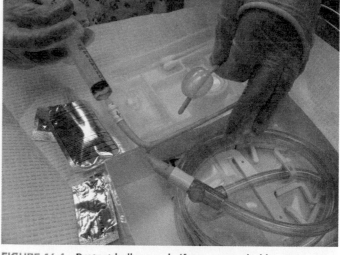

FIGURE 16.4 Pretest balloon only if recommended by manufacturer.

8. Place the sterile drapes.

- **FEMALE:** Cuff the underpad drape edges over your sterile gloves and tuck this drape beneath the patient's buttock. Place the fenestrated drape over the perineum.
- **MALE:** Place the underpad drape over the thighs, as indicated. Place the fenestrated drape (window) over the penis. The urethral meatus will be exposed. (see Figures 16.6 through 16.7).

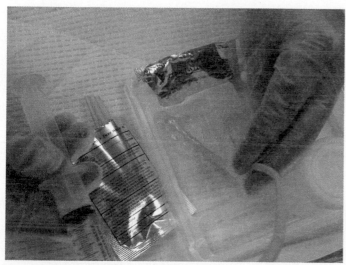

FIGURE 16.5 Lubricate catheter.

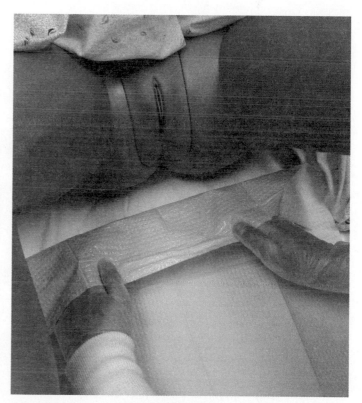

FIGURE 16.6 Place under buttock drape for a female.

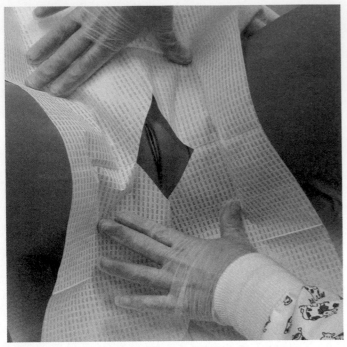

FIGURE 16.7 Place fenestrated drape for male and female patients.

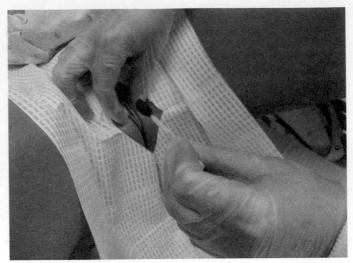

FIGURE 16.8 Clean periurethral mucosa for male and female patients.

9. Cleans the periurethra mucosa.

- **FEMALE:** Use your nondominant hand to hold open the labia minora.
- Grasp the sterile iodine swab in your dominant hand and wipe the periurethral mucosa and meatus. Wipe anterior to posterior, inner to outer. Use one pass/swipe per swab. Discard the swab. Repeat using all swabs.
- Hold the labia open, with your non-dominant hand through the next few steps and until you inflate the balloon.
- **MALE:** Place your nondominant hand on the symphasis pubis, then grasp the penis. Use a concentric, circular motion, beginning at the meatus to cleanse the glans penis, with a sterile swab. Discard the swab. Repeat using all swabs. Hold the penis in place, with your non-dominant hand and until you inflate the balloon.
- **MALE, UNCIRCUMCISED:** The foreskin is retracted, as performed in a previous step. Cleanse the glans penis (see Figure 16.8).

10. Perform catheterization.

- Place the sterile container (holding the catheter and attached bag) onto the sterile drape between the cooperative patient's legs.
- Secure the sterile lubricated catheter in your dominant hand (see Figures 16.9 through 16.12).
- Do not touch the sterile catheter with your nonsterile, nondominant hand.
- **FEMALE:** Insert and thread the catheter gently into the meatus, angling it in the direction of the umbilicus approximately three inches.
- Obtain a new sterile catheter if you accidently enter the vagina or pass the catheter over another nonsterile area.
- **MALE:** Hold the penis at a 90° angle to the body, and exert gently traction. Insert and thread the lubricated catheter—approximately 7–8 inches.
- Observe for urine flow.
- Hold the catheter in place with your nondominant hand.
- Use your dominant hand to fill the balloon with the sterile, water-filled syringe. You may now use both hands for any following tasks.
- Give a gentle tug on the catheter to seat it in the neck of the bladder.
- If supplied separately, attach the catheter to a sterile, closed drainage system (bag). Keep the system sterile. Do not allow the tubing, on either end, to become contaminated.
- **MALE, UNCIRCUMCISED:** Replace the foreskin over the glans penis.

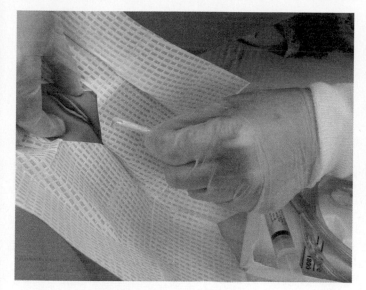

FIGURE 16.9   Perform female catheterization.

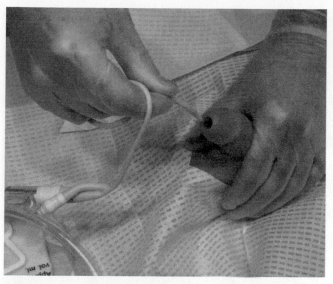

FIGURE 16.10   Perform male catheterization.

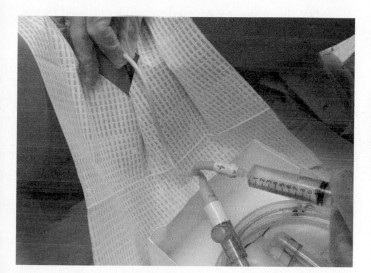

FIGURE 16.11   Inflate the balloon with sterile water.

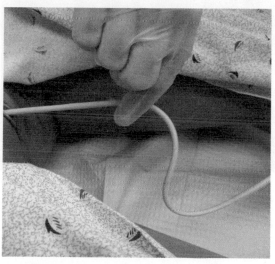

FIGURE 16.12   Secure into bladder neck with a gentle tug.

11. Position the drainage bag below the level of the bladder.

- Remove sterile gloves, perform hand hygiene, and don new non-sterile gloves.
- Secure the tubing to the patient's leg with an adhesive device or leg strap.
- Hook the drainage bag to a nonmovable portion of the OR bed frame.
- Observe the urine color and amount.
- Place the urine drainage spout into the holster; do not allow the drainage spout to drag on the floor (see Figure 16.13).

12. Clean up.

- Remove the drapes and discard.
- Wipe off excess prep solution to prevent skin excoriation.
- Remove your gloves and wash your hands.
- Document, examples provided:
  - type of catheter used-indwelling, double lumen,
  - size of the catheter-16 Fr.
  - amount of fluid inserted into the balloon-5 mL,
  - patient's response—tolerated and denies pain
  - color and amount of urine drainage-yellow and 250 mL

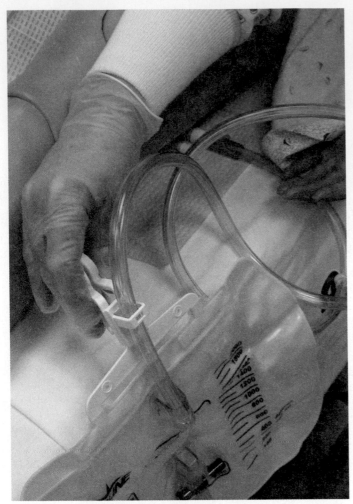

FIGURE 16.13 Secure bag below bladder level onto the nonmovable bed frame.

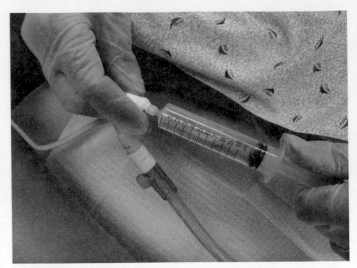

FIGURE 16.14 Discontinue: withdraw all sterile water.

13. Remove the catheter, at the end of the procedure or when the catheter is ordered to be discontinued by the physician.

- Don nonsterile gloves.
- Insert an empty 10 mL syringe into the catheter port.
- Withdraw the entire amount of sterile water from the balloon.
- Do not cut the catheter.
- Withdraw the catheter; observe for intactness.
- Wipe off any remaining solutions or lubricant. Dry the skin.
- Document: amount of fluid removed from the balloon, the patient's response, and the intactness of the catheter (see Figure 16.14).

Straight Catheterization

14. Perform a straight catheterization to drain the bladder or to obtain a sterile urine specimen.

    - Gather the supplies: straight catheter, size 14 or 16 Fr.; a catheter-insertion kit, which does not contain a drainage bag or indwelling catheter; and a sterile specimen container, if not supplied in the kit.
      - Note: The straight catheter is frequently red in color and contains only one lumen (see Figure 16.15).
    - Prepare the patient and the supplies, and place the collection container, or catheter kit tray, near the perineal area.
    - Perform the catheterization, and place the drainage end of the catheter into the collection container.
      - Hold the catheter in place with one hand.
      - Drain the bladder, allowing the urine to flow into the sterile collection container.
    - Obtain a urine specimen, if ordered. Place a sterile specimen container under the drainage end of the catheter to collect approximately 30 mL or more of urine.
    - Replace the catheter end into the collection container and drain the bladder.
    - Remove the catheter, measure the amount of urine drained, clean up the patient, and discard the kit.
    - Label and send the urine specimen to the laboratory for analysis. Place the sealed urine specimen container in a biohazard specimen bag.
    - Document.

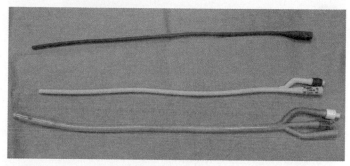

FIGURE 16.15 Urinary catheter lumens: 1 straight, 2 indwelling, and 3 Irrigation.

SKIN PREPARATION OR ANTISEPSIS

1. Perform the preliminary requirements before the skin preparation is initiated.

    - Recognize the importance of preventing surgical site infections (SSI's). Infections at the surgical site account for approximately 38% of all hospital-acquired infections.
      - All infections, including SSI's, are the fourth leading cause of death in the US.
      - The CDC advocates for prevention with education, hand hygiene, aseptic technique, appropriate antibiotics, and surgical site hair removal by clipping only. Refer to chapters 1 through 7 and 14.
    - Arrange the OR furniture.
    - Gather the required supplies: abdominal Providone-Iodine prep kit and prep table.
    - Check the expiration date of the solutions in the kit.
    - Place a waste disposal can within reach.
    - In the preop holding area:
      - Identify the patient and key components.
      - Remove any unnecessary hair according to the surgeon's order. Use an electric clipper. Shaving is not recommended because microabrasions are sites for infection.
      - The surgeon may request hair removal after the patient has received anesthesia. Hair removal is routinely performed by the circulator or first assistant.
      - Identify allergies.
    - Transport the patient to the operating room. Refer to Chapter 11.
    - Explain the procedure to the alert patient and place in the supine position.
    - Keep the patient warm with blanket.
    - Complete the urinary catheterization, if ordered.

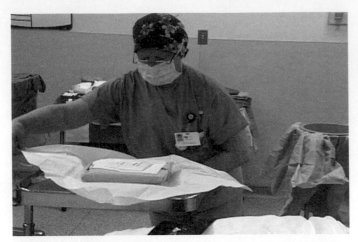

FIGURE 16.16 Open skin prep kit.

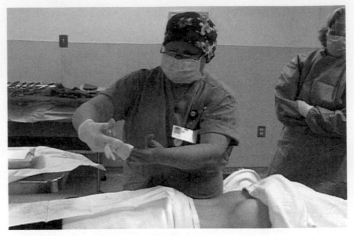

FIGURE 16.17 Perform open gloving.

2. Open the prep kit and follow the manufacturer's instructions and OR guidelines.

- Expose the area to be prepped. Include an area approximately 6 inches larger on all boarders to accommodate placement of sterile drapes. Refer to Chapter 17.
- Assess the patient's skin integrity. Report abnormalities, rashes, lesions, or burns to the surgeon. Remove any jewelry and label and secure it.
- Inspect the kit, remove the plastic dust cover, open the inner wrap, and prepare a sterile field on a prep stand or unused Mayo stand.
- Maintain aseptic technique.
- Perform open-gloving. Refer to Chapter 15 (see also Figures 16.16 and 16.17).

3. Prepare the sterile items in the kit.

- Pour the two solutions, scrub solution and paint solution, into separate wells in the kit (see Figure 16.18).

4. Drape each side of the abdomen, as if, for example, draping for a general surgery laparotomy.

- Cuff your sterile gloves under the corners of the drape.
- Tuck one drape along each side of the patient to absorb excess solution and prevent pooling (see Figures 16.19 and 16.20).

5. Clean the umbilicus. Dip the cotton-tipped applicators into the scrub solution and clean the umbilicus.

- Discard the contaminated applicators.
- Do not touch the patient's skin with your sterile gloves (see Figure 16.21).

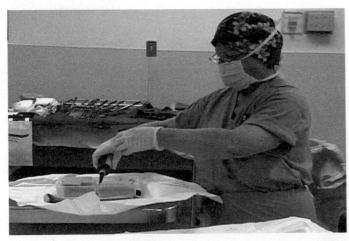

FIGURE 16.18 Pour solutions.

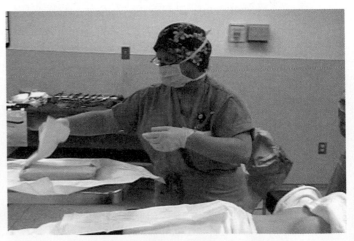

FIGURE 16.19 Prepare drapes.

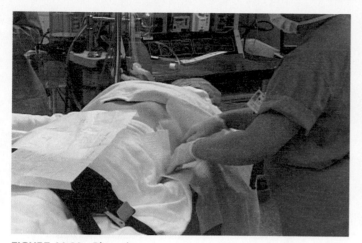

FIGURE 16.20 Place drape.

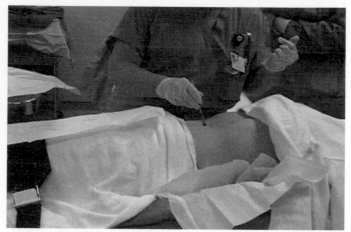

FIGURE 16.21 Clean umbilicus.

6. Prep the skin.

- Follow manufacturer's recommendations.
- Do not warm the solutions in the microwave.
- Soak winged-sponges in the scrub solution; squeeze out excess.
- Grasp the winged-handles on the sponge and scrub the skin, with friction, in a concentric pattern, beginning at the planned incision site and working toward the perimeter.
- Scrub over the area only once with the first sponge. Discard the sponge and repeat (see Figure 16.22).

7. Use the blotting towels.

- Open the blotting towel and place it onto the scrubbed skin.
- Allow time for the towel to absorb or wick away the excess skin prep solution.
- Grasp the towel edges opposite from you and roll or peel the towel towards you.
- Repeat blotting with a new sterile towel, as needed (see Figure 16.23).

8. Apply paint solution.

- Apply the second solution, concentrated Povidone-iodine paint, on a sponge stick from the planned incision site outward.
- Repeat with a fresh sponge stick (see Figure 16.24).

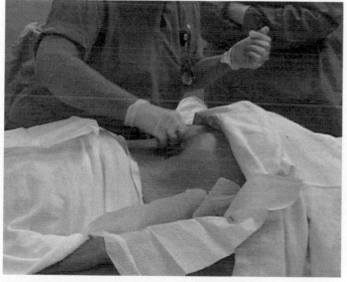

FIGURE 16.22 Use friction in a concentric pattern.

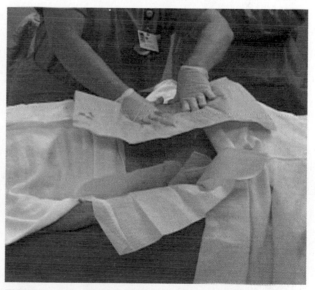

FIGURE 16.23 Blot, and lift towel up and off.

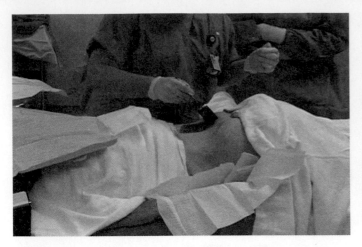

FIGURE 16.24 Apply concentrated paint solution.

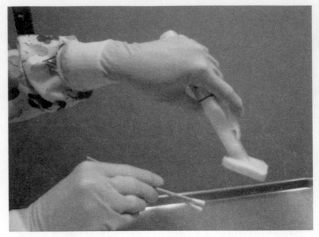

FIGURE 16.25 CHG wand prep.

9. Follow your facility's policy when prepping two anatomical areas:
   - Prepare and use separate prep kits or other prep solutions, such as Chlorhexidine Gluconate (CHG) wands for each area (see Figure 16.25).
   - This sequence varies among geographical regions. Routinely, the cleanest area is prepped first. For example, the skin on the abdomen is prepped first followed by a prep of a stoma. Follow your hospital policy.
   - Maintain aseptic technique.

10. Allow the prep solution to dry, based on the manufacturer's instructions before applying drapes. Prevent fires due to unintended ignition of pooled flammable solutions. Refer to Chapter 13.

11. Remove wet surgical supplies before continuing. Prevent extending the drying time of the prep solution, fuel for a fire, and hypothermia.
   - Remove wet blankets or drapes from the patient's sides.
   - Apply a new grounding pad if the original is accidently moistened by the skin prep solution. Dry the underlying skin before reapplying.

12. Assess the skin for a reaction to the prep solution, at the end of the procedure.
   - Compare the "before and after" appearance of skin surfaces. Povidone-iodine solution on the skin is removed to prevent excoriation.
   - If permitted, tilt the patient to one side and wipe excess solution from the patient's back (see Figure 16.26).

13. Documentation in the patient's record includes the following:
   - Preoperative instructions and compliance
   - Removal and disposition of jewelry
   - Skin condition preop and postop
   - Hair removal, per orders
   - Solution used
   - Site prepped
   - Name of person performing the prep
   - Fire prevention strategies used per facility policy
   - Postop removal of solutions

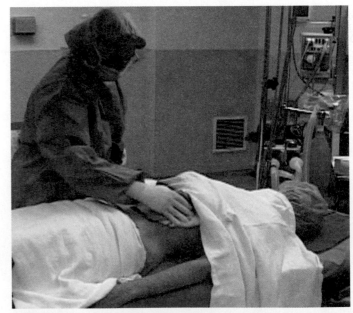

FIGURE 16.26 Postoperatively, remove to prevent excoriation.

STUDENT'S NAME: _____

CHAPTER 16 PERFORM URINARY CATHETERIZATION

PERFORMANCE RANK:

S or √ = Satisfactory: Competent—safe, accurate, sequential, and timely
U = Unsatisfactory: Unsafe—inaccurate and unprepared

PERFORMANCE RATING:

5   Independent: Expert—safe, confident, seamless performance; mentors others
4   Minimally monitored: Intermediate—safe, self-corrects few errors
3   Competent: Novice—safe, revises with evaluator cues, few errors
2   Remedial: Unsafe—critical errors, unable to implement evaluator cues consistently
1   Dependent: Unsafe—unacceptable, requires multiple evaluator interventions

PERFORMANCE CRITERIA	Performance Rank	Performance Rating
1. Perform Mutual Professional and Scholastic Criteria as appropriate (see the Preface or Appendix A).		1 2 3 4 5
2. Verify patient's allergy status to solutions in the kit; use kit only if not allergic.		1 2 3 4 5
3. Don nonsterile gloves.		1 2 3 4 5
4. Position the male or female manikin and the surgical overhead light.		1 2 3 4 5
5. Perform perineal hygiene; remove nonsterile gloves; perform hand hygiene.		1 2 3 4 5
6. Inspect and open the urinary catheter kit on a nonsterile prep table.		1 2 3 4 5
7. Perform open gloving with sterile gloves provided in kit (refer to Chapter 15).		1 2 3 4 5
8. Prepare sterile supplies and the catheter.		1 2 3 4 5
9. Place drapes.		1 2 3 4 5
10. Prep the periurethral area.		1 2 3 4 5
11. Perform the urinary catheterization.		1 2 3 4 5
12. Remove the drapes and place in appropriate receptacle.		1 2 3 4 5
13. Remove your gloves and don a pair of new nonsterile gloves.		1 2 3 4 5
14. Secure the drainage bag.		1 2 3 4 5
15. Don nonsterile gloves, use a 10 mL syringe, and discontinue/remove the catheter.		1 2 3 4 5
16. Clean up the patient and supplies, and reposition for comfort and safety.		1 2 3 4 5
17. Measure the urine output in a graduated-cylinder.		1 2 3 4 5
18. State the information to document in the patient's chart.		1 2 3 4 5

ADDITIONAL COMMENTS _____

PERFORMANCE EVALUATIONS AND RECOMMENDATIONS

❏ PASS: Satisfactory Performance
    ❏ Demonstrates professionalism
    ❏ Exhibits critical thinking
    ❏ Demonstrates proficient clinical performance appropriate for time in the program
❏ FAIL: Unsatisfactory Performance
    ❏ Critical criteria not met (see Performance Rank or Rating Above)
    ❏ Professionalism not demonstrated.
    ❏ Critical thinking skills not demonstrated.
    ❏ Skill performance unsafe or underdeveloped.
❏ REMEDIATION:
    ❏ Schedule lab practice. Date: _____
    ❏ Reevaluate by instructor. Date: _____
❏ DISMISS from lab or clinicals today.
❏ Program director notified. Date: _____

SIGNATURES

Date _____   Evaluator _____   Student _____

COMPETENCY ASSESSMENT

STUDENT'S NAME: _____

CHAPTER 16 PERFORM SKIN PREPARATION

PERFORMANCE RANK:

　　S or √ = Satisfactory: Competent—safe, accurate, sequential, and timely
　　U = Unsatisfactory: Unsafe—inaccurate and unprepared

PERFORMANCE RATING:

　　5　　Independent: Expert—safe, confident, seamless performance; mentors others
　　4　　Minimally monitored: Intermediate—safe, self-corrects few errors
　　3　　Competent: Novice—safe, revises with evaluator cues, few errors
　　2　　Remedial: Unsafe—critical errors, unable to implement evaluator cues consistently
　　1　　Dependent: Unsafe—unacceptable, requires multiple evaluator interventions

PERFORMANCE CRITERIA	Performance Rank	Performance Rating
1. Perform Mutual Professional and Scholastic Criteria as appropriate (see the Preface or Appendix A).		1　2　3　4　5
2. Obtain a skin prep kit with scrub and paint solutions; open after allergy status is verified.		1　2　3　4　5
3. Verify patient's allergy status to solutions in the prep kit.		1　2　3　4　5
4. State actions to take if the patient is allergic to skin prep solutions.		1　2　3　4　5
5. Position the patient in the supine position.		1　2　3　4　5
6. Open the prep kit on a nonsterile prep table and establish a sterile field (laparotomy example).		1　2　3　4　5
7. Don sterile gloves (refer to Chapter 15).		1　2　3　4　5
8. Prepare the sterile supplies and drapes in the kit.		1　2　3　4　5
9. Drape the patient.		1　2　3　4　5
10. Clean the umbilicus.		1　2　3　4　5
11. Scrub the abdomen.		1　2　3　4　5
12. Use blotting towels.		1　2　3　4　5
13. Apply the paint solution.		1　2　3　4　5
14. Dispose of the used supplies; doff gloves and prevent self-contamination.		1　2　3　4　5
15. Perform hand hygiene.		1　2　3　4　5
16. State information to document in the patient's chart.		1　2　3　4　5

ADDITIONAL COMMENTS _____

PERFORMANCE EVALUATIONS AND RECOMMENDATIONS

- ❑ PASS: Satisfactory Performance
    - ❑ Demonstrates professionalism
    - ❑ Exhibits critical thinking
    - ❑ Demonstrates proficient clinical performance appropriate for time in the program
- ❑ FAIL: Unsatisfactory Performance
    - ❑ Critical criteria not met (see Performance Rank or Rating Above)
    - ❑ Professionalism not demonstrated.
    - ❑ Critical thinking skills not demonstrated.
    - ❑ Skill performance unsafe or underdeveloped.
- ❑ REMEDIATION:
    - ❑ Schedule lab practice. Date: _____
    - ❑ Reevaluate by instructor. Date: _____
- ❑ DISMISS from lab or clinicals today.
- ❑ Program director notified. Date: _____

SIGNATURES

Date _____   Evaluator _____   Student _____

ACTIVITIES AND DISCUSSION QUESTIONS

Activities

1. View the Complete Perioperative Process and Focus on Skills video, Skill # 16 (video can be found at www.myhealthprofessionskit.com).
2. Observe the instructor perform the skills.
3. Practice the skills in this chapter by using a manikin in the lab setting.
4. Select and teach one skill to your lab partner, then observe and critique the performance.
5. Refer to your ST textbook and this lab manual to answer the Discussion Questions (see next column).
6. Review the video and the information in this lab manual when you prepare for your certification examination.

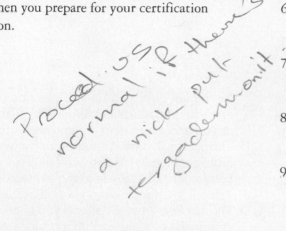

Discussion Questions

1. What is the difference between a straight catheter and a retention, or indwelling, catheter?
2. The surgeon orders the indwelling catheter to be removed. You cannot find a 10 mL syringe. What is your next action?
3. Name the essential steps in the skin prep skill.
4. State two tasks performed that promote patient safety during the skin prep.
5. The patient is in preop holding, has an umbilicus body piercing, and refuses to have the jewelry removed. What should you do?
6. The patient states that he shaved the hair on his abdomen yesterday in preparation for a laparoscopic herniorraphy. What should you do?
7. The patient states that he is very cold. Your classmate decides to warm up the prep kit in a microwave. What should you do?
8. You have just completed the skin prep. The surgeon states that he is in a hurry and wants to drape immediately. What should you do?
9. Note here any questions that you need your instructor to clarifyy.

Apply Surgical Drapes

17

INTRODUCTION

Surgical drapes establish a barrier against pathogenic microorganisms. Patients are shielded from endogenous and exogenous species. Drapes, and gowns, provide protection to health care workers from exposure to the patient's potentially infectious blood or body fluids. Manufacturers supply drapes in various sizes and shapes to accommodate anatomy and the surgeon's requirements.

- Before performing the following skill, your lab instructor will discuss some of the principles for practice and objectives involved in this chapter as well as the importance of following the skill sequence and instructions.
- In the sterile role, practice draping anatomical areas on a manikin for a laparotomy procedure, a procedure on an extremity, and a pelviscopy. In the nonsterile role, practice applying a pneumatic

tourniquet on a manikin and describe the application parameters. Work with a lab partner as you encourage and critique each other. Your instructor will offer strategies for success. Appendix E highlights the value of teaching others as a component of active learning strategies. Refer to Appendix C for an overview of the chapter.
- The lab instructor will advise you of any additional criteria to be evaluated. At a designated time, demonstration of these skills will be evaluated and graded by your lab instructor using the competency assessment tool.
- When in the clinical setting, your instructor may once again assess your performance using the same tool. Refer to Appendix A for clinical evaluation and documentation.

Team Member	Type of Role		Timing		
	Nonsterile	Sterile	Preop	Intraop	Postop
Surgical Technologist		X	X		
Assistant Circulator	X		X		
Operating Room Team		X	X		

OBJECTIVES

The learner will demonstrate the following with 100 percent accuracy each time the skill is performed.

1. State the rationale for using drapes on OR furniture and the operative field.
2. Apply the principles of aseptic technique.

3. Select, organize, and prepare drapes.
4. Drape for a laparotomy procedure.
5. Assist with the application of a pneumatic tourniquet.
6. Drape for an extremity procedure.
7. Drape for a pelviscopy procedure in lithotomy position.

Principles for Practice

The foundation and rationale for our practice, in the perioperative environment, stem from evidence provided by professionals, organizations, and governmental agencies. Refer to the Bibliography, Glossary of Terms, and the following documents or developmental agencies:

- Manufacturers' product guidelines
- Operating room policy
- Surgeon's preference card
- Safe Medical Devices Act of 1990 (SMDA)
- Food and Drug Administration (FDA)
- Occupational Safety and Health Administration (OSHA)
- Centers for Disease Control and Prevention (CDC)
- The American Society of Anesthesiologists (ASA)
- Association of Surgical Technologists (AST)
- Association of periOperative Registered Nurses (AORN)

SKILL SEQUENCE AND INSTRUCTIONS
APPLY LAPAROTOMY DRAPES

1. Provide a physical barrier to protect patients and health care workers from potentially harmful microbes or blood-borne pathogens.

   - Reference the surgeon's preference card, and select and prepare in the order of use, drapes appropriate for the surgical procedure.
   - Follow manufacturer's instructions. Drapes cover the back table, Mayo stand, the patient, and additional equipment that will be incorporated into the sterile field.
   - Refer to Chapters 4 and 7 (see also Figures 17.1 through 17.7).

2. Prepare and pass laparotomy drapes and clamps, as requested.

   - Select four nonpenetrating, or blunt, towel clips for use with the textile towels. Clips are not used with paper towels manufactured with adhesive strips. Clips are not used when plastic, adhesive incisional drapes are used over the towels.
   - Grasp and pass the folded towels to the surgeon according to the placement order.
   - Do not reach over the undraped area. The surgeon will place three towels from one side of the patient, walk to the opposite side, and place the fourth towel. Follow the surgeon.
   - Pass the clips, as needed (see Figures 17.8 through 17.10).

3. Obtain the laparotomy (fenestrated) drape.

   - Remove the paper tape covering the adhesive, according to the surgeon's preference. Discard the paper covering.
   - Orient the drape by following any preprinted instructions or diagrams.
   - Carry the folded drape to the operative field.
   - Pass the "lap" drape to the surgeon. The fenestration or opening will be placed over the planned incision site (see Figures 17.11 and 17.12).

4. Grasp and open the fan-folded laparotomy drape.

   - Perform this with two sterile team members: the ST and the surgeon, or the surgeon and the first assistant.
   - Hold all portions of the folded drape until it is time to release the edges.
   - Grasp the superior edge of the drape and form a cuff around your sterile glove.
   - Follow the lead of the surgeon. Drape from the planned incision site outward towards the periphery.
   - Drape smoothly and simultaneously. Use a gliding motion to unfold the superior edge and pass it off to the anesthesia care provider, who will fasten the edge to IV poles or a frame.
   - Do not shake the drape to open it.
   - Unfold the inferior edge over the patient's legs and feet. Drop the drape. Keep your sterile gloves at or above waist level (see Figures 17.13 through 17.17).

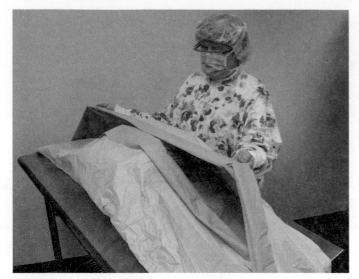

FIGURE 17.1   Whole or plain sheet drape.

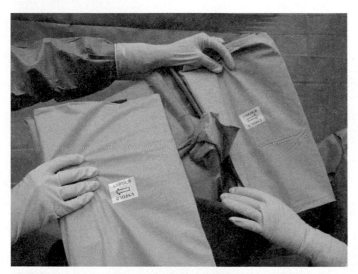

FIGURE 17.3   Fenestrated or slit sheet drape.

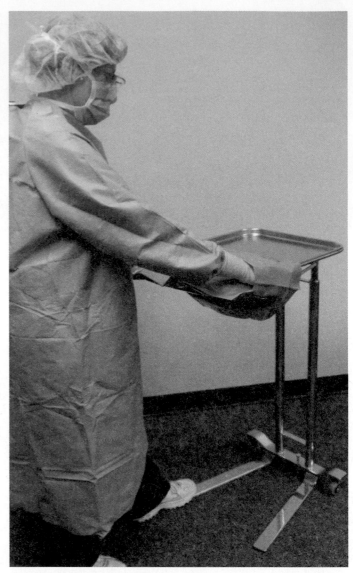

FIGURE 17.2   Mayo stand drape.

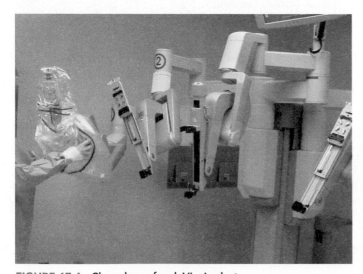

FIGURE 17.4   Clear drape for daVinci robot.

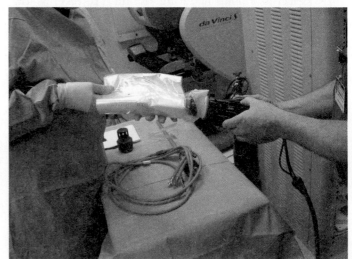

FIGURE 17.5   Clear drape for camera and cord.

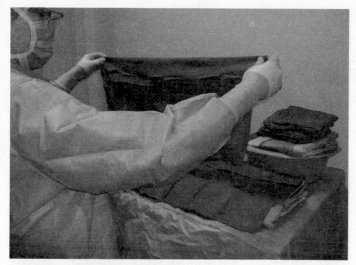

FIGURE 17.6   OR towels used for draping.

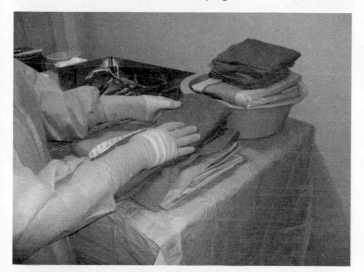

FIGURE 17.8   Four towels for laparotomy draping.

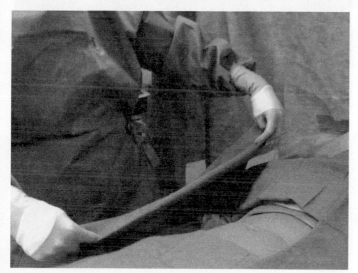

FIGURE 17.10   Surgeon places fourth towel.

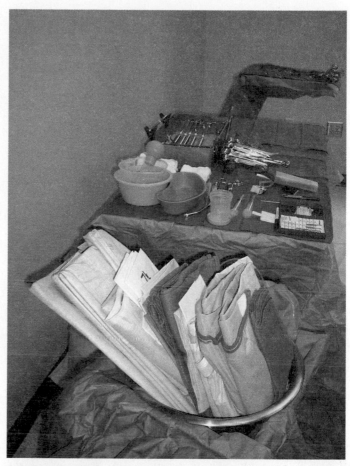

FIGURE 17.7   Layer gowns and drapes in a ring stand.

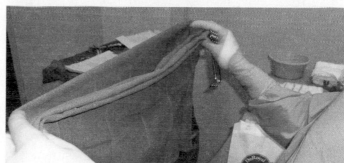

FIGURE 17.9   Pass towels, individually, to the surgeon.

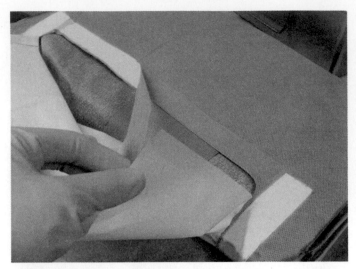
FIGURE 17.11 Prepare fenestrated "lap" drape.

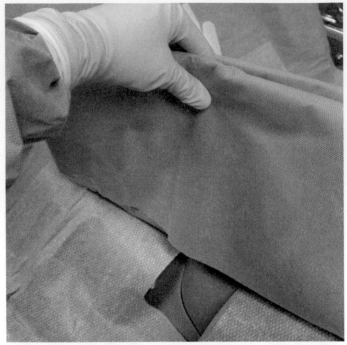
FIGURE 17.12 Position drape over the planned incision site.

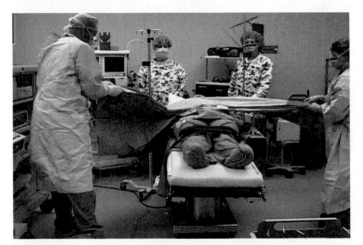
FIGURE 17.13 Grasp and unfold "lap" drape.

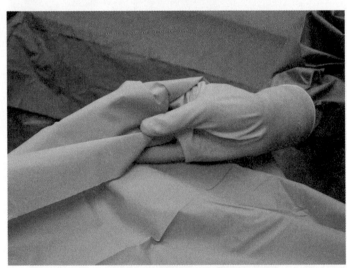
FIGURE 17.14 Make a cuff; protect your sterile glove.

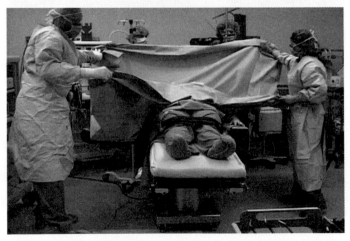
FIGURE 17.15 Follow the surgeon's lead.

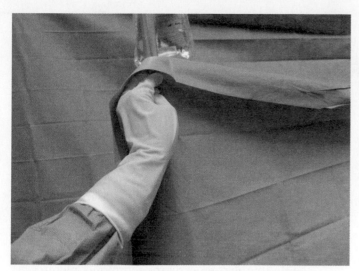

FIGURE 17.16   Protect gloves from attachment location.

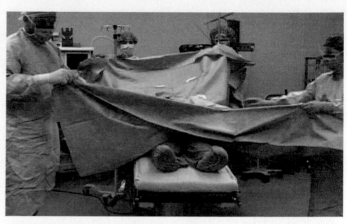

FIGURE 17.17   Drop inferior drape segment over patient's lower extremities.

5. Perform additional tasks as indicated.

    • Request a new drape, if you accidently drop it before it is in position.
    • Complete the remaining preparatory tasks before the procedure begins. Refer to Chapter 18.
    • The surgeon will make the incision momentarily.

APPLY A PNEUMATIC TOURNIQUET AND DRAPE AN EXTREMITY

1. Prepare the patient and equipment for an extremity procedure (left forearm example).

   Pneumatic Tourniquet Nonsterile Role:

   - Verify proper function of the pneumatic tourniquet.
   - Place the patient in the supine position and use positioning aids, such as mechanical devices or gel pad bolsters, to isolate and elevate the left arm. Follow recommended practices and the manufacturer's guidelines for the selection and application of the tourniquet.
   - Protect the skin on the upper arm with smooth, wrinkle-free padding or a stockinette, and position the appropriately sized tourniquet cuff onto the upper left arm.
   - Allow the cuff to overlap approximately three inches but less than six inches.
   - Do not place the pneumatic tourniquet over boney prominences, skin folds, or wounds.
   - Poorly sized or improperly placed cuffs may negatively impact the surgical outcome. Refer to Table 17.1 (see also Figures 17.18 through 17.20).
   - Perform a skin prep and allow the solution to dry. Refer to Chapter 16.

   - Set the cuff pressure on the automatic unit based on the patient's limb occlusion pressure (LOP), systolic blood pressure reading, and instructions from the surgeon or anesthesia care provider. Recommended adult maximum cuff pressure limits are 300–350 mm Hg for a thigh cuff and 250–300 mmHg for the arm and lower leg.
   - Intraoperatively, monitor the continuous tourniquet pressure time, or "cuff-up time," and maintain the audible alert tones on the tourniquet monitor. Recommended practices for an adult indicate continuous pressure should be less than one hour on an upper extremity and less than two hours on a thigh (see Figures 17.21 and 17.22).

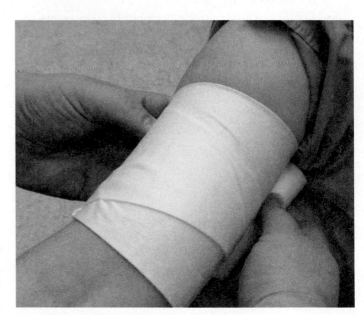

FIGURE 17.18   Protect the skin.

TABLE 17.1   Tourniquet Errors

Fit	Error	Problem
Cuff size	Too small	Loose when inflated; blood in operative field
Cuff size	Too large	Nerve or vessel damage
Cuff fit	Too loose	Need higher inflation pressures to occlude flow
Cuff fit	Too tight	Return of venous blood flow impeded

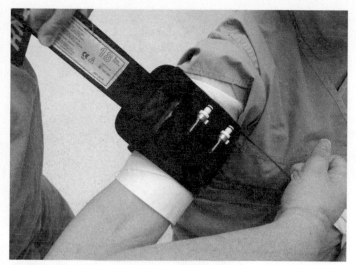

FIGURE 17.19 Select cuff size, encircle arm, and tie.

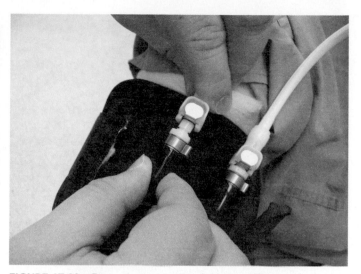

FIGURE 17.20 Connect pneumatic tubing to cuff.

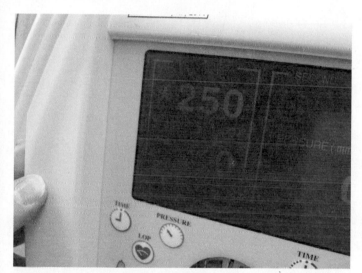

FIGURE 17.21 Set cuff pressure parameters.

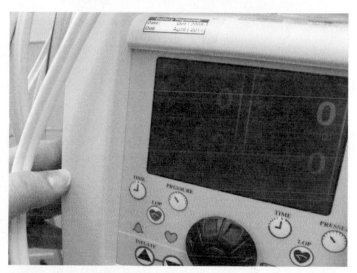

FIGURE 17.22 Set time parameters.

2. Orient and position extremity drapes, in the sterile role.

U-Drape or Split drape

- Unfold the fan-folded u-shaped split drape (u-drape), and secure it around the circumference of the upper arm. Do not touch the patient with your sterile gloves.
- Remove the paper backing and secure the drape edges together.
- Secure cloth drapes and OR towels with a nonpenetrating towel clamp (see Figures 17.23 through 17.29).

Impervious Stockinette Drape

- Place the cloth side of the tube-shaped impervious stockinette drape over the patient's left hand, and unfold it over the left arm. Continue to elevate the arm.

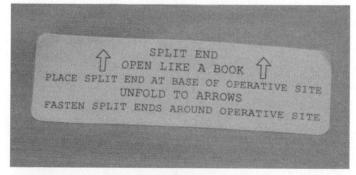

FIGURE 17.23 Follow u-drape directional cues.

- Do not contaminate your gloves or gown by touching the patient's arm (see Figures 17.30 and 17.31).

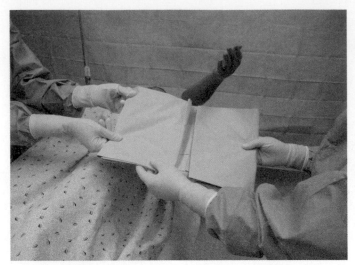

FIGURE 17.24 Orient and unfold u-drape laterally.

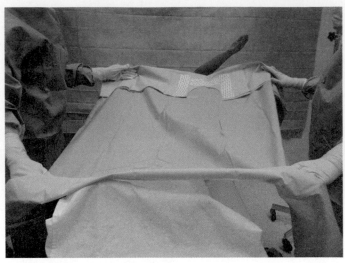

FIGURE 17.25 Unfold drape superiorly and inferiorly.

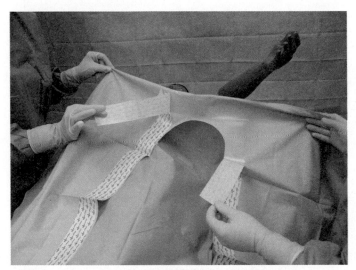

FIGURE 17.26 Remove adhesive strip backing.

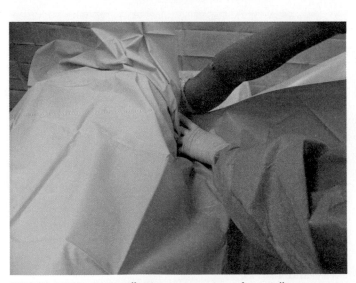

FIGURE 17.27 Press adhesive to arm, circumferentially.

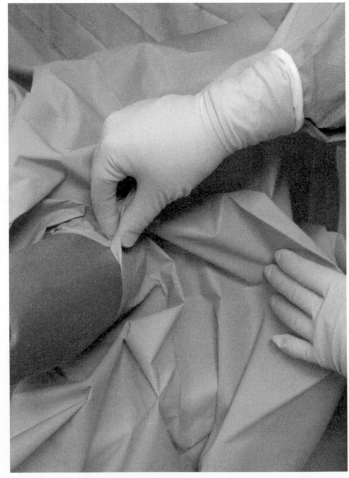

FIGURE 17.28 Seal drape edges.

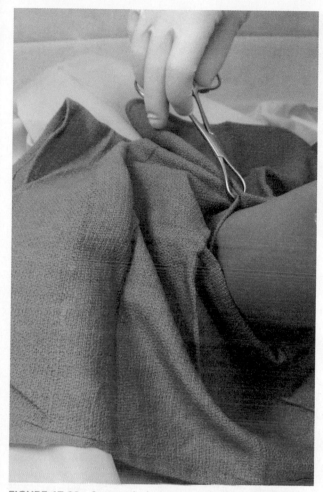

FIGURE 17.29 Secure cloth drapes with a towel clamp.

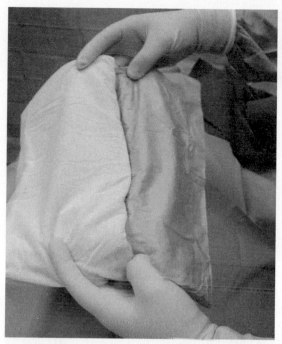

FIGURE 17.30 Place impervious stockinette.

Fenestrated Extremity Drape

- Obtain the fenestrated drape, orient the slit of this drape over the patient's hand, and pass the arm through it. Continue to elevate the patient's (draped) arm.
- Hold the extremity drape edges and begin to unfold the drape. Make a cuff over your glove, and pass the superior edge to the anesthesia care provider. Unfold the inferior drape edge, and allow it to drop over the patient's legs and feet.
- Pass scissors to the surgeon who will then cut a window in the stockinette drape (see Figures 17.32 through 17.36).

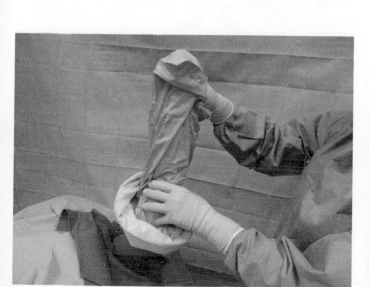

FIGURE 17.31 Unfold the extremity stockinette.

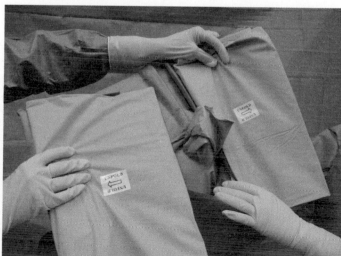

FIGURE 17.32 Position the fenestrated drape.

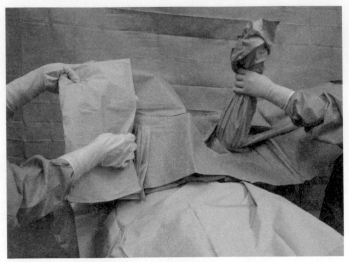

FIGURE 17.33 Unfold the drape laterally.

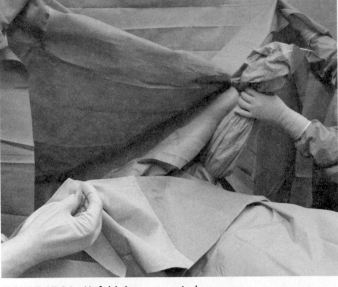

FIGURE 17.34 Unfold drape superiorly.

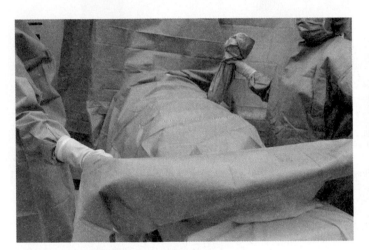

FIGURE 17.35 Unfold drape over legs.

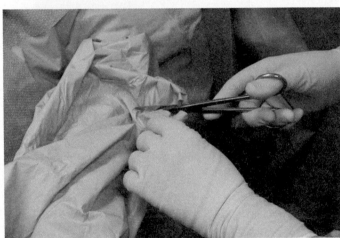

FIGURE 17.36 Pass Mayo scissors to the surgeon.

Plastic Incisional Drape

- Prepare a plastic incisional drape also known as an "incise or I drape." This sheet-like drape is impregnated with an antimicrobial iodophor and is yellow in color. This optional drape will be noted on the surgeon's preference card.

  ○ Pass this drape with the tacky side facing the operative site.

  ○ Assist the surgeon to unfold and pull open this drape—use traction. Assist to apply the drape over the incision site.

  ○ Gather and discard the paper backing. Return the scissors to your back table (see Figures 17.37 through 17.38)

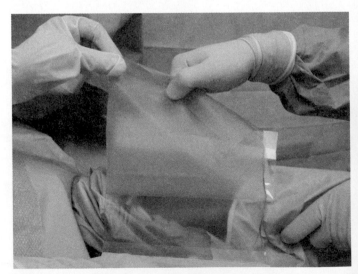

FIGURE 17.37 Orient and position the plastic sheeting.

3. Pass the Esmarch rubber bandage to the surgeon who will wrap the arm, distally to proximally. This exsanguination action along with the use of a tourniquet will achieve the goal of a nearly bloodless surgical field.

4. The pneumatic tourniquet pressure limits are verified with the surgeon and the circulator adjusts the settings.

   • The tourniquet is inflated.
   • The surgeon unwraps the Esmarch bandage.
   • Return the Esmarch to the back table; rewind it at an appropriate time.

• Pass a nonpenetrating towel clip to the surgeon, if requested, for positioning the arm. The circulator will document the "cuff up" time, monitor and announce the limb exsanguination time, and at the conclusion of the procedure document the "cuff-down" time (see Figures 17.39 through 17.41).

5. Perform additional preparatory skills.
   • Refer to Chapter 18.

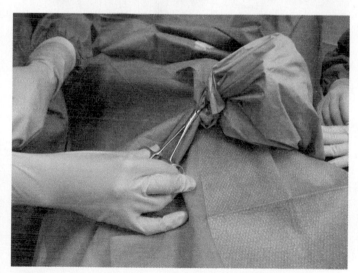

FIGURE 17.38 Remove paper backing and discard.

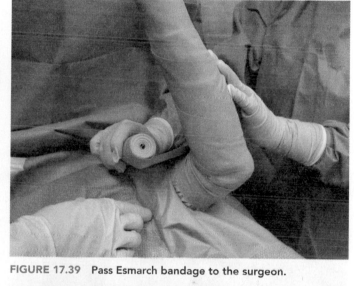

FIGURE 17.39 Pass Esmarch bandage to the surgeon.

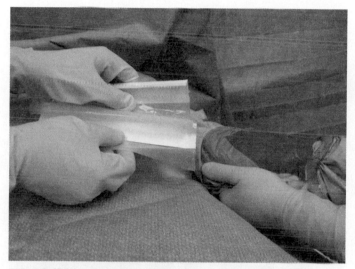

FIGURE 17.40 Pass instruments to assist with positioning.

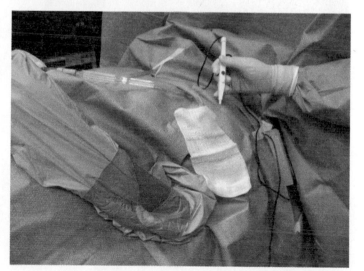

FIGURE 17.41 Left forearm draped for the procedure.

APPLY PELVIC, LITHOTOMY DRAPES

1. Prepare the patient, equipment, supplies, and drapes for the selected procedure (example follows).

   Nonsterile Role:

   - Attach two stirrups onto the OR bed. Adjust symmetrically.
   - Position the patient on the OR bed. Use two team members to simultaneously raise (or lower) the legs and place them into the stirrups. Adjust to protect the patient's skin and to prevent nerve injury and vascular changes.
   - Remove the lower portion of the OR bed to allow the surgeon to access the perineal area (see Figures 17.42 and 17.43).

   - Prepare two skin-prep kits. Drape the patient for the skin preps. Use one prep on the abdomen and the second on the perineal or vaginal area. Refer to Chapters 15 and 16.

     ○ Recommended practices advocate for prepping the cleanest area first, followed by the least-clean area. Follow your OR policy.
     ○ Do not allow cross-contamination between the areas by aerosolization of prep solution originating at the least-clean area.
     ○ Remove prepping drapes (see Figure 17.44).

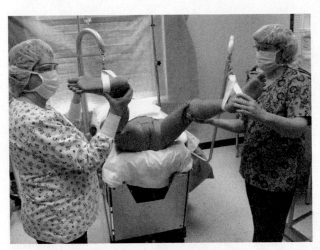

FIGURE 17.42 Simultaneously raise the manikin's legs.

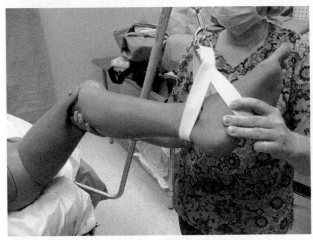

FIGURE 17.43 Adjust and ensure optimal positioning.

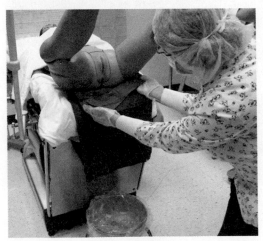

FIGURE 17.44 Perform abdominal and vaginal preps, and remove drapes.

2. Drape the patient for the procedure. Use three separate drape components for this skill. Alternatively, a one-piece pelviscopy drape with attached leggings may be preferred by your facility or surgeon.

Sterile Role: Perineal or Under-buttock Drape

- Prepare in order of use: the under-buttock drape, two leggings, and the lithotomy-pelviscopy drape (laparoscopy drape with abdominal and perineal fenestrations); place into a sterile basin in the ring stand for convenient access.
- Move the ring stand close to the operative field.
- Grasp and orient the under-buttock drape according to the preprinted cues. Cuff your sterile gloves under the drape.
- Place under the patient's buttock. Allow the plastic fluid collection bag to fall below the OR table level (see Figures 17.45 and 17.46).

Triangular Leggings

- Grasp the first triangular leggings drape. Follow any preprinted instructions. Cuff your hands while holding onto the tail end of the leggings.
- Maintain control of the drape. Slide the drape over the patient's right leg. Do not contaminate your gown.
- Repeat with the second leggings (see Figures 17.47 through 17.53).

Fenestrated Pelviscopy Drape

- Grasp the pelviscopy drape. Follow the preprinted instructions. Remove the adhesive strip backing.
- Orient and place the fenestration over the surgical site on the abdomen; use the umbilicus as a guide.
- Open the fan-folded segments according to the preprinted directions.
- Open two segments laterally.
- Release the third segment inferiorly over the perineal area. This segment is opened towards the sterile ST.
- Pass the fourth, superior segment to the anesthesia care provider.
- Fold down the perineal shield.
- Remove and discard the paper separator covering the abdomen (see Figures 17.54 through 17.60).

3. Perform additional preoperative sterile skills.

- Attach equipment and prepare supplies.
- Refer to Chapter 18 (see Figure 17.61).

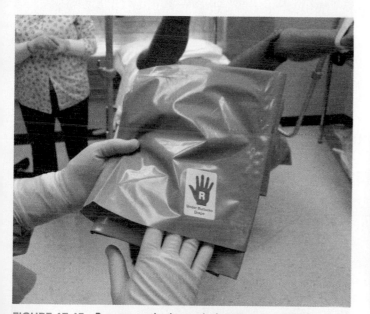

FIGURE 17.45   Prepare under-buttock drapes; view clues.

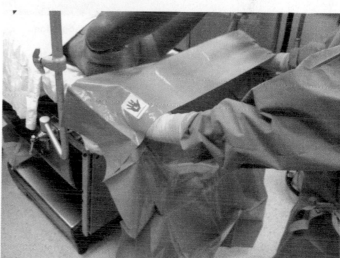

FIGURE 17.46   Cuff hands, place under buttocks.

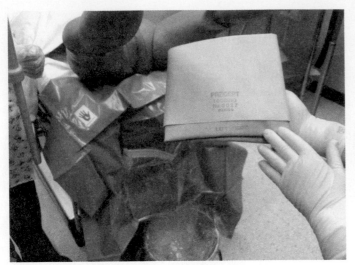

FIGURE 17.47 Orient leggings for right leg.

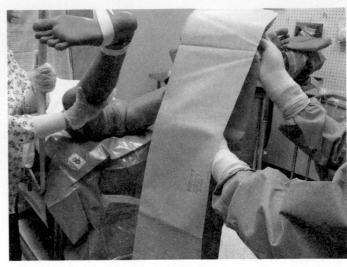

FIGURE 17.48 Open leggings and keep elevated.

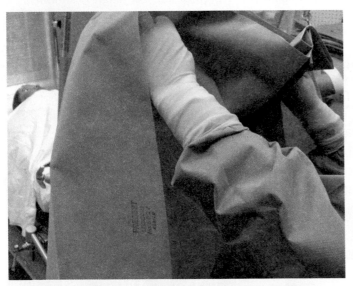

FIGURE 17.49 Hold tail in left hand, along with drape edge.

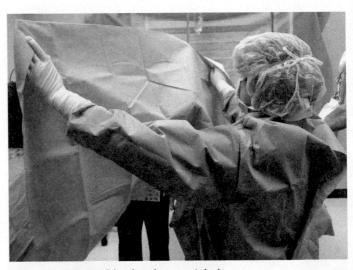

FIGURE 17.50 Hold tail and cover right leg.

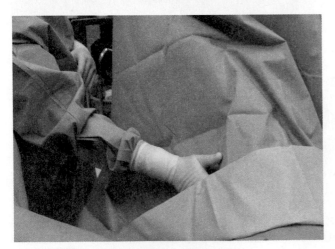

FIGURE 17.51 Cover upper leg with leggings.

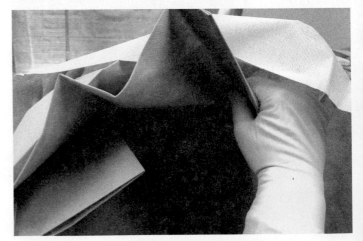

FIGURE 17.52 Orient second leggings; hold tail in right hand.

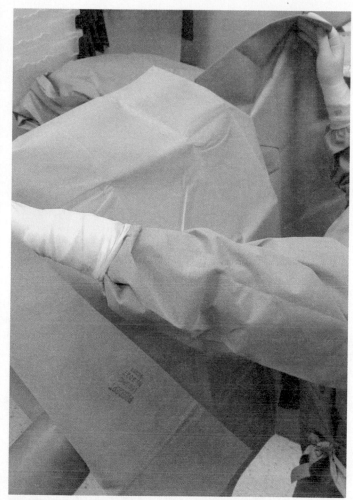

FIGURE 17.53 Unfold drape, keep tail elevated, and cover left leg.

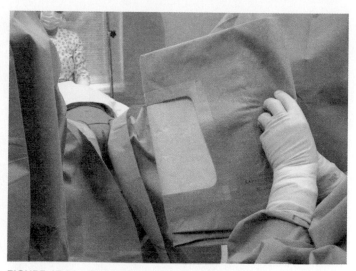

FIGURE 17.54 Orient the pelviscopy drape.

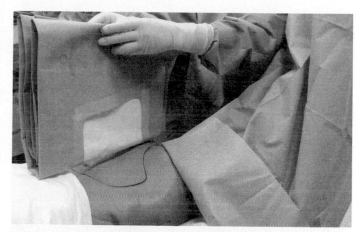

FIGURE 17.55 Position fenestration over abdomen.

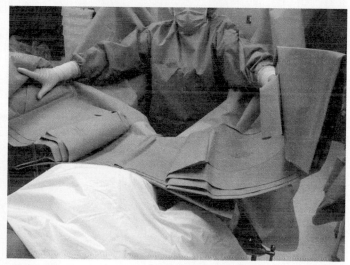

FIGURE 17.56 Open fan-folded drape laterally.

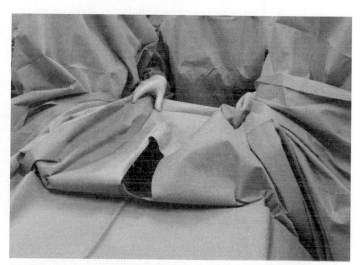

FIGURE 17.57 Pull lower half of drape over perineal area.

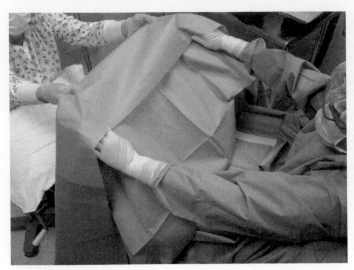

FIGURE 17.58 Pass upper half of drape to anesthesia care provider.

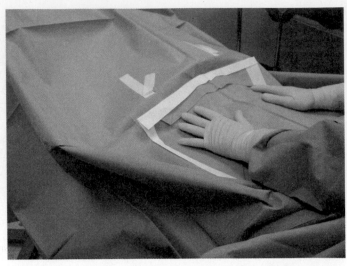

FIGURE 17.59 Secure the drape over the abdomen.

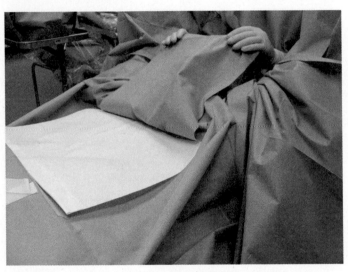

FIGURE 17.60 Fold down the perineal shield, and discard the paper.

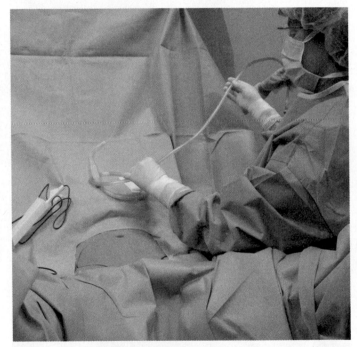

FIGURE 17.61 Draping complete.

STUDENT'S NAME: *Manjula*

CHAPTER 17 LAPAROTOMY DRAPES

PERFORMANCE RANK:

S or √ = Satisfactory: Competent—safe, accurate, sequential, and timely

U = Unsatisfactory: Unsafe—inaccurate and unprepared

PERFORMANCE RATING:

5   Independent: Expert—safe, confident, seamless performance; mentors others

4   Minimally monitored: Intermediate—safe, self-corrects few errors

3   Competent: Novice—safe, revises with evaluator cues, few errors

2   Remedial: Unsafe—critical errors, unable to implement evaluator cues consistently

1   Dependent: Unsafe—unacceptable, requires multiple evaluator interventions

PERFORMANCE CRITERIA	Performance Rank	Performance Rating
1. Perform Mutual Professional and Scholastic Criteria as appropriate (see the Preface or Appendix A).		1 2 3 4 (5)
2. State the rationale for draping after the prep solution has dried.		(1) 2 3 4 5
3. Present prepared OR towels to surgeon (refer to Chapter 7).		(1) 2 3 4 5
4. Pass towel clamps, when requested.		1 2 3 4 (5)
5. Prepare laparotomy drape.		1 2 (3) 4 5
6. Pass laparotomy drape. *contaminated*		1 2 (3) 4 5
7. Assist to drape the patient; work in tandem with the surgeon; cuff-protect gloves and gown.		(1) 2 3 4 5

ADDITIONAL COMMENTS _____

PERFORMANCE EVALUATIONS AND RECOMMENDATIONS

❑ PASS: Satisfactory Performance

    ❑ Demonstrates professionalism

    ❑ Exhibits critical thinking

    ❑ Demonstrates proficient clinical performance, appropriate for time in the program

❑ FAIL. Unsatisfactory Performance

    ❑ Critical criteria not met (see Performance Rank or Rating above)

    ❑ Professionalism not demonstrated.

    ❑ Critical thinking skills not demonstrated.

    ❑ Skill performance unsafe or underdeveloped.

☑ REMEDIATION:

    ☑ Schedule lab practice. Date: _____

    ☑ Reevaluate by instructor. Date: _____

❑ DISMISS from lab or clinicals today.

❑ Program director notified. Date: _____

19/35

SIGNATURES

Date ___11/4/13___   Evaluator _____   Student _____

COMPETENCY ASSESSMENT

STUDENT'S NAME: _____

CHAPTER 17 EXTREMITY DRAPES AND TOURNIQUET

PERFORMANCE RANK:

S or √ = Satisfactory: Competent—safe, accurate, sequential, and timely

U = Unsatisfactory: Unsafe—inaccurate and unprepared

PERFORMANCE RATING:

5   Independent: Expert—safe, confident, seamless performance; mentors others

4   Minimally monitored: Intermediate—safe, self-corrects few errors

3   Competent: Novice—safe, revises with evaluator cues, few errors

2   Remedial: Unsafe—critical errors, unable to implement evaluator cues consistently

1   Dependent: Unsafe—unacceptable, requires multiple evaluator interventions

PERFORMANCE CRITERIA	Performance Rank	Performance Rating
1. Perform Mutual Professional and Scholastic Criteria as appropriate (see the Preface or Appendix A).		1 2 3 4 5
2. State the safety parameters for tourniquet use.		1 2 3 4 5
3. State the rationale for draping after the prep solution has dried.		1 2 3 4 5
4. Nonsterile role: Position the patient for a forearm, extremity procedure.		1 2 3 4 5
5. Nonsterile role: Prepare the equipment, pad the patient's upper arm, and apply the pneumatic tourniquet.		1 2 3 4 5
6. Sterile role: Arrange all selected extremity drapes in order of use.		1 2 3 4 5
7. Sterile role: Apply drapes; work in tandem with a second, sterile team member; cuff-protect gloves and gown.		1 2 3 4 5

ADDITIONAL COMMENTS _____

PERFORMANCE EVALUATIONS AND RECOMMENDATIONS

❑ PASS: Satisfactory Performance

     ❑ Demonstrates professionalism

     ❑ Exhibits critical thinking

     ❑ Demonstrates proficient clinical performance appropriate for time in the program

❑ FAIL: Unsatisfactory Performance

     ❑ Critical criteria not met (see Performance Rank or Rating above)

     ❑ Professionalism not demonstrated.

     ❑ Critical thinking skills not demonstrated.

     ❑ Skill performance unsafe or underdeveloped.

❑ REMEDIATION:

     ❑ Schedule lab practice. Date: _____

     ❑ Reevaluate by instructor. Date: _____

❑ DISMISS from lab or clinicals today.

❑ Program director notified. Date: _____

SIGNATURES

Date _____   Evaluator _____   Student _____

COMPETENCY ASSESSMENT

STUDENT'S NAME: _____

CHAPTER 17 PELVIC LITHOTOMY DRAPES

PERFORMANCE RANK:

S or √ = Satisfactory: Competent—safe, accurate, sequential, and timely

U = Unsatisfactory: Unsafe—inaccurate and unprepared

PERFORMANCE RATING:

5   Independent: Expert—safe, confident, seamless performance; mentors others

4   Minimally monitored: Intermediate—safe, self-corrects few errors

3   Competent: Novice—safe, revises with evaluator cues, few errors

2   Remedial: Unsafe—critical errors, unable to implement evaluator cues consistently

1   Dependent: Unsafe—unacceptable, requires multiple evaluator interventions

PERFORMANCE CRITERIA	Performance Rank	Performance Rating
1. Perform Mutual Professional and Scholastic Criteria as appropriate (see the Preface or Appendix A).		1 2 3 4 5
2. State the rationale for safely positioning the patient in the lithotomy position.		1 2 3 4 5
3. State the rationale for draping after the skin prep has dried.		1 2 3 4 5
4. Nonsterile role: Position the patient in stirrups; work in tandem with another team member.		1 2 3 4 5
5. Sterile role: Prepare and place the under buttock drape; cuff-protect gloves and gown.		1 2 3 4 5
6. Sterile role: Prepare and place triangular leggings drapes; cuff-protect gloves and gown.		1 2 3 4 5
7. Sterile role: Prepare and place fenestrated pelviscopy drape; cuff-protect gloves and gown.		1 2 3 4 5

ADDITIONAL COMMENTS _____

PERFORMANCE EVALUATIONS AND RECOMMENDATIONS

❑ PASS: Satisfactory Performance
- ❑ Demonstrates professionalism
- ❑ Exhibits critical thinking
- ❑ Demonstrates proficient clinical performance appropriate for time in the program

❑ FAIL: Unsatisfactory Performance
- ❑ Critical criteria not met (see Performance Rank or Rating above)
- ❑ Professionalism not demonstrated.
- ❑ Critical thinking skills not demonstrated.
- ❑ Skill performance unsafe or underdeveloped.

❑ REMEDIATION:
- ❑ Schedule lab practice. Date: _____
- ❑ Reevaluate by instructor. Date: _____

❑ DISMISS from lab or clinicals today.

❑ Program director notified. Date: _____

SIGNATURES

Date _____   Evaluator _____   Student _____

ACTIVITIES AND DISCUSSION QUESTIONS

Activities

1. View the Complete Perioperative Process and Focus on Skills video, Skill #17 (video can be found at www.myhealthprofessionskit.com).
2. Observe the instructor perform the skills.
3. Practice with your lab partner by using a student actor or lab manikin as the patient.
4. Select and teach one skill to your lab partner, then observe and critique the performance.
5. Refer to your ST textbook and this lab manual to answer the Discussion Questions (see next column).
6. Review the video and the information in this lab manual when you prepare for your certification examination.

Discussion Questions

1. Why is the time-out protocol performed before the patient is positioned, prepped, and draped for the procedure?
2. Identify the steps and/or supplies that are missing from this list to drape for a laparotomy procedure.

   - Time-out protocol
   - Aseptic technique
   - Four OR towels
   - Cuff sterile gloves
   - Hold fan-folded drape at or above waist level

3. If you had to name one essential step, what might it be?
4. You pass a sharp towel clip to the surgeon, and he uses it to secure the drapes. What should you do?
5. The last time you assisted with draping, you dropped the fan-folded drape below waist level, and it had to be discarded. Formulate a plan to perform this skill correctly.
6. You are just entering the OR as a nonsterile team member, and the patient is in a lithotomy position. There is an abdominal drape wrapped in a sterile package sitting on a supply table. The first assistant is almost finished with the skin prep. Should you open the drape and pass it to the scrubbed ST? Explain.
7. You are assisting the circulator today. You are assigned to apply the pneumatic tourniquet cuff to the patient's right thigh. When you begin to place the padding on the patient's thigh, you notice a two-inch round, oozing, foul-smelling wound on the posterior thigh. What should you do next?
8. Note here any questions that you need your instructor to clarify.

18 Perform Postdraping and Preincision Preparation

INTRODUCTION

After draping the incision site, the surgeon is ready to begin the procedure. The surgical technologist places the Mayo stand and back table near the patient. The ST works with other sterile team members to position and make ready supplies, instruments, and equipment. This can be a stressful time, just prior to the incision. Confidence and efficiency are facilitated with practice in the lab setting.

- Before performing the following skill, your lab instructor will discuss some of the principles for practice and objectives involved in this chapter as well as the importance of following the skill sequence and instructions.
- Practice this skill with your lab partner. Encourage and critique each other. Your instructor will offer strategies for success. Appendix E highlights the value of teaching others as a component of active learning strategies. Refer to Appendix C for an overview of the chapter.
- The lab instructor will advise you of any additional criteria to be evaluated. At a designated time, demonstration of these skills will be evaluated and graded by your lab instructor using the competency assessment tool.
- When in the clinical setting, your instructor may once again assess your performance using the same tool. Refer to Appendix A for clinical evaluation and documentation.

Team Member	Type of Role		Timing		
	Nonsterile	Sterile	Preop	Intraop	Postop
Surgical Technologist		X	X		
Assistant Circulator	X		X		
Operating Room Team		X	X		

OBJECTIVES

The learner will demonstrate the following with 100 percent accuracy each time the operative environment is entered.

1. Uphold aseptic technique.
2. Move the Mayo stand and back table to the surgical field in preparation for the surgical procedure.
3. Position sterile light handle covers.
4. Attach tubing and cords to the drapes.
5. Pass distal ends of tubing and cords to the circulator.
6. Prepare marking pen, sponges, scalpel, and electrocautery.
7. Demonstrate occupational and patient safety awareness.

Principles for Practice

The foundation and rationale for our practice, in the perioperative environment, stem from evidence provided by professionals, organizations, and governmental agencies. Refer to the Bibliography, Glossary of Terms, and the following documents or developmental agencies:

- Manufacturers' product guidelines
- Operating room policies
- Surgeon's preference card
- Occupational Safety and Health Administration (OSHA)
- Centers for Disease Control and Prevention (CDC)
- Association of Surgical Technologists (AST)
- Association of periOperative Registered Nurses (AORN)

SKILL SEQUENCE AND INSTRUCTIONS

1. Collaborate with sterile team members to position the Mayo stand and back table immediately before the surgical incision.
   - Move the Mayo stand and back table to the surgical field.
     - Position the Mayo stand over the draped patient (usually over the feet for an abdominal procedure) so that you can easily reach the instruments and pass them to the surgeon.
     - Anticipate standing across the OR table, or opposite the surgeon.
     - Position the postend of the Mayo stand so that you can easily reach and control it to accommodate a requested height change in the OR bed.
     - Move the back table with your hands on the horizontal surface. Position it in a convenient location, usually near the foot of the OR bed (see Figures 18.1 through 18.3).

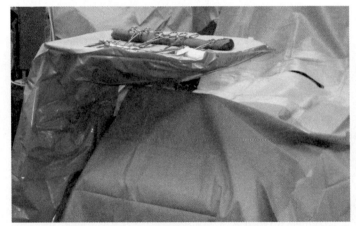

FIGURE 18.1 **Move and place the Mayo stand in position.**

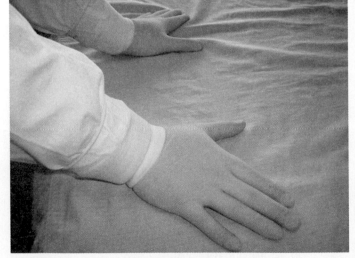

FIGURE 18.3 **Move table, hands on top.**

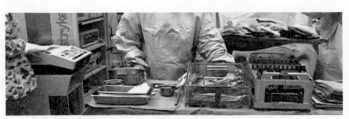

FIGURE 18.2 **Move and position the back table.**

2. Secure light handle covers onto the overhead lights. Direct the light beam to illuminate the operative field.

- Appropriate light handle covers were opened onto the sterile field in Chapter 4. Covers are disposable or may be reprocessed. Fenestrated covers allow for digital photography during the procedure.
- Secure covers so that they do not accidently fall into the sterile field. Sterile team members will grasp the light handles to adjust illumination during the procedure (see Figure 18.4).

3. Stand on step stools, positioned for use by team members next to the OR bed.

- Stools are positioned by the circulator, as needed, to assist the sterile team member with visualization of the operative field.
- Prevent falls from the stool. Remain attentive to your location. Slips, trips, and falls are major causes of injury for health care workers (see Figure 18.5).

4. Attach the suction tubing and electrocautery (Bovie) cord to the sterile drapes. Pass the distal ends to the circulator.

- Attach tubes and cords to the sterile drapes with the Velcro tabs or by using nonpenetrating clips. Estimate the amount of tubing that will be required to work on the sterile field. Attach approximately a fourth to a half of the proximal length of the tube or cord.
- Attach the electrocautery holster, or box, to the sterile drapes or to another preferred location. Use Velcro tabs or nonpenetrating clips. Do not coil the cord around metal instruments because this is a fire hazard. Refer to Chapter 13 .
- Place the electrocautery pencil tip (Bovie) into the holster. Place the scratch pad in the preferred location.
- Secure the tip onto a metal Yankauer wand (styles in plastic have an integral tip), and attach the wand onto the suction tubing.
- Pass the distal 3-foot length of the suction tube to the circulator. Pass the distal 3-foot length of the electrocautery cord to the circulator. The circulator will attach the tube to the suction canister and the cord to the electrocautery generator located off the sterile field.
- If you miscalculate and pass off too much of the sterile tubes or cords to the circulator, then you will not have enough to use on the sterile field. Discard the entire length. The circulator will open and present new sterile tubes or cords to you.
- Do not attempt to retrieve a tube or cord back onto the sterile field once they have been passed to the circulator. The distal ends of the tube and cord are no longer sterile (see Figures 18.6 through 18.9).

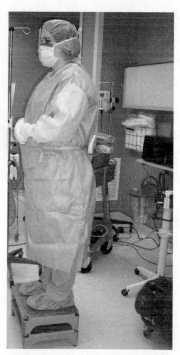

FIGURE 18.5 Use step stools to improve access to the surgical field.

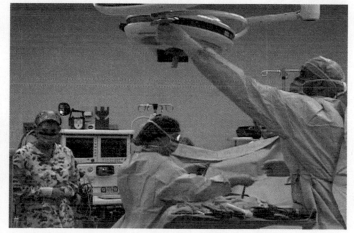

FIGURE 18.4 Securely attach light handle covers.

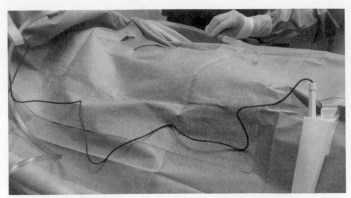

FIGURE 18.6 Secure working lengths of suction tube and Bovie cord.

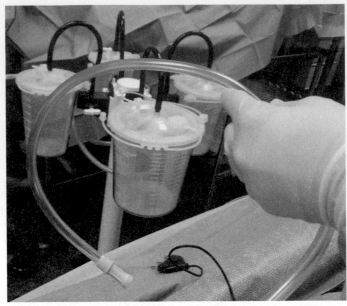

FIGURE 18.7 Pass distal ends to the circulator.

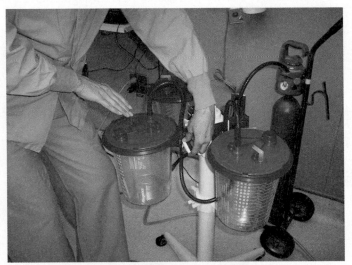

FIGURE 18.8 Ensure function of mechanical suction.

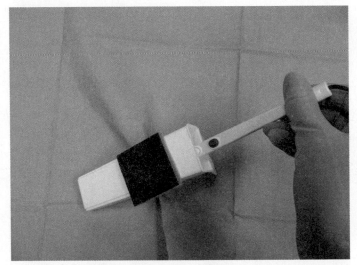

FIGURE 18.9 Electrocautery pencil, holster, and scratch pad.

5. The circulator will verify and adjust the cut and coagulation settings for the electrosurgical unit generator (ESU). If used, a foot-operated control pad is placed on the floor, under the OR bed for the surgeon to control the flow of current. Handheld controls for the electrosurgical pencil do not require a foot pad.

6. Prepare for the skin incision.

   • Place two RayTec sponges at the field.
   • Remove the cap from the marking pen; place the cap on the back table, and pass the pen when requested by the surgeon.
   • Anticipate passing the skin scalpel using a hands-free transfer method such as a no-touch basin, pad, or zone. The surgeon may use the scalpel in addition to the electrosurgical pencil to make the incision. Refer to Chapter 19.
   • Remain attentive and anticipate the needs of the surgeon.
   • The intraoperative phase of surgery begins with the incision (see Figures 18.10 and 18.11).

7. Adjust the height of the Mayo stand to correspond with any position changes in the OR bed as requested by the surgeon. (A Trendelenburg position will elevate the patient's legs and feet.)

   • Prevent injury to the patient.

     ○ Raise the height of the Mayo stand; manipulate the controls on the stand and secure the new height.
     ○ Do not allow the Mayo stand to rest on the patient's legs, feet, or other areas.
     ○ Do not rest your arms or any upper body weight on the Mayo stand. An accidental position change in the Mayo stand will cause you to fall onto the patient.

8. Assess the suction tubing on the sterile field for twists or kinks if the suction action is malfunctioning. The circulator will assess the suction source on the wall or the canisters for integrity during nonfunction episodes.

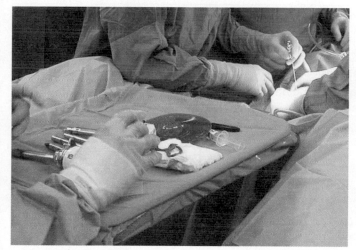

FIGURE 18.11 ST, left, focused on the surgical progression and the surgeon's requirements.

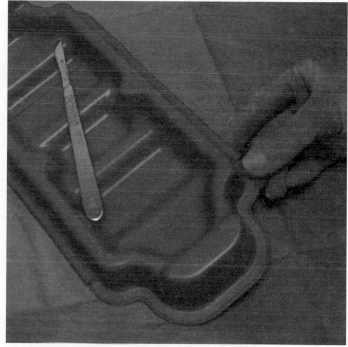

FIGURE 18.10 Hands-free transfer method.

STUDENT'S NAME: _____

CHAPTER 18 PERFORM POSTDRAPING AND PREINCISION PREPARATION

PERFORMANCE RANK:

> S or √ = Satisfactory: Competent—safe, accurate, sequential, and timely
> U = Unsatisfactory: Unsafe—inaccurate and unprepared

PERFORMANCE RATING:

> 5   Independent: Expert—safe, confident, seamless performance; mentors others
> 4   Minimally monitored: Intermediate—safe, self-corrects few errors
> 3   Competent: Novice—safe, revises with evaluator cues, few errors
> 2   Remedial: Unsafe—critical errors, unable to implement evaluator cues consistently
> 1   Dependent: Unsafe—unacceptable, requires multiple evaluator interventions

PERFORMANCE CRITERIA	Performance Rank	Performance Rating
1. Perform Mutual Professional and Scholastic Criteria as appropriate (see the Preface or Appendix A).		1 2 3 4 5
2. Move and position the Mayo stand to the correct side of the OR bed for the designated surgical procedure (laparotomy example).		1 2 3 4 5
3. Move and position the back table to the designated location.		1 2 3 4 5
4. Secure light handle covers and adjust the light to illuminate the surgical site.		1 2 3 4 5
5. Attach the Yankauer suction wand to the tubing, and secure the tubing onto the drapes; use nonpenetrating clips or the Velcro tubing tabs.		1 2 3 4 5
6. Attach the ESU pencil holster to the drapes; place the pencil inside; attach the scratch pad, in designated location.		1 2 3 4 5
7. Alert the circulator to grasp the distal ends of the suction tube and cord; pass the tube and cord.		1 2 3 4 5
8. Place two sponges at the surgical field, and prepare the marking pen and scalpel.		1 2 3 4 5
9. Adjust the height of the Mayo stand positioned at the OR bed.		1 2 3 4 5
10. Stand on a step stool positioned next to the OR bed, as needed.		1 2 3 4 5

ADDITIONAL COMMENTS _____

PERFORMANCE EVALUATIONS AND RECOMMENDATIONS

❑ PASS: Satisfactory Performance
    ❑ Demonstrates professionalism
    ❑ Exhibits critical thinking
    ❑ Demonstrates proficient clinical performance appropriate for time in the program

❏ FAIL: Unsatisfactory Performance
  ❏ Critical criteria not met (see Performance Rank or Rating above)
  ❏ Professionalism not demonstrated.
  ❏ Critical thinking skills not demonstrated.
  ❏ Skill performance is unsafe or underdeveloped.
❏ REMEDIATION:
  ❏ Schedule lab practice. Date: _____
  ❏ Reevaluate by instructor. Date: _____
❏ DISMISS from lab or clinicals today.
❏ Program director notified. Date: _____

SIGNATURES

Date _____   Evaluator _____   Student _____

ACTIVITIES AND DISCUSSION QUESTIONS

Activities

1. View the Complete Perioperative Process and Focus on Skills video, Skill #18 (video can be found at www.myhealthprofessionskit.com).

2. Observe the instructor perform the skill.

3. Practice with your lab partner by using a student actor or lab manikin.

4. Select and teach one skill to your lab partner, then observe and critique the performance.

5. Refer to your ST textbook and this lab manual to answer the Discussion Questions (see next column).

6. Review the video and the information in this lab manual when you prepare for your certification examination.

Discussion Questions

1. Name at least three essential patient safety measures included in this skill.

2. How will you maintain aseptic technique when you pass the suction tube and the ESU cord off the field to the circulator?

3. The Yankauer tip and the tubing are attached at the field, but there is no suction action. Why do you think this is?

4. In addition to the no-touch basin, how else can you communicate that a sharp is on the field?

5. You need to use a step stool for this procedure; how will you keep yourself safe while standing on it?

6. At the start of the procedure, the surgeon asked the anesthesia care provider to put the patient into a Trendelenburg position. What should the ST do at once?

7. Note here any questions that you need your instructor to clarify.

Unit II

Surgery Fundamentals

Identify, Prepare, and Pass Instruments

19

INTRODUCTION

During surgery, the surgical technologist will assess, identify, prepare, and pass selected instruments to right- and left-handed surgeons. The ST can participate in the second assisting surgical technologist's role which may include sponging, suctioning, retracting, manipulating the endoscopic camera, and cutting suture. The Association of Surgical Technologist's refers to this skill set as the second scrub role in its sixth edition of the *Core Curriculum for Surgical Technology.*

- Before performing the following skills, your lab instructor will discuss some of the principles for practice and objectives involved in this chapter as well as the importance of following the skill sequence and instructions.
- Practice instrument skills with your lab partner. Your instructor will work in tandem with you during simulations of surgical procedures. Use a manikin and practice the first and second scrub skills together with your lab partner. Encourage and critique each other. Your instructor will offer strategies for success. Appendix E highlights the value of teaching others as a component of active learning strategies. Refer to Appendix C for an overview of the chapter.
- The lab instructor will advise you of any additional criteria to be evaluated. At a designated time, demonstration of these skills will be evaluated and graded by your lab instructor using the competency assessment tool.
- When in the clinical setting, your instructor may once again assess your performance using the same tool. Refer to Appendix A for clinical evaluation and documentation.

Team Member	Type of Role		Timing		
	Nonsterile	Sterile	Preop	Intraop	Postop
Surgical Technologist		X		X	
Assistant Circulator	X			X	
Second Assisting or Second Scrub ST Role		X		X	
Operating Room Team		X		X	

OBJECTIVES

The learner will demonstrate this skill with 100 percent accuracy each time performing in the operative environment.

1. Maintain aseptic technique.
2. Pass instruments to the surgeon in the position of use for right- and left-handed surgeons.
3. Promote safety when handling and passing sharps.

 Principles for Practice

The foundation and rationale for our practice, in the perioperative environment, stem from evidence provided by professionals, organizations, and governmental agencies. Refer to the Bibliography, Glossary of Terms, and the following documents or developmental agencies:

4. Use hands-free transfer methods when passing sharp instruments.
5. Load a stapler cartridge.
6. Recognize frequently used hand signals.
7. Perform point-of-use instrument care during the surgical procedure.
8. State policy for reporting and impounding malfunctioning instruments.
9. Perform second scrub skills.

- State practice acts
- Manufacturers' product instructions
- Operating room policies
- Surgeon's preference card
- Occupational Safety and Health Administration (OSHA)
- Centers for Disease Control and Prevention (CDC)
- The American Society of Anesthesiologists (ASA)
- Association of Surgical Technologists (AST)
- Association of periOperative Registered Nurses (AORN)

SKILL SEQUENCE AND INSTRUCTIONS

Scalpels and Handling

1. Prepare a variety of scalpels for use by the surgeon. Pass using a hands-free transfer method.

   - There are choices in blade and handle sizes depending on the requirements of the surgical procedure, surgeon's preferences, and OR policy. Preloaded, retractable safety scalpels are also available. Refer to Chapter 10.

   - Load a #3 handle with any of the corresponding sized blades: #10, #11, #12, and #15.
   - Load a #4 handle with: #20 or #21 blade.
   - Load a #7 handle with: #11 or #15 blade.
   - Pass the scalpel using a hands-free method: emesis basin, no-touch basin, designated area, or pad (see Figures 19.1 through 19.5).

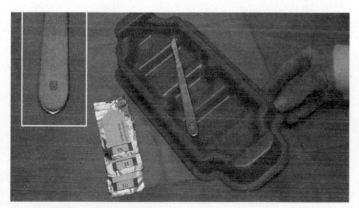

FIGURE 19.1   Handle #3.

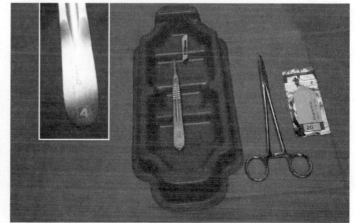

FIGURE 19.2   Handle #4.

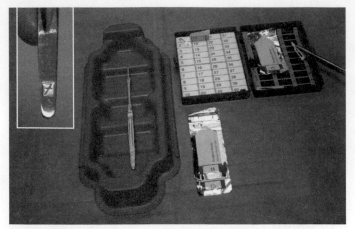

FIGURE 19.3 Handle #7.

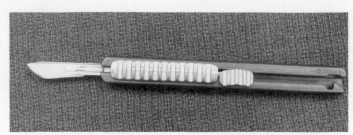

FIGURE 19.4 Retractable blade on a reusable handle.

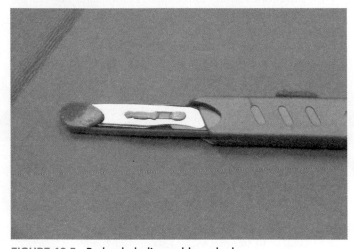

FIGURE 19.5 Preloaded, disposable scalpel.

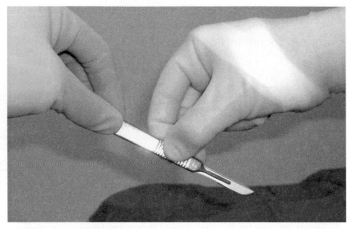

FIGURE 19.6 Hand-to-hand passing is not recommended by AST or AORN.

2. For the hand-to-hand pass, verbal and visual communication with acknowledgement is essential before passing.

- Grasp the handle from above, with the blade tip facing the ST. Point the tip downward as it is passed to the surgeon.
- This method of passing a scalpel is not recommended by AST or AORN (see Figure 19.6).

Scissors and Handling

3. Identify and pass a variety of scissors. Scissors are available in various sizes and functions to cut tissue, suture, dressing materials, or wire. The Metzenbaum scissors, with blunt ends, will cut and dissect delicate tissue. They are available in straight or curved.

- Identify instruments by the working ends and the overall shape.
- Assess all instruments for proper functioning. Do not pass misaligned or dull instruments.
- Pass the scissors by placing the ring handles in the surgeon's palm. Pass a curved instrument with the point facing toward the surgeon's midline.
- Pass instruments to right- and left-handed surgeons.
- Indicate the instrument names that you will be required to know on the lines below each instrument picture (see Figure 19.7).

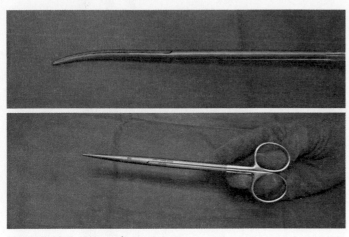

FIGURE 19.7   Metzenbaum scissors.

Name: _____

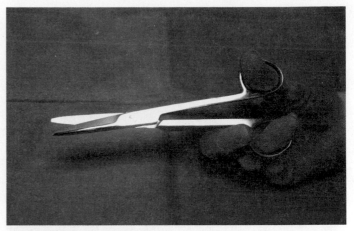

FIGURE 19.8   Mayo scissors.

Name: _____

4. Identify Mayo scissors. They are thicker in design, have blunt ends, and are commonly used for cutting suture and heavy tissue. The nickname for straight Mayo scissors may be "suture scissors." The nickname for curved Mayo scissors may be "Mayos" (see Figure 19.8).

5. Pass scissors in the position of use to the surgeon.

   • Grasp the scissors near the working end.

• Pass by rotating your wrist and place the instrument's ring handles firmly into the surgeon's palm. You will hear a "snap" sound as the instrument meets the surgeon's glove. Use a firm pass so that the surgeon is aware that the pass has occurred.

• Recognize hand signals indicating the type of instrument that you will pass to the surgeon.

• Pass Metzenbaum scissors for cutting or dissecting delicate tissue.

• Pass straight Mayo scissors for cutting suture.

• Recognize patterns and anticipate. If you pass suture material, such as a suture tie or suture on a needle, then the next instrument you should have in your hand and ready to pass is a pair of suture scissors (see Figures 19.9 through 19.11).

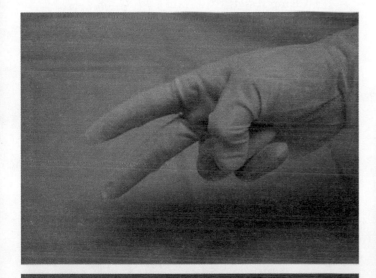

Surgeon's Signal to pass

FIGURE 19.9   Hand signal by surgeon.

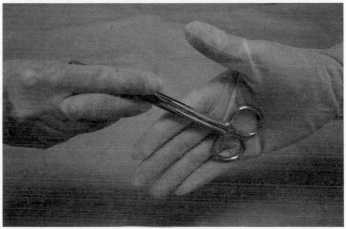

FIGURE 19.10   Pass scissors.

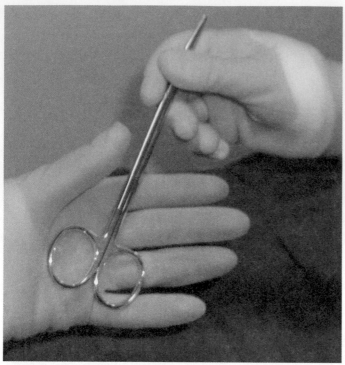

FIGURE 19.11 Pass.

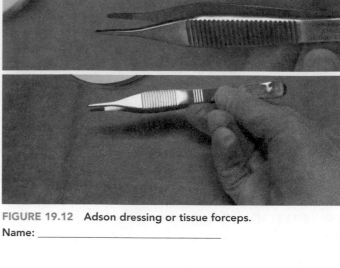

FIGURE 19.12 Adson dressing or tissue forceps.
Name: _____

Forceps and Handling

6. Identify and pass a variety of forceps.

- Designed so that they can perform specific functions on tissue, this category includes hemostats, clamps, and pickups.
- Examine the working ends of the instruments—rat-tooth, atraumatic, or multitoothed. Jaws are designed with horizontal or longitudinal serrations. Handle styles include fluted, serrated, or pyramidal.

- Forceps will:
  - Grasp tissue.
  - Tag the end of a sponge.
  - Approximate tissue for stapling.
  - Clamp vessels.
  - Assist with dissection (see Figures 19.12 through 19.15).

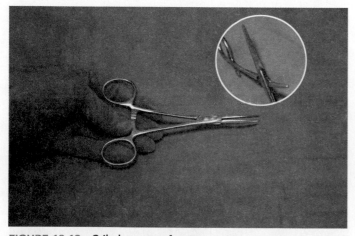

FIGURE 19.13 Crile hemostat forceps.
Name: _____

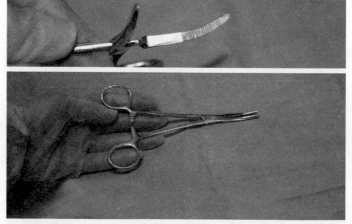

FIGURE 19.14 Curved kelly forceps.
Name: _____

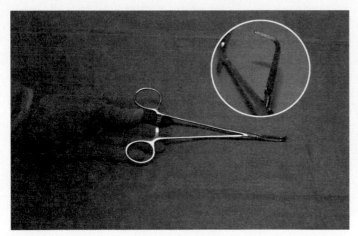

FIGURE 19.15 Meeker dissecting forceps.

Name: _____

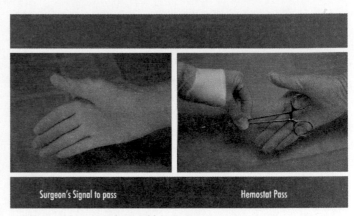

Surgeon's Signal to pass   Hemostat Pass

FIGURE 19.16 Hand signal by surgeon.

7. Pass ringed forceps with the ratchet closed to the first tooth or step. The surgeon will open the ratchet before use. Pass pickup designed forceps with the two sides squeezed closed.

- Pass with the working end positioned for immediate use by the surgeon.
- Pass curved instruments with the point facing the surgeon's midline.
- Recognize your error in passing because the surgeon will make an orientation adjustment before using it.
- Observe and correct any errors (see Figures 19.16 through 19.18).

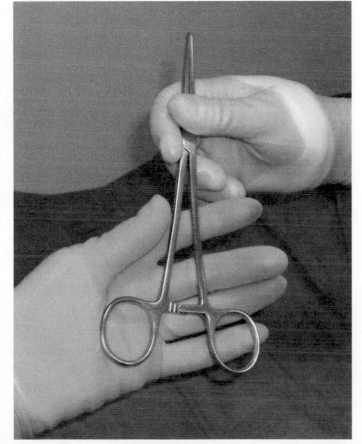

FIGURE 19.17 Pass ringed forceps.

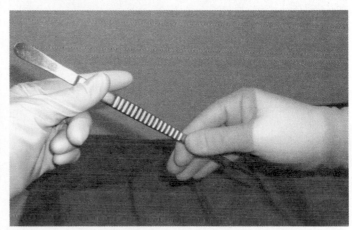

FIGURE 19.18 Pass forceps.

Retractors and Handling

8. Identify and pass a variety of retractors.

   - Retractors assist the surgeon to access and visualize the incisional area. They may be handheld or self-retaining. The handle grip end of retractors can vary in design to aid in the ergonomics for those performing the tissue retraction.
   - Variations include ringed, horned, lamb, open-ended, or ankh shaped.
   - Retractors may be double-ended like the Army Retractor, also known as an "Army-Navy."
   - Pass the working end of the retractor so it is available for immediate use by the surgeon. The surgeon will position the retractor and may ask a scrubbed team member to retract according to their instructions (see Figures 19.19 through 19.22).

9. Identify and pass a variety of self-retaining retractors.

   - Adjust the ratchet in the self-retaining retractors, and pass the retractor to the surgeon in the closed position.
   - The Weitlaner retractor is also known as a "Weitlander," or Cerebellar.
   - Identify the Balfour abdominal retractor and all of the parts: bladder, or accessory, blade, arm blades, wing nut, and screws. Prepare to pass in two segments.

     - Pass the retractor/arm blades in the closed position for placement in the patient's body.
     - Pass the bladder, or accessory blade, to the surgeon with the ringed end facing the surgeon.
     - The surgeon will adjust the tension, and position and secure the parts. (see Figures 19.23 through 19.27).

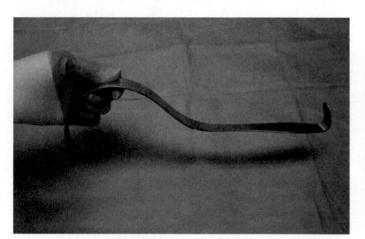

FIGURE 19.19 Deaver retractor.
Name: _____

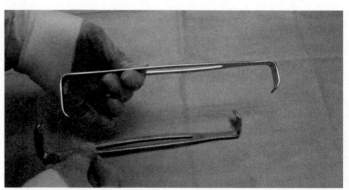

FIGURE 19.20 Army retractor.
Name: _____

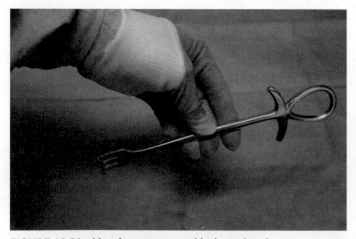

FIGURE 19.21 Murphy retractor, ankh shaped end.
Name: _____

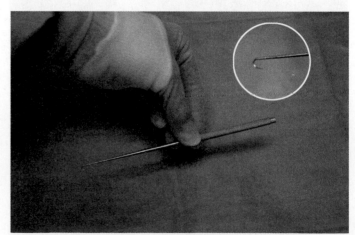

FIGURE 19.22 Joseph single skin hook retractor.
Name: _____

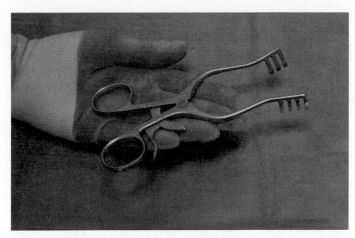

FIGURE 19.23 Weitlaner, blade ends open.
Name: _____

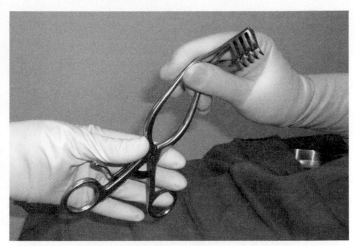

FIGURE 19.24 Pass, blade ends closed.

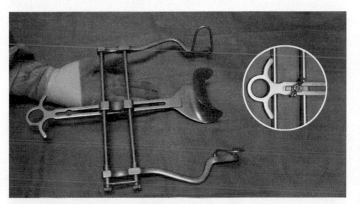

FIGURE 19.25 Balfour retractor, open.
Name: _____

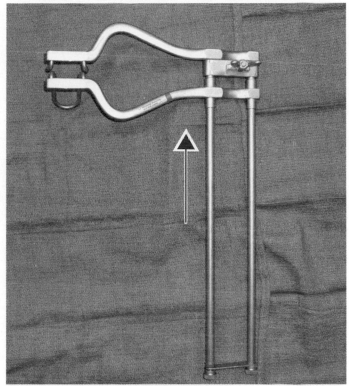

FIGURE 19.26 Close arms and pass.

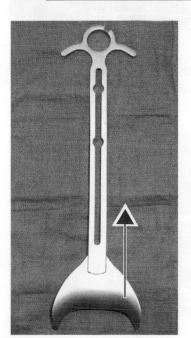

FIGURE 19.27 Hold bladder, or accessory blade, and pass.

Needle Holders and Handling

10. Identify, load, and pass needle holders. Needle holders, or drivers, grasp suture needles. The designs vary depending on the thickness of the tissue to be approximated and the size of the suture needle.

- Load the needle holder with the surgeon-selected suture needle. Refer to Chapter 20 for specific instructions on loading and passing.
- Ensure the needle holder is firmly ratcheted closed.
- Advocate for patient safety.
  - Do not pass the loaded needle holder to the surgeon if the suture needle does not seat securely into the needle holder.
  - Select another needle holder and tag or separate the nonfunctioning instrument for repair (see Figures 19.28 through 19.31).

Accessory Instruments

11. Identify, assemble, and pass additional instruments and equipment.

- Assemble the abdominal Poole suction. Secure the inner cannula into the outer, perforated cannula. Attach assembled instrument to the plastic suction tubing.
- Pass the prepared sponge stick in the position of function. Refer to Chapter 10.
- Identify and pass a Backhaus towel forceps, used to secure surgical towels prior to draping the patient. Close the ratchet to the first step and pass finger-rings facing the surgeon.
- Assemble the stapler with a staple cartridge, used to assist with wound closure. Follow the manufacturer's instructions, and insert the cartridge into the stapler.
- Place a magnetic instrument pad near the surgical site per OR policy. The mat will hold instruments until exchanged (see Figures 19.32 through 19.39).

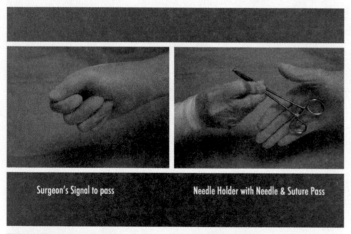

Surgeon's Signal to pass   Needle Holder with Needle & Suture Pass

FIGURE 19.28 Pass loaded needle holder.

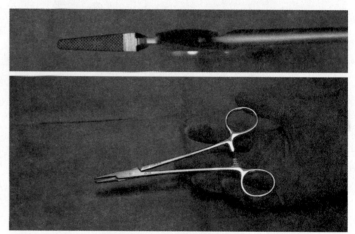

FIGURE 19.29 Crile wood needle holder.
Name: _____

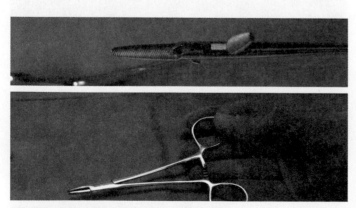

FIGURE 19.30 Brown plastic needle holder.
Name: _____

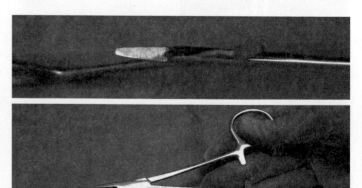

FIGURE 19.31 Webster needle holder.
Name: _____

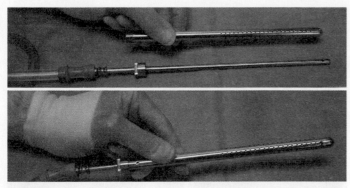

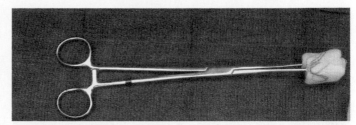

FIGURE 19.32   Poole abdominal suction: inner and outer cannula in 30 Fr. size.
Name: _____

FIGURE 19.33   "Sponge stick."
Name: _____

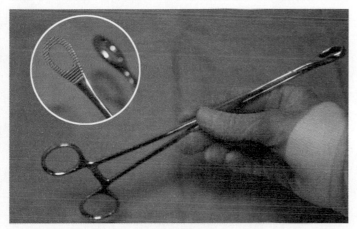

FIGURE 19.34   Foerster sponge forceps.
Name: _____

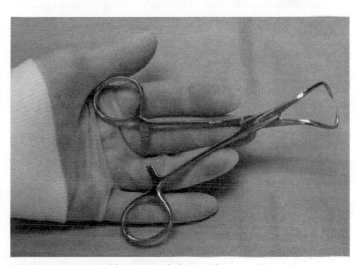

FIGURE 19.35   Backhaus towel clamp; close ratchet to pass.
Name: _____

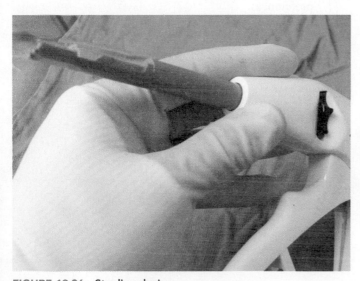

FIGURE 19.36   Stapling device.

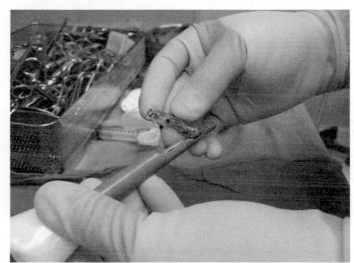

FIGURE 19.37   Insert staple cartridge.

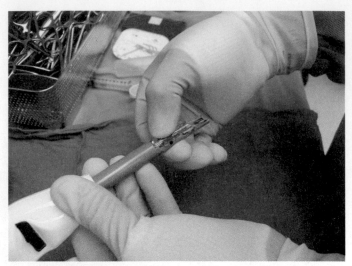

FIGURE 19.38 Secure cartridge.

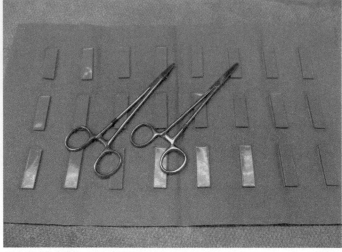

FIGURE 19.39 Magnetic instrument pad.

Point-of-Use Cleaning and Maintenance

12. Clean instruments at the point-of-use. Remove surgical debris, blood, and tissue to promote proper function and to enhance the ease of cleaning and decontamination after the procedure.

   • Wipe off instruments during the procedure.
   • Moisten sponges or instruments with sterile water. Normal saline harms the finish or pits the stainless steel instruments.
   • Flush instrument lumens to remove debris.

13. Follow your OR policy for tagging and impounding malfunctioning instruments.

   • Assess all instruments for proper function and parts before the procedure begins.
   • Tag and isolate malfunctioning instruments on the sterile field or pass to the circulator.

   • Transport items in need of repair to the decontamination area and isolation them, at the end of the procedure.

Intraoperative Use of Instruments

14. Integrate instrument skills into the sequence or progression of surgical procedures.

   • Obtain a general laparotomy instrument set or another set of choice. Identify and pass these instruments as they are used during a surgical procedure. Refer to Table 19.1.
   • Identify instruments using additional texts and resources, and seek guidance for your facility's preferences.

TABLE 19.1 Instrument Identification and Surgical Procedures

Surgical Procedure: _____

Surgical Progression	Selected Instruments
Post-draping and pre-incision preparation	Prepare skin knife, sponges Suction wand Bovie ESU Light handle covers Other
Incise skin	Skin knife Bovie ESU Forceps Other
Achieve hemostasis	Forceps or clamps Bovie ESU Sponges Other
Extend incision	Skin knife Mayo scissors Other
Retract	Army/navy retractors Richardson or Kelly retractors Other
Incise additional layers	Kocher or Kelly, to hold peritoneum Metzenbaum scissors Other
Achieve hemostasis	Forceps or clamps Bovie ESU Other
Retract	Large Richardson Balfour retractor Other
Explore, repair, or excise pathology	Longer instruments Clamp, cut, tie, Kelly, Kocher, Metzenbaum Scissors Suture ties or tie on passer (Chapter 20) Other
Obtain specimen	Labels Other
Irrigate/suction	Saline and bulb syringe Suction wand Other
Counts Medication	Count instruments (Chapter 8) Tabulate Medications (Chapter 9) Other
Close incision by layers	Needle holders Suture material (Chapter 20) Other

(Continued)

TABLE 19.1   Instrument Identification and Surgical Procedures (*Continued*)

Surgical Progression	Selected Instruments
Skin closure	Suture Stapler Glue Other
Dressing	Dressing sponges Mayo scissors Steri-strips and forceps Other

15. Perform in the second assisting or second-scrub surgical technologist's role under the direction of the surgeon and according to state practice acts.

   - Sponge the operative field.
     - Use a sponge-stick, RayTec sponge, or laparotomy sponge, according to the surgeon's preferences and one that is appropriate for the size of the wound.
     - Use pressure to wick fluids, without damaging tissues. Use pressure on the skin during closure to promote hemostasis.
   - Suction the operative field to clear blood or irrigation fluids.
     - Use the Yankauer suction wand to grasp fluids without damaging tissue.

   - Hold instrumentation to retract the surgical wound edges.
     - The surgeon will place the retractor and you will retract the wound edges according to the surgeon's demonstration and instructions. Follow instructions to maintain tissue integrity and prevent damage.
     - Use the design of the instrument handles to assist you.
   - Cut suture material.
     - Use Mayo scissors to cut the suture strands during wound closure or hemostasis. Routinely strands are cut at an angle, approximately ¼ inch above the knot and always as directed according to the surgeon's preferences. Refer to Chapter 20.
     - Manipulate the endoscopic camera used during minimally invasive endoscopic procedures. Capitalize on your eye-hand coordination in this skill. Refer to Chapter 25 (see Figures 19.40 through 19.44).

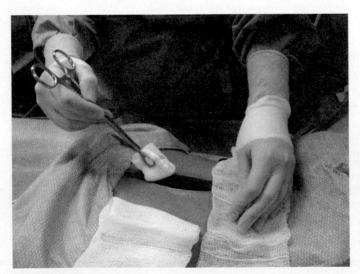

FIGURE 19.40   Sponge the wound to wick blood.

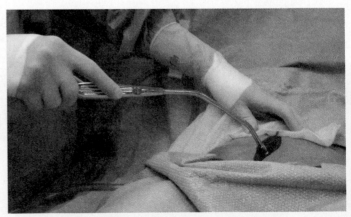

FIGURE 19.41   Suction blood or irrigation solutions.

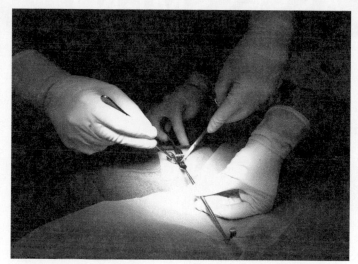

FIGURE 19.42   Hold retractors for the surgeon.

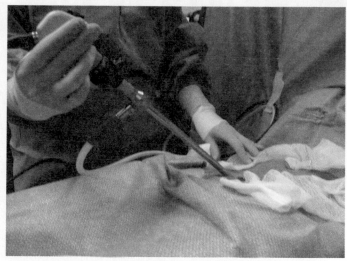

FIGURE 19.43   Steadily manipulate the endoscopic camera.

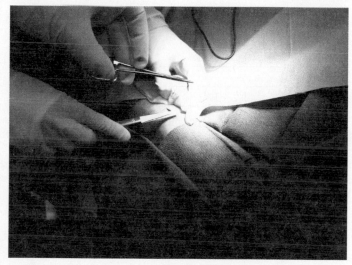

FIGURE 19.44   Cut suture as directed by the surgeon.

COMPETENCY ASSESSMENT

STUDENT'S NAME: _____

CHAPTER 19 IDENTIFY, PREPARE, AND PASS INSTRUMENTS

PERFORMANCE RANK:

S or √ = Satisfactory: Competent—safe, accurate, sequential, and timely
U = Unsatisfactory: Unsafe—inaccurate and unprepared

PERFORMANCE RATING:

5   Independent: Expert—safe, confident, seamless performance; mentors others
4   Minimally monitored: Intermediate—safe, self-corrects few errors
3   Competent: Novice—safe, revises with evaluator cues, few errors
2   Remedial: Unsafe—critical errors, unable to implement evaluator cues consistently
1   Dependent: Unsafe—unacceptable, requires multiple evaluator interventions

PERFORMANCE CRITERIA	Performance Rank	Performance Rating
1. Perform Mutual Professional and Scholastic Criteria as appropriate (see the Preface or Appendix A).		1 2 3 4 5
2. Transfer scalpels; use selected transfer method.		1 2 3 4 5
3. Identify and pass scissors to right- and left-handed surgeons.		1 2 3 4 5
4. Identify and pass forceps to right- and left-handed surgeons.		1 2 3 4 5
5. Identify and pass handheld and self-retaining retractors to right- and left-handed surgeons.		1 2 3 4 5
6. Identify needle holders (refer to Chapter 20).		1 2 3 4 5
7. Identify, assemble, and pass instructor-selected instrumentation.		1 2 3 4 5
8. Demonstrate (state) point-of-use instrument cleaning.		1 2 3 4 5
9. Demonstrate (state) appropriate method to isolate, tag, and remove from service any malfunctioning instrument.		1 2 3 4 5
10. Demonstrate the second assisting or second scrub role: sponge, suction, retract, and cut suture; manipulate the endoscopic camera in Chapter 25.		1 2 3 4 5

ADDITIONAL COMMENTS _____

PERFORMANCE EVALUATIONS AND RECOMMENDATIONS

❑ PASS: Satisfactory Performance
   ❑ Demonstrates professionalism
   ❑ Exhibits critical thinking
   ❑ Demonstrates proficient clinical performance appropriate for time in the program
❑ FAIL: Unsatisfactory Performance
   ❑ Critical criteria not met (see Performance Rank or Rating Above)
   ❑ Professionalism not demonstrated.
   ❑ Critical thinking skills not demonstrated.
   ❑ Skill performance unsafe or underdeveloped.

❏ REMEDIATION:
    ❏ Schedule lab practice. Date: _____
    ❏ Reevaluate by instructor. Date: _____
❏ DISMISS from lab or clinicals today.
❏ Program director notified. Date: _____

SIGNATURES

Date _____   Evaluator _____   Student _____

ACTIVITIES AND DISCUSSION QUESTIONS

Activities

1. View the Complete Perioperative Process and Focus on Skills video, Skill #19 (video can be found at www.myhealthprofessionskit.com).
2. Observe the instructor perform the skill.
3. Handle sharps under the direct supervision of your instructor.
4. Practice identifying, preparing, and passing instruments in a general laparotomy set.
5. Select and teach one skill to your lab partner, such as assembling and passing a balfour retractor, then observe and critique the performance.
6. Obtain an instrument set, and identify instruments used for selected surgical procedures. Refer to Table 11.1 and additional ST resources.
7. Demonstrate and discuss the second scrub role with your lab partner. Select sponging, suctioning, retracting, or cutting suture. Manipulate an endoscopic camera in Chapter 25.
8. Refer to your ST textbook and this lab manual to answer the Discussion Questions (see next column).
9. Review the video and the information in this lab manual when you prepare for your certification examination.

Discussion Questions

1. List the essential steps in passing any instrument.
2. What may be your first clue that you did not pass the instrument correctly to the surgeon?
3. If you are not identifying and passing the instruments in a timely manner, what can you do to improve the speed of your identification and passing?
4. Formulate methods to learn nicknames for instruments.
5. Note here any questions that you need your instructor to clarify.

20 Prepare, Load, and Pass Suture for Right- and Left-Handed Surgeons

INTRODUCTION

During wound closure, the surgical technologist will identify, load, and pass suture material to the surgeon. Anticipation, critical thinking, precise communication, multitasking, and consistent application of sharps safety are paramount to success with this skill. In a recent study reported in the Journal of the American College of Surgeons, most sharp injuries occur to the scrubbed team member, ST or RN, during use or passing of suture needles, scalpel blades, and syringes. You will learn to practice safety in the lab setting.

- Before performing the following, your lab instructor will discuss some of the principles for practice and objectives involved in this chapter as well as the importance of following the skill sequence and instructions.

- Practice with your lab partner. Encourage and critique each other. Your instructor will offer strategies for success. Appendix E highlights the value of teaching others as a component of active learning strategies. Refer to Appendix C for an overview of the chapter.
- The lab instructor will advise you of any additional criteria to be evaluated. At a designated time, demonstration of these skills will be evaluated and graded by your lab instructor using the competency assessment tool.
- When in the clinical setting, your instructor may once again assess your performance using the same tool. Refer to Appendix A for clinical evaluation and documentation.

Team Member	Type of Role		Timing		
	Nonsterile	Sterile	Preop	Intraop	Postop
Surgical Technologist		X		X	
Assistant Circulator	X			X	
Operating Room Team		X		X	

OBJECTIVES

The learner will demonstrate this skill with 100 percent accuracy each time performed.

1. Demonstrate aseptic technique.
2. Read and interpret the information on the suture packages.
3. Load and pass suture to a right- or left-handed surgeon.
4. Load and pass ties: free hand and with an instrument.
5. Place used needles into magnetic or foam counter.
6. Monitor the working environment and promote safety.
7. Account for broken parts.
8. State the policy for needlestick injuries.

 Principles for Practice

The foundation and rationale for our practice, in the perioperative environment, stem from evidence provided by professionals, organizations, and governmental agencies. Refer to the Bibliography, Glossary of Terms, and the following documents or developmental agencies:

- Manufacturers' product instructions
- Operating room policies
- Surgeon's preference card
- Needlestick Safety and Prevention Act of 2000
- United States Pharmacopeia (USP)
- International Sharps Injury Prevention Society (ISIPS)

- American College of Surgeons (ACS)
- American Academy of Orthopaedic Surgeons (AAOS)
- Federal Drug Administration (FDA)
- National Institute for Occupational Safety and Health (NIOSH)
- Occupational Safety and Health Administration (OSHA)
- Centers for Disease Control and Prevention (CDC)
- The American Society of Anesthesiologists (ASA)
- Association of Surgical Technologists (AST)
- Association of periOperative Registered Nurses (AORN)

SKILL SEQUENCE AND INSTRUCTIONS

Suture Packages

1. Select, validate, and open suture, in the nonsterile role.

   - Select the appropriate suture materials based on the surgeon's preference card.
   - Validate the type of suture and needle, and validate the package expiration date.
   - Open the outer peel packs and present the inner, sterile suture packages onto the sterile field. Refer to Chapter 4.
   - Determine and follow your OR's guidelines for opening suture packs.
   - Contain cost and prevent waste of unused suture. The circulator may open and pass suture to the ST just prior to use (see Figures 20.1 through 20.3).

2. Organize suture packs on the sterile field and count.

   - Organize suture materials in a location with other countable items. Use a standardized set-up, or use personal preference. Refer to Chapter 7.
   - Develop a plan; for example, organize by tissue layer.
   - Perform counts with the circulator. Refer to Chapter 8 (see also Figures 20.4 and 20.5).

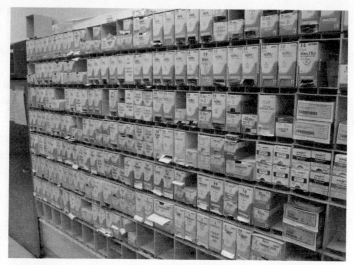

FIGURE 20.1   Select suture from storage boxes.

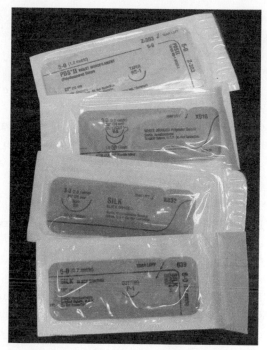

FIGURE 20.2   Individual suture in peel-packages.

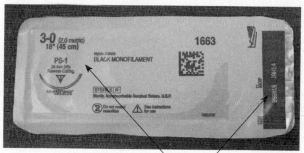

FIGURE 20.3   Identification information and expiration date viewed on each suture pack.

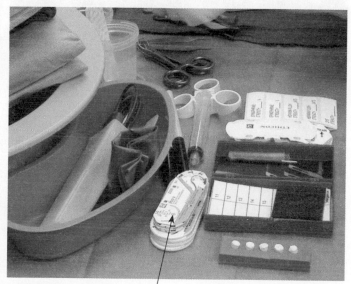

FIGURE 20.4   Arrange suture on the sterile field and prepare for the initial count.

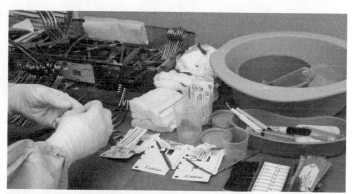

FIGURE 20.5   Count the sharps, including the suture, with the circulator.

Free Tie or Tie On a Passer

3. Identify and prepare a free tie or strand of suture, used to ligate blood vessels.

   Pass a free tie or "free-hand tie."

   - Remove one strand of suture from the package (no needle attached).
   - Gently stretch the strand horizontally between both hands, and then present it to the surgeon. The surgeon will grasp it in the middle of the strand (see Figures 20.6 and 20.7).

   Pass a tie on an instrument (passer):

   - Load one end of a free suture strand onto a curved clamp or "passer."
   - Orient the curve pointing toward the surgeon's midline.
   - Pass the loaded instrument and grasp the suture tail so it does not drag across the drapes, the wound, or the surgeon's glove (see Figures 20.8 through 20.10).

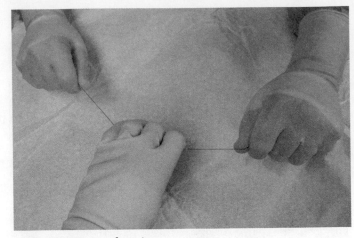

FIGURE 20.7 Pass free tie.

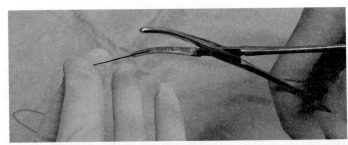

FIGURE 20.8 Clamp suture strand with instrument.

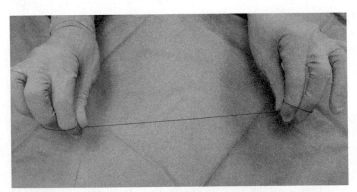

FIGURE 20.6 Free tie.

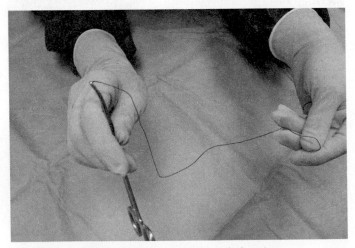

FIGURE 20.9 Orient for pass to right-handed surgeon.

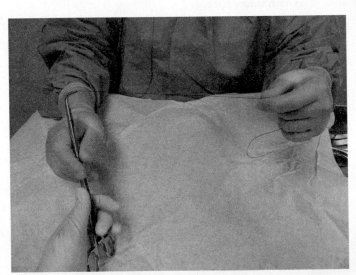

FIGURE 20.10 Pass the tie on a "passer" to the left-handed surgeon.

Suture Loaded on a Needle Holder

4. Identify, prepare, and pass a suture loaded onto a needle holder for the right-handed surgeon.

   • Identify the suture pack. Tear open the right side of the pack at the perforation and place the appropriately sized needle holder perpendicular to the needle.

   • The manufacturer orients the suture and the needle for the right-handed surgeon.

   • Needles are supplied in various sizes and edge types. View the example of a sweged needle, meaning it is attached to the suture strand (see Figures 20.11 through 20.12).

5. Position the tip of the needle holder to grasp the needle approximately a fourth to a third of the distance from the swage. Close the ratchet on the needle holder after the needle is correctly positioned in its jaws (see Figure 20.13).

6. Pull the suture out of the pack; be careful not to disengage the suture strand from the needle.

   • Be attentive to prevent a needlestick injury.

   • Prepare to pass the loaded needle holder to the right-handed surgeon (see Figure 20.14).

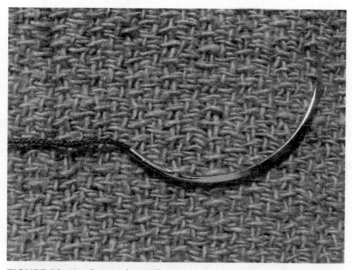

FIGURE 20.11   Sweged needle.

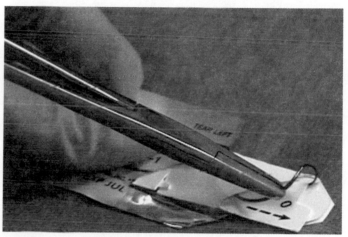

FIGURE 20.12   Grasp needle with needle holder.

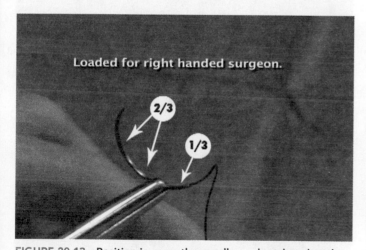

FIGURE 20.13   Position jaws on the needle, and ratchet closed.

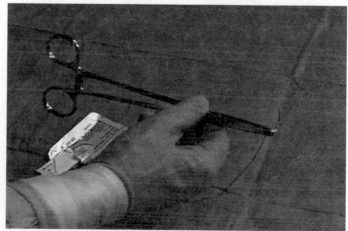

FIGURE 20.14   Needle holder with needle, prepared for the right-handed surgeon.

The Right-Handed Surgeon

7. Pass the suture using the hand-to-hand method.

   - Grasp the needle holder at the box lock area, hold from below, and snap-pass the finger rings into the surgeon's palm.
   - Pass so that the needle point faces the midline of the surgeon. "Needle to nose" may help you remember the orientation.
   - Control the suture strand.
   - Place the strand near the surgeon's working hand or place into the hand of the assistant. The strand should stay at or above table level.
     - The surgeon may make a minor adjustment to the angle of the needle on the needle holder.
     - Pay attention and perform the same adjustment before you pass subsequent suture.
   - Pass a pair of forceps for grasping tissue to the assistant.
   - Prepare straight Mayo scissors (additional information to follow) for cutting the suture (see Figures 20.15 through 20.17).

8. Pass a loaded needle holder using the hands-free transfer method including a no-touch basin, mat, or designated area.

The Left-Handed Surgeon

9. Prepare and pass suture to a left-handed surgeon.

   - Load suture from the front or the back of the package.
     - From the front of the package:
       - Use a needle holder to grasp and remove the needle from the package.
       - Rotate the needle 180° or reorient it on the needle holder so that the needle will point to the midline of the surgeon from his or her left hand.
     - From the back of the package:
       - Open the back of the package and load the suture onto a needle holder. Due to the orientation of the needle in the package, you will not need to rotate the needle.
   - Pass the loaded needle holder to the surgeon's left hand (see Figures 20.18 through 20.21).

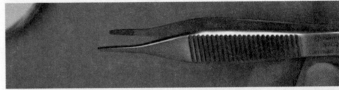

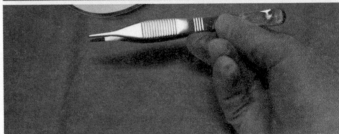

FIGURE 20.16 Select and pass Adson tissue forceps.

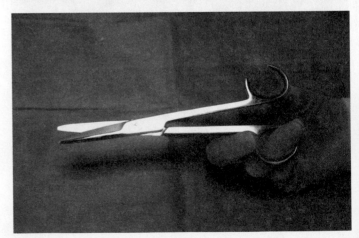

FIGURE 20.17 Mayo "suture" scissors are used to cut suture strands.

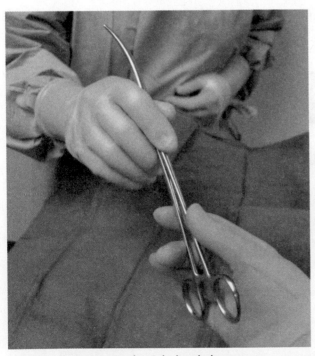

FIGURE 20.15 Pass to the right-handed surgeon.

Forceps and Suture Scissors

10. Prepare and pass Adson forceps during skin closure to assist with approximating the tissue. Be prepared to pass instruments to both the surgeon and the first assistant.

11. Identify and prepare to pass a pair of suture scissors, such as straight Mayo scissors. Refer to Chapter 19.

    • Cut the suture strand, if asked by the surgeon.

    • The surgeon will direct your performance.

○ Routinely, the cut will be made at a slight angle with the sharp tip of the suture scissors (straight Mayo scissors) above the knot.

○ Skin suture will typically have longer ends (tags) left above the knot, and deeper layer suture will be cut close to the knot.

○ Do not cut too close to the knot because it will unravel.

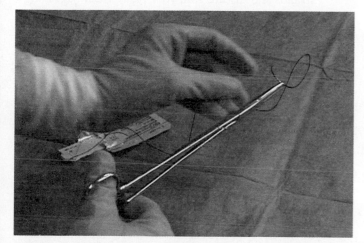

FIGURE 20.18   Reposition needle for a left-handed surgeon.

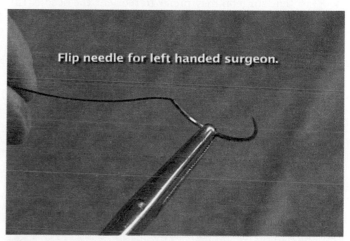

FIGURE 20.19   Secure the needle.

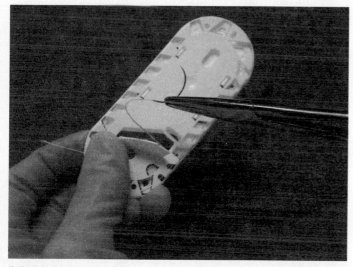

FIGURE 20.20   Load from the back of the suture package for the left-handed surgeon.

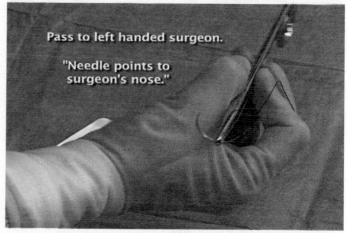

FIGURE 20.21   Pass to the surgeon's left hand.

Surgeons' Preferences

12. Prepare for each surgeon's preferences.

- Occasionally, the right-handed surgeon may have a preference for using a back-handed stitching technique for approximating tissue.
    - In this circumstance, you will load a Heaney needle holder for a left-handed surgeon, but you will pass it to the right hand. The surgeon will use a motion that resembles hitting a tennis ball or ping-pong ball back-handed.
    - The surgeon may prefer to reorient the needle. In this situation, load and pass the needle holder in the traditional manner.
- Load an eyed Keith needle with a suture strand, according to the surgeon's preferences.
    - Grasp the needle with a needle holder and pull the suture strand through the eye. Pull about 2 to 3 inches, and gently wrap the needle holder with the long end to prevent dislodging the strand.
    - Pass to the surgeon (see Figure 20.22).

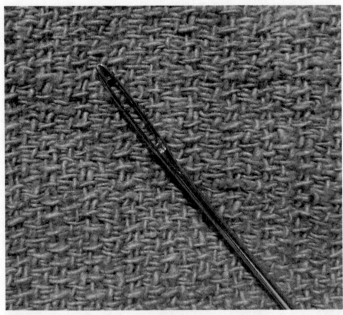

FIGURE 20.22 Load a keith needle with a suture strand.

Communicate and Anticipate

13. Use organization and clear communication when handling sharps.

- The surgeon may say "needle back" when passing back the used needle and holder into the no-touch or neutral zone.
- Remain attentive.
- Place used suture needles neatly into the magnetic or foam counter on your back table.
- Use suture scissors to snip off the remaining suture strands and discard into your paper trash bag. Long strands can become caught in other instruments and may pull the needles out of the counter, causing them to become misplaced.
- Save long pieces of suture, according to the surgeon's instructions, so they can be used later in the case. If you have a long piece, tidy the strand to keep it from being misplaced.
- Establish a system to identify suture especially when the surgeon alternates between sizes.
- Account for all parts of a broken suture needle. Place all parts into the needle mat, and count each piece.
- Alert the surgeon to the amount of suture on-hand at the back table. Ask the circulator for additional suture according to the surgeon's instructions.
- Arrange the needles in the needle mat with the tip of an instrument. Anticipate and call for intraoperative counts with the circulator according to your OR's policy related to the timing of anatomical closing.
- Participate in the final count, at the conclusion of the procedure. Refer to Chapter 8.

Needlestick Injury

14. If a needle accidently punctures your glove, pass the contaminated needle to the circulator on a needle holder.

    - Stretch out your hand so that the circulator can remove your top glove. Assess for a puncture to your skin through the second pair of gloves. Refer to Chapter 21.
    - If there is a puncture to your skin, step away from the sterile field, remove the glove, and wash the puncture area with soap and water.
    - Follow the facility's policy for follow-up care, laboratory studies, reporting, and surveillance for percutaneous injuries.
    - In response to the 2000 Needlestick Safety and Prevention Act (NSPA), in 2001 OSHA updated the Bloodborne Pathogens Standard, requesting employers to select safer needle devices and to maintain a log of contaminated sharps injuries.
    - Report-off to the ST replacing you. Identify the location of all sharps on the sterile field, and perform a count with the circulator.

Postoperative Skills

15. Dispose of sharps according to your OR policy, during room turnover.

    - Close the needle mat, and dispose of it into a large, leakproof red sharps disposal unit. Refer to Chapter 23 and see Figure 20.23.
    - Do not reach into the container.

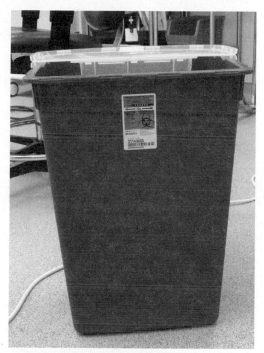

FIGURE 20.23   Large sharps container.

STUDENT'S NAME: _____

CHAPTER 20 PREPARE, LOAD, AND PASS SUTURE FOR RIGHT- AND LEFT-HANDED SURGEONS

PERFORMANCE RANK:

S or √ = Satisfactory: Competent—safe, accurate, sequential, and timely
U = Unsatisfactory: Unsafe—inaccurate and unprepared

PERFORMANCE RATING:

5   Independent: Expert—safe, confident, seamless performance; mentors others
4   Minimally monitored: Intermediate—safe, self-corrects few errors
3   Competent: Novice—safe, revises with evaluator cues, few errors
2   Remedial: Unsafe—critical errors, unable to implement evaluator cues consistently
1   Dependent: Unsafe—unacceptable, requires multiple evaluator interventions

PERFORMANCE CRITERIA	Performance Rank	Performance Rating
1. Perform Mutual Professional and Scholastic Criteria as appropriate (see the Preface or Appendix A).		1 2 3 4 5
2. Validate the name, size of the suture, type of needle, and expiration date of the required suture materials (refer to Chapter 4), Instructor Selects Suture Samples.		1 2 3 4 5
3. Organize the suture for a baseline count. (refer to Chapter 8)		1 2 3 4 5
4. Select the appropriate size needle holder; prepare suture for a right-handed surgeon.		1 2 3 4 5
5. Pass to the right-handed surgeon.		1 2 3 4 5
6. Select the appropriate size needle holder; prepare suture for a left-handed surgeon.		1 2 3 4 5
7. Pass to the left-handed surgeon.		1 2 3 4 5
8. Prepare and pass a free tie: free-hand and on an instrument.		1 2 3 4 5
9. Identify and pass Adson forceps and Mayo scissors.		1 2 3 4 5
10. State the policy for care and reporting in the event of a needlestick injury.		1 2 3 4 5
11. Place used sharps in the needle mat; arrange for the final count.		1 2 3 4 5

ADDITIONAL COMMENTS _____

PERFORMANCE EVALUATIONS AND RECOMMENDATIONS

❏ PASS: Satisfactory Performance
    ❏ Demonstrates professionalism
    ❏ Exhibits critical thinking
    ❏ Demonstrates proficient clinical performance appropriate for time in the program
❏ FAIL: Unsatisfactory Performance
    ❏ Critical criteria not met (see Performance Rank or Rating above)
    ❏ Professionalism not demonstrated.

❏ Critical thinking skills not demonstrated.
❏ Skill performance unsafe or underdeveloped.
❏ REMEDIATION:
　❏ Schedule lab practice. Date: _____
　❏ Reevaluate by instructor. Date: _____
❏ DISMISS from lab or clinicals today.
❏ Program director notified. Date: _____

SIGNATURES

Date _____　　　Evaluator _____　　　Student _____

ACTIVITIES AND DISCUSSION QUESTIONS

Activities

1. View the Complete Perioperative Process and Focus on Skills video, Skill #20 (video can be found at www.myhealthprofessionskit.com).
2. Observe the instructor perform the skill.
3. Handle sharps under the direct supervision of your instructor.
4. Practice identifying, preparing, and passing suture and ties.
5. Select and teach one skill to your lab partner, then observe and critique the performance.
6. Refer to your ST textbook and this lab manual to answer the Discussion Questions (see next column).
7. Review the video and the information in this lab manual when you prepare for your certification examination.

Discussion Questions

1. List the essential steps in preparing and passing suture to the surgeon.
2. What do you do if the expiration date has passed on the suture package?
3. Name at least two other instruments that you need to pass along with the suture.
4. What steps will you take if the suture needle punctures your glove? Will you do anything differently if the needle punctures your skin?
5. Develop a strategy or plan for learning the most frequently requested suture.
6. Note here any questions that you need your instructor to clarify.

21 Maintain Aseptic Technique

INTRODUCTION

Aseptic technique is a broad term representing a tremendous commitment to excellence. The standards of practice require all personnel, in all related roles and departments, to perform their duties consistently. Complacency is unacceptable. The surgical technologist and all team members implement aseptic technique throughout the three phases of surgery—pre- intra- and postoperative. In this chapter, focus on demonstrating compliance during the intraoperative phase of surgery.

- Before performing the following skill, your lab instructor will discuss some of the principles for practice and objectives involved in this chapter as well as the importance of following the skill sequence and instructions.

- Role-play with your lab partner; demonstrate maintaining aseptic technique, and simulate breaks in aseptic technique, correct the errors, and describe the rationale. Your instructor will offer strategies for success. Appendix E highlights the value of teaching others as a component of active learning strategies. Refer to Appendix C for an overview of the chapter.
- The lab instructor will advise you of any additional criteria to be evaluated. At a designated time, demonstration of this skill will be evaluated and graded by your lab instructor using the competency assessment tool.
- When in the clinical setting, your instructor may once again assess your performance using the same tool Refer to Appendix A for clinical evaluation and documentation.

Team Member	Type of Role		Timing		
	Nonsterile	Sterile	Preop	Intraop	Postop
Surgical Technologist		X		X	
Assistant Circulator	X			X	
Operating Room Team		X		X	

OBJECTIVES

The learner will demonstrate this skill with 100 percent accuracy each time the operative environment is entered.

1. Evaluate compliance with aseptic technique.
2. Demonstrate safe and precise management of a surgical specimen.
3. Identify selected contamination errors—gown, glove, and back table set-up.

4. Demonstrate correction of selected contamination errors.
5. Appraise the functions of various departments and staff members in supporting aseptic technique.
6. Recognize the relationship between the wound classification system and the risk of a surgical site infection.

Principles for Practice

The foundation and rationale for our practice, in the perioperative environment, stem from evidence provided by professionals, organizations, and governmental agencies. Refer to the Bibliography, Glossary of Terms, and the following documents or developmental agencies:

- Operating room policies
- American Society of Hearing, Refrigeration, and Air Conditioning Engineers (ASHRAE)
- Facility Guidelines Institute (FGI)
- Occupational Safety and Health Administration (OSHA)
- Centers for Disease Control and Prevention (CDC)
- Association of Surgical Technologists (AST)
- Association of periOperative Registered Nurses (AORN)

SKILL SEQUENCE AND INSTRUCTIONS

Fundamentals of Aseptic Technique

1. Demonstrate assimilation of the principles of aseptic technique during the intraoperative phase of surgery. Refer to Chapters 1 through 7.
2. Prevent, identify, and correct contamination errors.
3. Communicate with responsibility and assertiveness, and use professional verbal and body language.
4. Accept only validated sterile items onto your sterile field.
5. Respect your sterile parameters, and monitor the actions of other team members (see Figures 21.1 through 21.5).

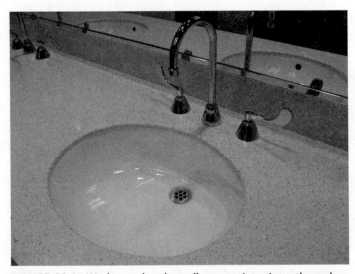

FIGURE 21.1 Wash your hands at all appropriate times throughout the day.

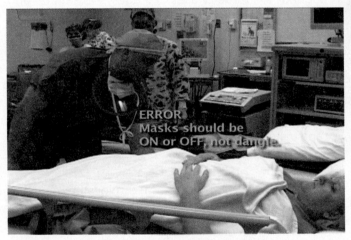

FIGURE 21.2 Remind colleagues; secure the face mask.

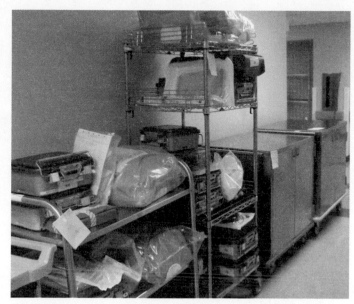
FIGURE 21.3 Use new sterile supplies for each patient.

Surgical Specimens

6. Focus on your intermediary role when receiving specimens from the surgeon, and when transferring specimens to the circulator.

- Receive the specimen from the surgeon, and verbally repeat the identification.
- Place the specimen in a basin, the Mayo stand or back table, and label it as "right" or "left" and include other identification information.
- Request permission from the surgeon to transfer, or pass the specimen to the circulator.
- State the identification of the specimen to the circulator. The circulator verifies the ordered laboratory examination.
- Depending on the size and type of specimen, and the examination to be performed, the container type and method of transfer will vary.
- Label the container, and not the lid with patient and specimen identification information. The label can be pre-printed from the database, or handwritten. (Circulator role.)

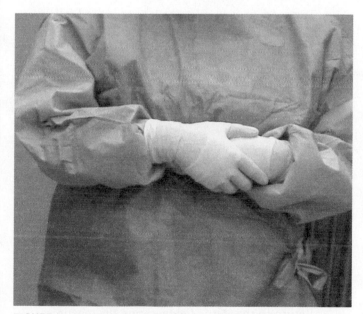
FIGURE 21.4 Use only acceptable hand positions.

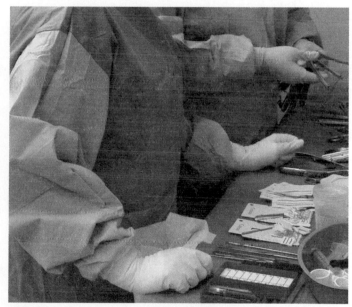
FIGURE 21.5 Keep hands in the sterile zone.

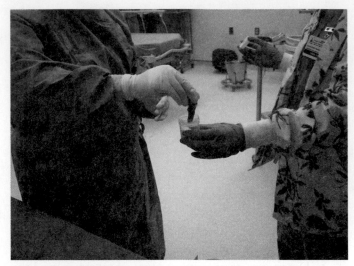

FIGURE 21.6 Maintain aseptic technique when passing specimens.

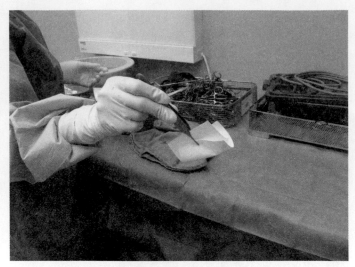

FIGURE 21.7 Pass specimen safely to the circulator.

- Transfer a permanent specimen into saline or a chemical fixative to be examined in the laboratory. Do not cause splashing of chemicals out of the container during the transfer.
- Transfer a small, fresh specimen to be examined by frozen section in a moisten towel or nonstick pad. Do not immerse this specimen.
  - ○ Alternately, grasp the specimen with a saline-moistened glove or an instrument, and place it into a specimen cup. Do not touch the cup with the instrument or your gloves (see Figures 21.6 and 21.7).
  - ○ This specimen is transported to the pathology lab for immediate examination and reporting.
- Transfer stones, or teeth in a dry, sterile container.
- Transfer body fluids or washings in the syringe or trap used for collection. A Luken's trap is placed into the suction line to collect bronchial or peritoneal washings. The cirulator will arrange immediate transportation to the lab.
- Transfer swabbings for aerobic or anerobic microorganisms in the original tubes. Place the tube into the biohazard bag, held by the circulator.
- Transfer products of conception, per the hospital policy.
- Transfer a fetus off the sterile field, according to your hopital's policy.
- Transfer amputated body parts, limbs, in a fluid impervious bag or size-appropriate container. These specimens may go to the lab for examination or to the morgue for refrigeration.

- Transfer foreign bodies for forensic examination based on legal and hospital policies.
- Contain specimens in biohazard bags, appropriately sized, so that the outside of the bag remains uncontaminated. Affix specimen examination orders. (Circulator role.)
- Transport specimens to the laboratory and follow storage and sign-in protocols for that department. (Transporter or nonsterile team member role.)

Contamination Errors

7. Correct a contamination error—remove a contaminated glove, obtain new sterile supplies, or regown and reglove.

- Use proper technique to remove a contaminated glove.
- Move away from the sterile field.
- Communicate with the circulator who will don a pair of nonsterile gloves to remove your glove.
- Stretch out your hand covered with the contaminated glove. Hold your gown sleeve at the forearm with your opposite sterile glove. The circulator will remove your contaminated top glove. Return to the sterile field wearing the remaining sterile glove.
- When time permits, the circulator will place another pair of sterile gloves onto your back table, and you will perform assisted-gloving with another sterile team member. Refer to Chapter 14.
- Perform open gloving to don new sterile gloves if another sterile team member is unavailable. Refer to Chapter 15 (see Figures 21.8 through 21.12).

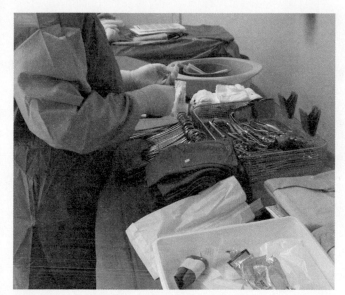

FIGURE 21.8 Glove contamination due to a tear.

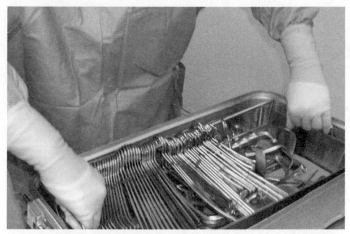

FIGURE 21.9 Gloves are contamination if you touch the sides of an instrument pan.

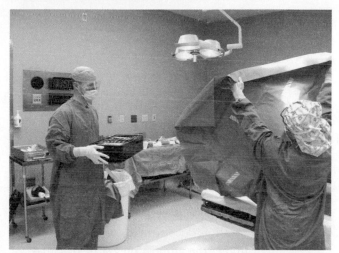

FIGURE 21.10 Validate integrity of the wrapper before placing the instrument pan onto your back table.

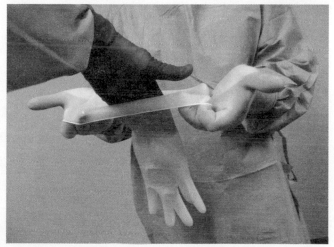

FIGURE 21.12 Regown with assisted gloving by another sterile team member.

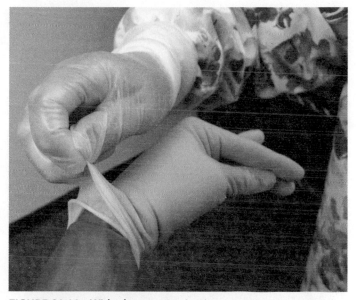

FIGURE 21.11 With glove contamination, present your contaminated glove to the circulator for removal.

8. Correct major contamination errors, in the sterile role, by regowning and regloving or by establishing an entirely new back table set up.

9. Obtain new sterile supplies, in the nonsterile role, whenever a sterile supply is contaminated by a nonsterile surface. Obtain a new urinary catheter if the sterile catheter touches a nonsterile surface or a surface of the skin (see Figures 21.13 through 21.15).

10. Adhere to prescribed movement patterns within the sterile field—sterile to sterile and nonsterile to nonsterile.

   • Monitor your movement. Stay within the sterile field to prevent contamination by nonsterile team members or equipment.

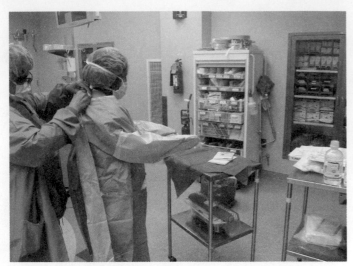

FIGURE 21.13 Regown and reglove.

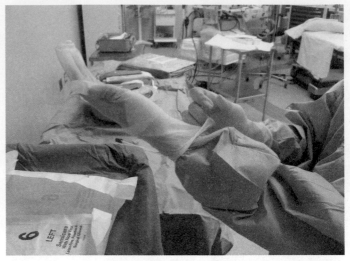

FIGURE 21.14 Regown, reglove, and new set-up.

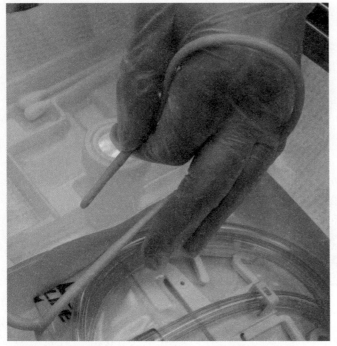

FIGURE 21.15 Obtain a new urinary catheter.

- Monitor the traffic patterns and nonsterile team members.
- Pass sterile team members front-to-front or back-to-back.
- Pass nonsterile team members facing them.

Wound Classification

11. At the end of the surgical procedure, the surgeon assigns a wound classification rank to the patient based on variables that influence microbial contamination. Intraoperative factors, such as a break in sterile technique, can increase the rank and risk of a SSI.

- The classification is documented in the patient's chart. The higher the number on a scale of 1 to 4, the greater the risk of infection.
- Refer to Table 21.1.
- Identifying risk and analyzing data aids in planning for prevention, interventions, and medications.

TABLE 21.1 Prediction of Surgical Site Infection Risk
Centers for Disease Control and Prevention Wound Classification System

Title	SSI Risk	Characteristics	Example
Class I	1–5 %	Clean: Uninfected wounds. Not entered: Respiratory, alimentary, or GI tracts.	Breast biopsy
Class II	3–11 %	Clean-contaminated: Uninfected, no breaks in surgical technique; controlled entry into the respiratory, alimentary, GI, GU, or GYN tracts.	Hysterectomy
Class III	11–17 %	Contaminated: Acute inflammation, new trauma, major break in aseptic technique.	Appendectomy with a ruptured appendix.
Class IV	> 27%	Dirty or Infected: Chronic infection, devitalized tissue, perforated viscera.	Incision and drainage of an abscess.

Perioperative Aseptic Technique

12. Promote aseptic technique throughout the perioperative environment.

- Clean, process, and sterilize instruments in the sterile processing department. Specialized training is required to perform these skills.
- Use wrapped sterile supplies, fluids, and medications provided by companies licensed for this purpose.
- Monitor the work of room turnover staff members who are responsible for cleaning floors and equipment.
- Perform a more thorough cleaning every 24 hours, including all walls, floors, and equipment. Hospital housekeeping staff members clean according to a schedule and use FDA approved disinfectants.
- Ensure standardized parameters for the indoor temperature, relative humidity, sequential filters, room air exchanges, and positive pressure gradients in the OR suite, performed by hospital environmental department staff.
- Give instructions and proper OR attire to visitors and vendors who venture into the OR on approved business.
- Support the patient in surgery through collaboration and implementation of professional guidelines (see Figure 21.16)

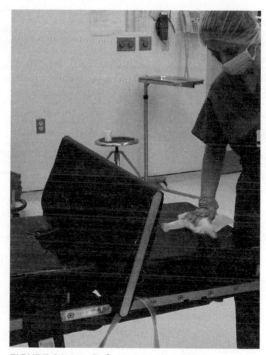

FIGURE 21.16 Enforce aseptic technique.

STUDENT'S NAME: _____

CHAPTER 21 MAINTAIN ASEPTIC TECHNIQUE

PERFORMANCE RANK:

> S or √ = Satisfactory: Competent—safe, accurate, sequential, and timely
> U = Unsatisfactory: Unsafe—inaccurate and unprepared

PERFORMANCE RATING:

5	Independent: Expert—safe, confident, seamless performance; mentors others
4	Minimally monitored: Intermediate—safe, self-corrects few errors
3	Competent: Novice—safe, revises with evaluator cues, few errors
2	Remedial: Unsafe—critical errors, unable to implement evaluator cues consistently
1	Dependent: Unsafe—unacceptable, requires multiple evaluator interventions

PERFORMANCE CRITERIA	Performance Rank	Performance Rating
1. Perform Mutual Professional and Scholastic Criteria as appropriate (see the Preface or Appendix A.).		1 2 3 4 5
2. Obtain permission from the surgeon then prepare and pass a surgical specimen to the circulator.		1 2 3 4 5
3. Identify and correct a contaminated sterile glove.		1 2 3 4 5
4. Identify and correct a contaminated sterile gown.		1 2 3 4 5
5. Identify and correct a contaminated back table set-up.		1 2 3 4 5
6. Describe the relationship between the wound classification and the risk of an SSI.		1 2 3 4 5

ADDITIONAL COMMENTS _____

PERFORMANCE EVALUATIONS AND RECOMMENDATIONS

❑ PASS: Satisfactory Performance
    ❑ Demonstrates professionalism
    ❑ Exhibits critical thinking
    ❑ Demonstrates proficient clinical performance appropriate for time in the program
❑ FAIL: Unsatisfactory Performance
    ❑ Critical criteria not met (see Performance Rank or Rating above)
    ❑ Professionalism not demonstrated.
    ❑ Critical thinking skills not demonstrated.
    ❑ Skill performance unsafe or underdeveloped.
❑ REMEDIATION:
    ❑ Schedule lab practice. Date: _____
    ❑ Reevaluate by instructor. Date: _____
❑ DISMISS from lab or clinicals today.
❑ Program director notified. Date: _____

SIGNATURES

Date _____   Evaluator _____   Student _____

ACTIVITIES AND DISCUSSION QUESTIONS

Activities

1. View the Complete Perioperative Process, The Laparoscopic Process, and Focus on Skills video, Skill #21 (video can be found at www.myhealthprofessionskit.com).
2. Observe the instructor perform the skills.
3. Practice the skills with your lab partner.
4. Select and teach one skill to your lab partner, such as correcting a contaminated sterile glove while in the sterile role, then observe and critique the performance.
5. Refer to your ST textbook and this lab manual to answer the Discussion Questions (see next column).
6. Review the video and the information in this lab manual when you prepare for your certification examination.

Discussion Questions

1. List the essential steps used by the ST to maintain aseptic technique.
2. Explain the relationship between microbes and infections.
3. What steps will you take if you touch the top of the back table drape with your bare, ungloved hands?
4. Using communication etiquette, what will you say to the circulator who states that you contaminated the left sleeve of your gown by touching the back of the surgeon's gown? Select from the following. Explain.

   a. I know I didn't touch his gown; I did not feel it.
   b. How could you see if I touched his gown? You are sitting next to your computer?
   c. Ask your preceptor if he saw you touch the surgeon's gown.
   d. Ask the surgeon if he felt you touch his gown.
   e. Reenact your movements.
   f. Move away from the sterile field.
   g. Ask for assistance to correct the error.
   h. Hold out your left arm so that another sterile team member can cover it with a new sterile sleeve.

5. Compare your response in #4 with the method described to correct a glove contamination error.
6. Develop a strategy or plan to prevent contamination of your gloves when helping with a laparotomy drape.
7. Note here any questions that you need your instructor to clarify.

Prepare Dressings and Drains, and Facilitate Postanesthesia Care

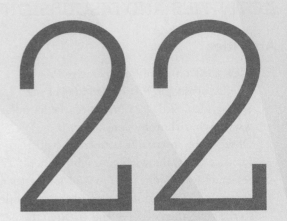

INTRODUCTION

The surgical technologist assists the surgeon, and other team members, to cover or dress the surgical wound and to prepare wound drainage systems. In the nonsterile role, the ST supports the team during transfer of the patient to the postanesthesia care unit (PAUC).

- Before performing the following skill, your lab instructor will discuss some of the principles for practice and objectives involved in this chapter as well as the importance of following the skill sequence and instructions.
- Practice preparing various wound dressings and drainage systems, along with your lab partner. Encourage and critique each other. Your instructor

will offer strategies for success. Appendix E highlights the value of teaching others as a component of active learning strategies. Refer to Appendix C for an overview of the chapter.
- The lab instructor will advise you of any additional criteria to be evaluated. At a designated time, demonstration of this skill will be evaluated and graded by your lab instructor using the competency assessment tool.
- When in the clinical setting, your instructor may once again assess your performance using the same tool. Refer to Appendix A for clinical evaluation and documentation.

Team Member	Type of Role		Timing		
	Nonsterile	Sterile	Preop	Intraop	Postop
Surgical Technologist	X	X		X	X
Assistant Circulator	X			X	X
Operating Room Team	X	X		X	X

OBJECTIVES

The learner will demonstrate this skill with 100 percent accuracy each time the operative environment is entered.

1. Demonstrate aseptic technique.
2. State the rationale for using various types of surgical wound dressings.
3. Receive wound dressings after the final, closing count.
4. Prepare and pass dressing and instruments on the sterile field.
5. Prepare adhesive strips.
6. Prepare a three-layer dressing.
7. Prepare and apply an ostomy bag.
8. Facilitate establishing wound drainage systems—active and passive.
9. Assist with removal of drapes.
10. Clean the skin in preparation for adhesives or final dressing layers.
11. Assist with the transfer and transportation of the patient to the postanesthesia care unit (PACU) at the conclusion of the procedure.
12. Discuss essential components of the PACU experience for the patient.

 ## Principles for Practice

The foundation and rationale for our practice, in the perioperative environment, stem from evidence provided by professionals, organizations, and governmental agencies. Refer to the Bibliography, Glossary of Terms, and the following documents or developmental agencies:

- Manufacturers' product instructions
- OR policies
- State practice acts
- Occupational Safety and Health Administration (OSHA)
- Centers for Disease Control and Prevention (CDC)
- Association of Surgical Technologists (AST)
- Association of periOperative Registered Nurses (AORN)

SKILL SEQUENCE AND INSTRUCTIONS
PREPARE DRESSINGS AND DRAINS

Timing of Dressing Supplies

1. Gather the required dressing supplies according to the surgeon's preference card. Dressings are applied for absorption, aesthetics, moisture, phamaceuticals, protection, and support.

   - Place unopened supplies on a separate table in the OR, preoperatively.
   - The circulator will add dressing supplies to the sterile field following wound closure and the final count. Dressing supplies, which do not contain x-ray detectable stripes, pose a retention risk to the patient (see Figures 22.1 and 22.2).

2. Prepare the dressing supplies.

   - Clear your Mayo stand of instruments and supplies no longer needed for the procedure.
   - Moisten a lap sponge in the basin of sterile saline solution on your back table, squeeze out the excess, and open up the layers.
     - Your surgeon will express a preference for how moist or wet the lap sponge should be. A surgeon may ask for a "sloppy" wet sponge or just a "moist" sponge.
   - Pass the opened lap sponge, then a dry sponge to the surgeon or first assistant who will wipe off and dry the skin surrounding the wound.
   - Prepare and pass the initial dressings materials, such as Steri-strips.
     - Cut strips in half, as indicated.
     - Pull off the backing from the top portion of the strips.
     - Pass the strips to the surgeon. Prepare to pass forceps, if used (see Figures 22.3 and 22.4).

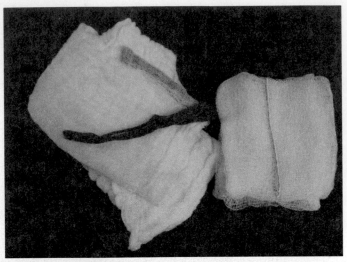

FIGURE 22.1 Countable sponges are not used for dressings.

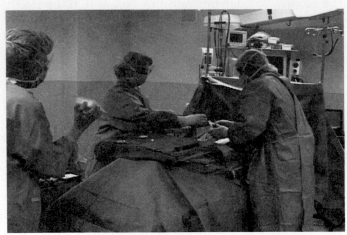

FIGURE 22.2 Dressing sponges are added after wound closure.

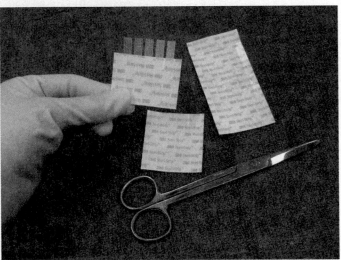

FIGURE 22.3 Prepare Steri-strips.

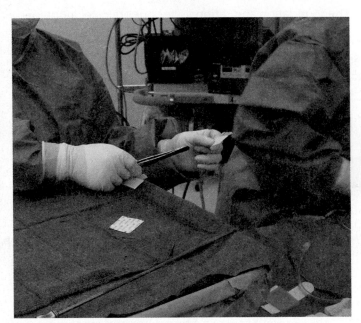

FIGURE 22.4 Pass forceps and strips.

3. Prepare and apply a three-layer dressing for wound coverage.

- Prepare and pass the first layer, such as a non-adherent pad or petrolatum dressing (Bismuth Tribromophenate).
- Prepare and pass the second layer which will absorb any drainage, such as gauze or pads.
- Prepare the third top layer—tape or gauze wrap—and apply this layer after the drapes are removed.
- Keep the dressing and other components clean and visually pleasing. Patients may judge the quality of the surgery by the neatness of the dressing.
- Use a Band-Aid—a miniature three-layer dressing—to cover small incisions resulting from a laparoscopy procedure (see Figures 22.5 through 22.8).

4. Move the Mayo stand away from the surgical field.

- Assess the position of the Mayo stand over the patient.
- Elevate the stand's height to allow clearance before pulling the stand away. Prevent injury to the patient.
- Roll the Mayo stand away from the field.
- Check the drapes for any remaining items (see Figure 22.9).

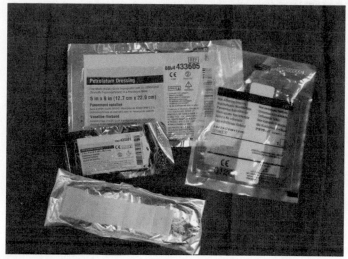

FIGURE 22.5   First layer variations include petrolatum gauze.

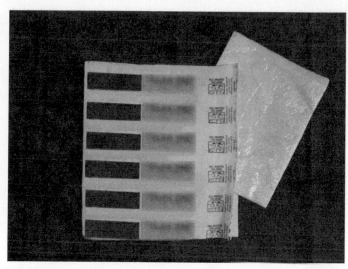

FIGURE 22.6   First or second layer variations include nonadherent pads.

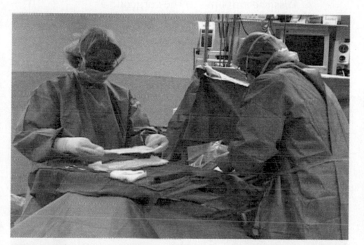

FIGURE 22.7   Prepare dressings according to the purpose.

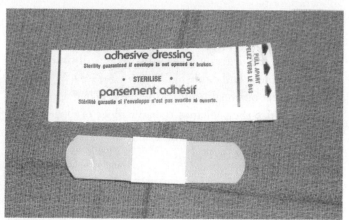

FIGURE 22.8   A Band-Aid is a three layer dressing.

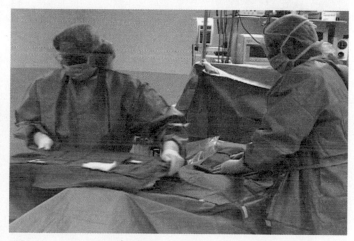

FIGURE 22.9   Move the Mayo stand away from the patient.

5. Cover the wound and any initial dressing layers with a sterile OR towel before removing the drapes.

- Hold the OR towel in place to protect the incision site.
- Be alert for wound drains or tubes so they are not unintentionally pulled out.
- Remove the drapes by rolling them off of the patient. Later place them into a red disposal bag, for incineration (see Figures 22.10 and 22.11).

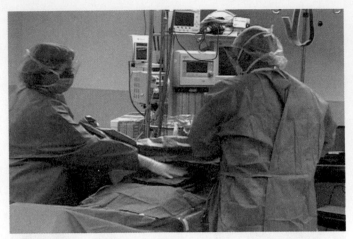

FIGURE 22.10 Cover the incision then remove the drapes.

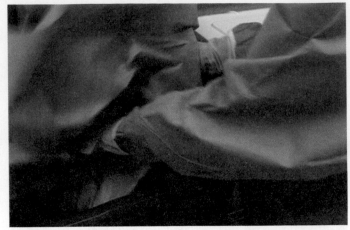

FIGURE 22.11 Dispose of drapes into a biohazard bag at the end of the procedure.

6. Apply the final dressing layer to clean, dry skin. This layer may consist of gauze wrap, ace wrap, stretch wrap, or tape.

   • Remove bloody gloves before the final, top dressing layer is applied to prevent contamination of the clean, top dressing layer. This layer will contact the bed linens and clothing.

   • Prepare optional liquid adhesives. When applied to the skin, they enhance the adherence of tape.

      ○ Wrap the glass ampoule in a gauze sponge, and squeeze to activate it.

      ○ Milk the liquid into the applicator tip.
      ○ Pass the ampoule to the surgeon.
      ○ Isolate the gauze; it may contain shards of glass. Do not use it a second time.

   • Limbs may be wrapped with tan stretch gauze or ace wrap to promote venous circulation and minimize edema; this covering layer is applied by the surgeon. (see Figures 22.12 through 22.14).

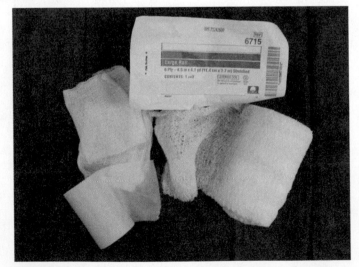

FIGURE 22.12 Gauze wrap is an example of an outer dressing layer.

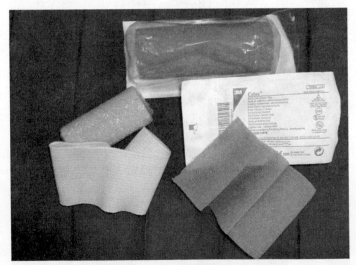

FIGURE 22.13 Support wrap is applied by the surgeon.

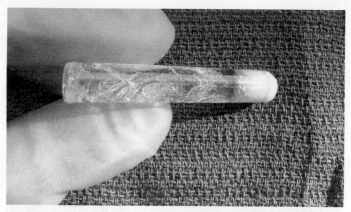

FIGURE 22.14 Ampoule contains a liquid adhesive which is applied to the skin before placing selected dressing material.

7. Remove excess skin prep solution from the patient's skin to prevent excoriation. The circulator may perform this skill.

- Follow manufacturer's instructions; some solutions are created to remain on the skin.
- Gently roll the patient side-to-side, as indicated, to wipe off any remaining solution posteriorly (see Figure 22.15).

8. Document the patient care provided and the supplies used during the intraoperative phase of surgery in the patient's electronic record, which is performed by the circulator.

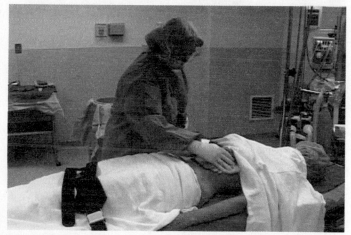

FIGURE 22.15 Remove prep solution per manufacturer's guidelines.

Stoma Site Collection Bag

1. Prepare the colostomy bag which functions to collect intestinal drainage and protect the peristomal skin from digestive enzymes. Various collection pouches are available for intestinal or urinary drainage surgically diverted to the abdominal surface. The stoma, or intestinal opening to the surface, is covered by the collection pouch, or bag.

- Remove the drapes, and wipe off and dry the peristomal skin.
- Obtain the colostomy bag, sizing guide, and the sleeve clip from the circulator.
  - Pouches and supplies vary among manufacturers.
- Place a marking pen and Mayo scissors on your Mayo stand.
- Measure the patient's stoma with the manufacturer-supplied sizing guide.
- Draw a circle or oval on the bag wafer to match the sizing guide.
- Cut an opening in the wafer about 1/8 inch larger than the measurement.
- Do not cut into the plastic bag.

2. Apply the colostomy bag over the stoma.

- Verify the opening by placing it over the stoma; customize the fit, as needed.
- If the opening is too large, the peristomal skin will not be protected and will become excoriated from the intestinal enzymes.
- Apply additional skin protecting solutions to the skin before placing the wafer.
- Plan to position the colostomy bag so that the bag sleeve is angled towards the patient's hip to facilitate emptying contents postoperatively.
- Remove the central paper backing, place the opening over the stoma, and gently smooth or press on the adhesive wafer.
- Remove the outer paper strip and smooth the wafer edge in place.
- Position the clamp onto the bag sleeve so that the bowed-side is closest to the patient's body.
- Secure the clamp to close the collection pouch (see Figures 22.16 through 22.20).

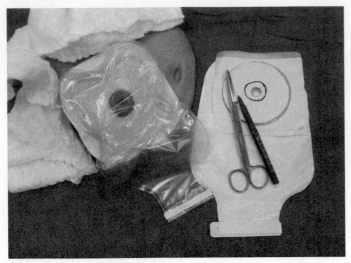

FIGURE 22.16 Prepare wafer backing.

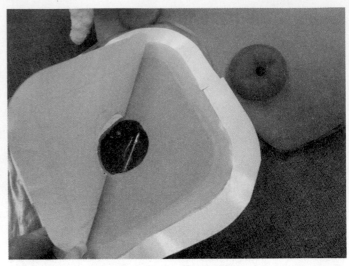

FIGURE 22.17 Remove central paper backing.

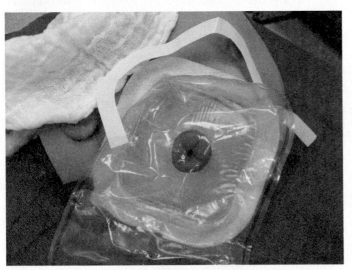

FIGURE 22.18 Apply to peristomal skin; remove outer paper backing.

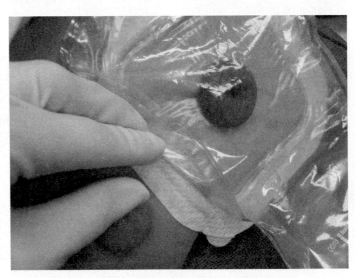

FIGURE 22.19 Seal wafer edges onto the abdomen.

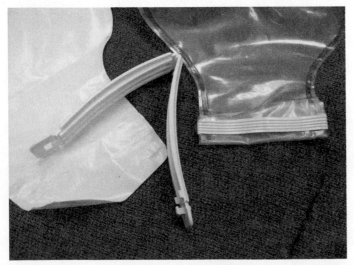

FIGURE 22.20 Secure the sleeve edge with the manufacturer's clip.

Closed Wound Drainage System

1. Assist the surgeon to place wound drains and connect the drains to a closed wound drainage system, such as the Hemovac or Jackson-Pratt.

   - Wound drains and collection devices are used to collect and measure postoperative drainage. Systems are selected according to the anticipated amount of draining. Example capacities include 100 mL drainage in the Jackson-Pratt system (JP) and 400 mL in the Hemovac system. Exudate that is allowed to pool in the wound and surrounding tissue is a source for infection and pain, and wound healing is delayed.

   - Pass supplies and instruments used by the surgeon to make a stab wound. The drainage tube has a sharp trocar attached and is used to make the stab wound. Drains are inserted in a location adjacent to, but not in, the surgical wound. The perforated end of the drain remains in the patient.

   - After drain insertion, return the instruments and trocar to your back table.

   - Place the trocar in a designated location or into a sterile sharps container on the back table for safety.

   - Pass suture to the surgeon, as requested, to secure the drain to the skin. Surgical wound closure is completed by the surgeon, initial dressings are placed, and drapes are removed.

   - Remove your outer pair of gloves to prevent cross-contamination of blood onto the collection device.

   - Obtain the collection device from your back table, and attach the patient's drainage tube into the suction port (see Figures 22.21 through 22.23).

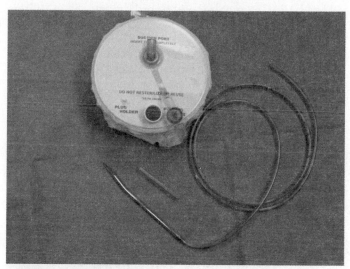

FIGURE 22.21   Pass tubing with trocar to the surgeon.

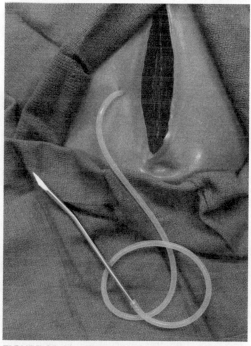

FIGURE 22.22   Trocar used to insert Jack-Pratt drain in the abdomen.

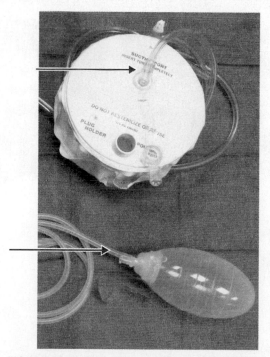

FIGURE 22.23   Attach the drain tube from the patient into the suction port.

2. Activate the manual suction-action of the drainage system.

Jackson-Pratt system

- Hold the empty collection bulb, and turn the open drain port away from your face.
- Compress the collection bulb between your thumb and forefinger. Use your hand to compress larger bulbs.
- Insert the plug into the drain port. Drainage will flow into the collection bulb.
- In PACU, monitor and record drainage in milliliters (mL). Don nonsterile gloves. Empty and reactivate the collection device according to the manufacturer's directions and hospital policy for time intervals.
- Keep the system sterile; do not touch the drain port.
- Notify the surgeon of excessive drainage, or no drainage (see Figures 22.24 and 22.25).

Hemovac collection system

- Compress the top and bottom surfaces of the evacuator together.
- Insert the plug into the pouring spout and seal securely.
- Observe the drainage. In PACU, don nonsterile gloves, empty the evacuator according to your hospital's policy, reactivate suction-action, and record output.
- Keep the system sterile. Do not touch the open port.
- Notify the surgeon of excess drainage, or no drainage. (see Figures 22.26 and 22.27).

Open Drains

3. Assist with placement of a passive drain, such as the Penrose drain.

- Pass instruments and supplies, according to the surgeon's preference, to insert a wound drain. This type of hollow drain allows for evacuation of wound drainage by gravity or changes in patient positions. The drain is covered with a dressing composed of drainage sponges, and they are changed when moist, postoperatively.
- Apply the manufacturer-supplied sterile safety pin to prevent the migration of the drain into the abdomen (see Figure 22.28).

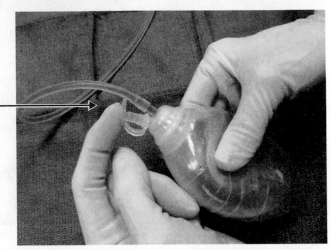

FIGURE 22.24 Squeeze bulb, hold, and insert the plug.

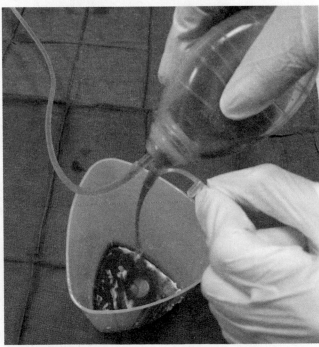

FIGURE 22.25 Empty and record drainage in the PACU.

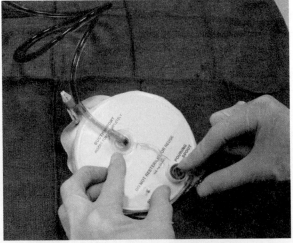

FIGURE 22.26 Compress evacuator, hold, and securely insert the plug.

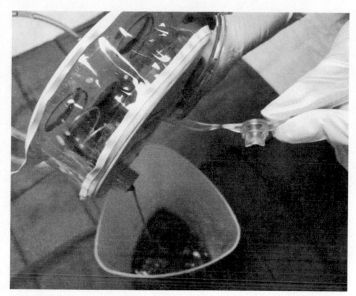

FIGURE 22.27 Empty and record, in the PACU.

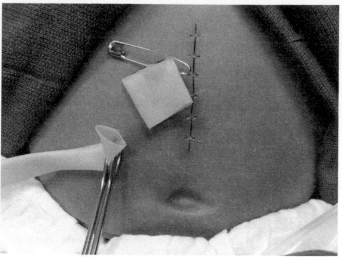

FIGURE 22.28 The penrose is an example of a passive drain.

FACILITATE POSTANESTHESIA CARE

1. Assist to transfer and transport the patient to the post anesthesia care unit at the conclusion of the procedure according to instructions from the anesthesia care provider, in the nonsterile role.

   - Don nonsterile gloves.
   - Use a transfer roller-board to assist four OR team members with a nonalert patient. Transfer the patient to a stretcher and elevate the side rails. Maintain proper body mechanics and ergonomics during the transfer.
   - Protect and place safely any tubing or drains connected to the patient.
   - Be cognizant of electrical cords, water, or equipment on the floor; prevent your own slips, trips, or falls.
   - Cover the patient with warm blankets (see Figures 22.29 through 22.31).

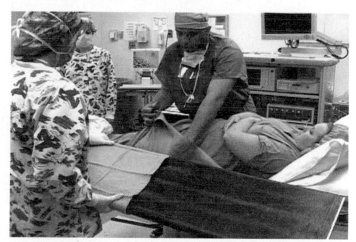

FIGURE 22.29 The OR team will use a transfer device such as the roller-board to facilitate moving the patient.

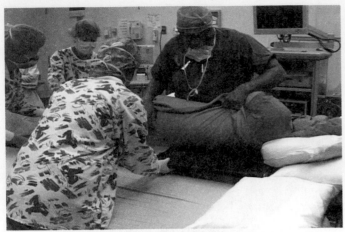

FIGURE 22.30 Maintain proper body mechanics when lifting or moving.

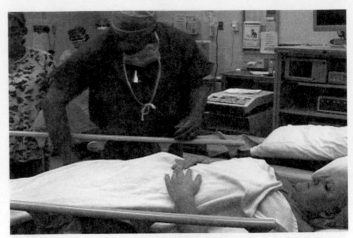

FIGURE 22.31 Elevate the side rails on the stretcher for patient safety.

2. Participate in the report or "hand-off" communication from OR personnel to the PACU nurse, according to state practice acts and hospital policy.

   • Communicate orally and in writing the essential elements of the intraoperative phase of care. This report is performed by the ACP and the circulator.
   • Communication formats vary. Refer to Table 22.1.

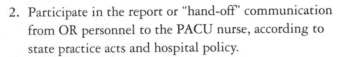

TABLE 22.1 Transfer of Care Communication

Category	Report
General	Patient information
	Procedure
	Surgeon
History	Diagnoses
	Allergies
	Routine medications
	Rational for procedure
Intraoperative dimensions	Vital signs
	Blood loss and fluid replacement
	Pain management
	Anesthetics and reversal agents
	Fluid intake and urine output
	Significant lab findings
	Outstanding events
Family or friends	Waiting location
	Contact information

3. Perform affiliated skills in the PACU, per state practice acts and hospital policy.

   • Obtain and document postoperative vital signs: T, P, B/P, pulse oximetry, and pain. Refer to Chapter 11.
   • Assist with patient position changes, as indicated.
   • Assist with wound drainage systems; empty and record drainage amounts.
   • Perform an ordered urinary catheterization due to urinary retention. Refer to Chapter 16 (see also Figure 22.32).

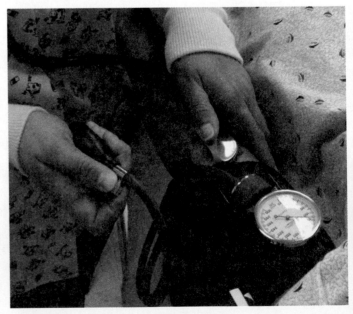

FIGURE 22.32 Obtain vital signs.

4. The PACU nurse assesses the patient for surgical or anesthesia complications and for routine recovery milestones.

- Assessment sequences vary and are conducted based on hospital policy. Refer to Table 22.2.
- Additional assessment parameters include:
  ○ Blood pressure
  ○ ECG
  ○ Intake and output
  ○ IV solutions
  ○ Level of consciousness
  ○ Nausea or vomiting
  ○ Orientation: person, place, time, situation
  ○ Oxygen use
  ○ Pulse oximetry reading
  ○ Skin color
  ○ Temperature
- Use the Aldrete Postanesthesia Recovery Score (APARS) to assess the patient's readiness for discharge from the PACU, according to your facility's policy. Refer to Table 22.3.
  ○ Five areas are assessed and scored with points 0–2.
  ○ A total score of 9–10 may support discharge from PACU.
  ○ Evaluate vital signs and pain along with emotional status, cognitive ability, chills, shivering, wound condition, intake and output, nausea or vomiting, and peripheral pulses.

5. Assist with patient discharge from PACU.

- A discharge order is given by the ACP or surgeon, once the recovery milestones have been reached.
- Assist the patient to exit PACU.
  ○ The PACU nurse reviews written discharge instructions with the patient and their significant other for those returning home.

  These instructions include:
  ○ Postoperative expectations
  ○ Postoperative doctor's appointment and contact number
  ○ Appropriate wound care
  ○ How to respond to unexpected symptoms
  ○ Activity limits
  ○ Medications
  ○ Transport the patient via a wheelchair to an outside vehicle, driven by a responsible adult. The patient may not drive themselves home due to the effects of general anesthesia.
  ○ Assist with transportation of the patient to an intensive care unit room via a hospital bed or to a hospital room.
  ○ Alert the hospital floor staff of the patient's arrival. Give any written orders to the floor clerk.
  ○ Transfer the patient onto an ambulance stretcher for transport to an extended care facility. Give the ambulance crew written documentation, per policy.

TABLE 22.2   Assessment by mnemonic: ABCD

Priority Assessment	
A	Airway: Patent
B	Breathing: Rate; Equal, clear breath sounds
C	Circulation: Apical HR; Peripheral pulses present
D	Drainage: Assess dressings and drains

TABLE 22.3 Aldrete Postanesthesia Recovery Score

Patient Response in Points		Initial Points	Time (minutes) in PACU				
			15	30	45	60	D/C
Activity							
Extremities							
Move 4	2						
Move 2	1						
Move 0	0						
Respiration							
Deep breath	2						
Limited	1						
Apnea	0						
Circulation							
Preanesthetic B/P							
+/− 20	2						
+/− 20–50	1						
+/− 50	0						
Consciousness							
Fully awake	2						
Open to call	1						
No response	0						
O_2 Saturation							
>92% room air	2						
>90% with O_2	1						
<90% with O_2	0						
Total							

COMPETENCY ASSESSMENT

STUDENT'S NAME: _____

CHAPTER 22 PREPARE DRESSINGS AND DRAINS, AND FACILITATE POSTANESTHESIA CARE

PERFORMANCE RANK:

S or √ = Satisfactory: Competent—safe, accurate, sequential, and timely
U = Unsatisfactory: Unsafe—inaccurate and unprepared

PERFORMANCE RATING:

5   Independent: Expert—safe, confident, seamless performance; mentors others
4   Minimally monitored: Intermediate—safe, self-corrects few errors
3   Competent: Novice—safe, revises with evaluator cues, few errors
2   Remedial: Unsafe—critical errors, unable to implement evaluator cues consistently
1   Dependent: Unsafe—unacceptable, requires multiple evaluator interventions

PERFORMANCE CRITERIA	Performance Rank	Performance Rating
1. Perform Mutual Professional and Scholastic Criteria as appropriate (see the Preface or Appendix A).		1 2 3 4 5
2. State the purpose for the selected dressing.		1 2 3 4 5
3. Receive dressing supplies after the final count.		1 2 3 4 5
4. Clean and dry the incision site and surrounding skin.		1 2 3 4 5
5. Prepare and pass steri-strips and instrumentation.		1 2 3 4 5
6. Cover the wound with a sterile towel, and remove the drapes.		1 2 3 4 5
7. Prepare and pass a three-layer dressing.		1 2 3 4 5
8. Prepare and pass an ostomy pouch.		1 2 3 4 5
9. Prepare and connect a wound drain and the collection system.		1 2 3 4 5
10. List at least four skills the ST may perfrom in the PACU.		1 2 3 4 5

ADDITIONAL COMMENTS _____

PERFORMANCE EVALUATIONS AND RECOMMENDATIONS

❑ PASS: Satisfactory Performance
    ❑ Demonstrates professionalism
    ❑ Exhibits critical thinking
    ❑ Demonstrates proficient clinical performance appropriate for time in the program
❑ FAIL: Unsatisfactory Performance
    ❑ Critical criteria not met (**see Performance Rank or Rating above**)
    ❑ Professionalism not demonstrated.
    ❑ Critical thinking skills not demonstrated.
    ❑ Skill performance unsafe or underdeveloped.

❑ REMEDIATION:
　　　❑ Schedule lab practice. Date: _____
　　　❑ Reevaluate by instructor. Date: _____
❑ DISMISS from lab or clinicals today.
❑ Program director notified. Date: _____

SIGNATURES

Date _____　　　Evaluator _____　　　Student _____

ACTIVITIES AND DISCUSSION QUESTIONS

Activities

1. View the Complete Perioperative Process, and Focus on Skills video, Skill #22 (video can be found at www.myhealthprofessionskit.com).
2. Observe the instructor perform the skills.
3. Practice transferring and transporting a manikin or student actor to the PACU. Role play with three other students and use a roller board.
4. Practice the sterile role skills in this chapter with your lab partner.
5. Select and teach one skill to your lab partner, such as covering a stoma with an ostomy pouch, then observe and critique the performance.
6. Refer to your ST textbook and this lab manual to answer the Discussion Questions (see next column).
7. Review the video and the information in this lab manual when you prepare for your certification examination.

Discussion Questions

1. List at least three purposes for dressings.
2. When preparing to move the Mayo stand away from the surgical field, what do you do first?
3. Why do you remove bloody gloves before applying the top dressing layer?
4. If you do not seal the wafer of the colostomy bag onto the skin of the patient securely, what may occur?
5. If you cut an opening in the colostomy bag wafer-backing that is more than 1/8-inch larger than the stoma, what may occur?
6. Would you consider the suction action of the Hemovac or Jack-Pratt systems to be mechanically or manually activated? Explain.
7. Note here any questions that you need your instructor to clarify.

Unit III

Essentials After Surgery

Dismantle the Sterile Field and Disrobe

23

INTRODUCTION

The surgical technologist dismantles the sterile field after the patient exits the operating room. A safe and efficient process prevents cross-contamination, and protects the function and integrity of surgical equipment and instruments. Items for disposal or reprocessing are sorted, contained, and transported to designated locations.

- Before performing the following skill, your lab instructor will discuss some of the principles for practice and objectives involved in this chapter as well as the importance of following the skill sequence and instructions.
- Practice the skills in this chapter with your lab partner. Encourage and critique each other. Your instructor

will offer strategies for success. Appendix E highlights the value of teaching others as a component of active learning strategies. Refer to Appendix C for an overview of the chapter.

- The lab instructor will advise you of any additional criteria to be evaluated. At a designated time, demonstration of this skill will be evaluated and graded by your lab instructor using the competency assessment tool.
- When in the clinical setting, your instructor may once again assess your performance using the same tool. Refer to Appendix A for clinical evaluation and documentation.

Team Member	Type of Role		Timing		
	Nonsterile	Sterile	Preop	Intraop	Postop
Surgical Technologist	X				X
Assistant Circulator					
Operating Room Team	X				X

OBJECTIVES

The learner will demonstrate this skill with 100 percent accuracy each time the operative environment is entered.

1. State the rational for point of use cleaning of instruments.
2. Sort and discard disposables.
3. Practice safe handling of all sharps.
4. Disrobe and prevent self contamination.
5. Prepare, label, and transport reusables—instruments and equipment—to the decontamination room.
6. Dispose of sorted trash bags.
7. Locate the eye wash station.

Principles for Practice

The foundation and rationale for our practice, in the perioperative environment, stem from evidence provided by professionals, organizations, and governmental agencies. Refer to the Bibliography, Glossary of Terms, and the following documents or developmental agencies:

- Manufacturers' product instructions
- Operating room policies
- State and local hazardous waste management laws
- The Association for the Advancement of Medical Instrumentation (AAMI)
- Occupational Safety and Health Administration (OSHA)
- Centers for Disease Control and Prevention (CDC)
- Association of Surgical Technologists (AST)
- Association of periOperative Registered Nurses (AORN)

SKILL SEQUENCE AND INSTRUCTIONS

Dismantle the Sterile Field

1. Dismantle the sterile field after the patient has exited the room

   - Secure sharp, hazardous items.
     - Remove the blades from the knife handles and place them into a red needle mat.
     - Do not leave loaded knife handles in the instrument tray.
     - Place hypos and electrocautery tips in a needle mat for disposal.
     - Discard sharp disposables per facility policy (see Figures 23.1 through 23.3).

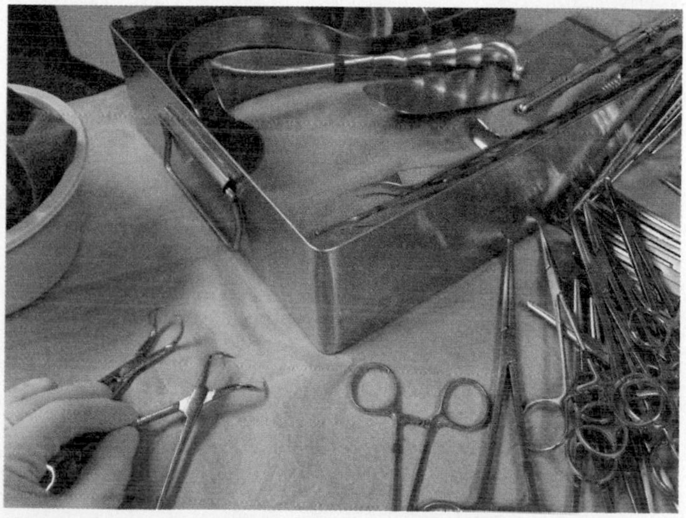

2. Sort and begin to clean and decontaminate instruments at the point of use, in the OR, to improve the efficiency and effectiveness of decontamination.

   - Continue to wear eye protection in anticipation of splashing or spraying of contaminants, and wear gloves.
   - Return all instruments for reprocessing, used or unused.
   - Wipe off gross debris from instruments to prevent development of biofilms. Use sterile water—not saline—to prevent corrosion, pitting, or discoloration of the stainless steel instruments.
   - Segregate sharp instruments in a separate container; protect the processing department staff.
   - Arrange instruments facing in the same direction to assist the processing department during cleaning.
   - Disassemble instruments with parts.
   - Open box locks completely.
   - Flush all instruments with lumens.
   - Protect delicate instruments in separate containers.
   - Stack lightweight instruments on top of heavier ones inside of a mesh-bottomed tray.
   - Remove your bloody top layer of gloves before you handle the trays for transportation. Prevent cross-contamination to the outside of the trays.
   - Cover instrument trays prior to transportation. Use leak-proof, puncture-resistant containers; biohazard labeling must be visible for staff safety and because of OSHA mandate.
   - Instruments and equipment may be transported to the decontamination area via a cart (see Figures 23.4 and 23.5).

FIGURE 23.1 Organize and secure sharp items.

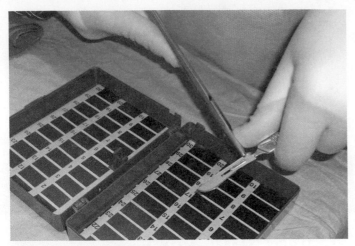

FIGURE 23.2 Remove blades from knife handles.

3. Sort all linens and disposables, and place into the proper bags.
- Bag reusable drapes and gowns separately for the laundry.
- Use red bags for biohazarous disposables for incineration—bloody drapes, gloves, gowns, and sponges.
- Secure bags and transport them to a larger holding area.
- Reusables, such as metal basins, cloth OR towels, drapes, and gowns, may be transported off site where they are washed, packaged, resterilized, and later returned to the facility.
- Place clean wrappers, trays, and paper into a recycling bag, per hospital policy (see Figure 23.6).

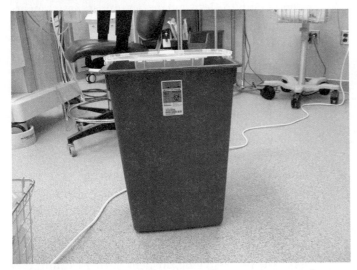

FIGURE 23.3 Dispose of sharps according to your protocol.

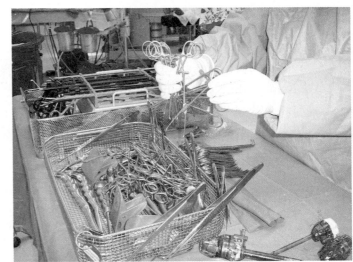

FIGURE 23.4 Sort and arrange instruments, and open box locks.

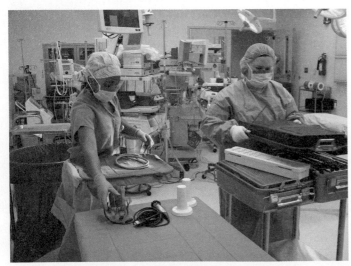

FIGURE 23.5 Return instruments to original containers.

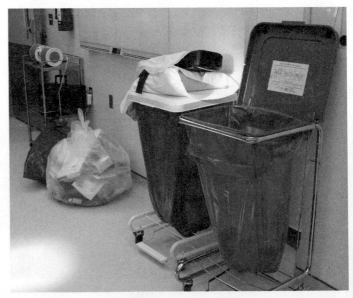

FIGURE 23.6 Sort disposables and reusables.

4. Dispose of liquids-solutions and secretions.
   - Dispose of unused solutions in an approved manner—solidify, absorb with towels, or remove with an automated collection device.
   - Solidify body fluids in the disposable canister with a gel agent, or remove them with an automated, electronic collection device.
   - Liquids are not disposed of in the scrub sink or in a substerile room sink (see Figures 23.7 through 23.10).

Disrobe

5. Doff or remove your gown in a manner preventing the outside from touching your skin or scrub attire (pants and top).

Disposable gown:

- Break the ties by pulling on the front of the gown.
- Lean forward and roll the gown up as you pull it off. Prevent contamination of your OR scrub attire.
- Place the rolled-up gown into the red bag.

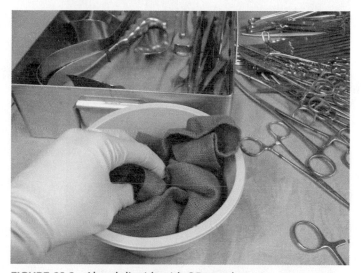

FIGURE 23.8   Absorb liquids with OR towels.

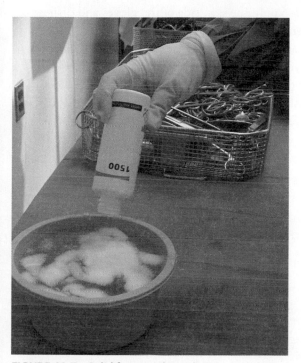

FIGURE 23.7   Solidify remaining solutions.

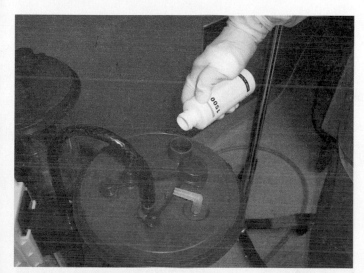

FIGURE 23.9   Solidify secretions.

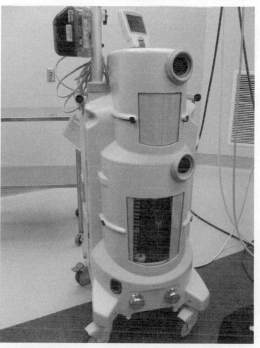

FIGURE 23.10   Automated fluid collection unit for liquid waste management.

Reusable gown:

- Ask a nongowned team member to untie the strings and unfasten the snaps in the back of your gown.
- Pull off your gown and roll it up. Prevent the soiled front of the gown from touching your OR scrub attire.
- Place the used gown into the laundry bag (see Figures 23.11 and 23.12).

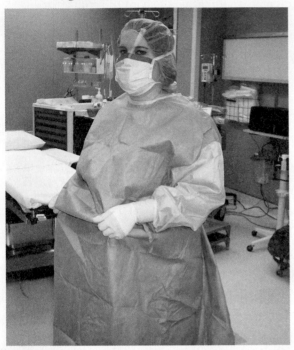

FIGURE 23.11   Remove gown.

6. Remove your gloves in a manner that prevents contamination of your bare skin with the used gloves. Think, "glove to glove, then skin to skin" as you remove the gloves. Refer to Chapter 15.

- Grasp glove in the palm area and pull off (glove to glove). Hold removed gloves in your other (gloved) hand.
- With your bare hand, place your index finger under the cuff of the remaining gloves (skin to skin); and push the gloves off as they turn inside out.
- Grasp only the skin side of the gloves and dispose of them in the red trash bag.
- There are other methods that are acceptable as long as you do not contaminate yourself.
- If your hands become contaminated with blood, wash your hands using soap and water (see Figure 23.13).

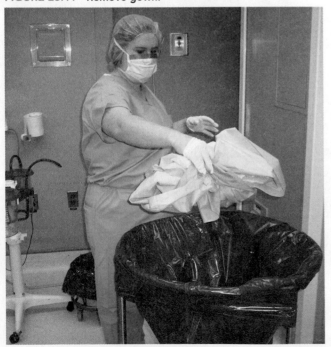

FIGURE 23.12   Prevent self-contamination; dispose of gown.

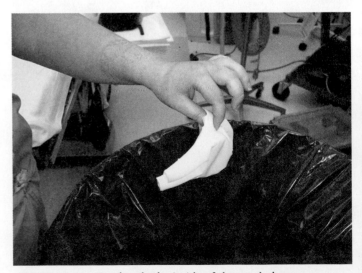

FIGURE 23.13   Touch only the inside of the used gloves.

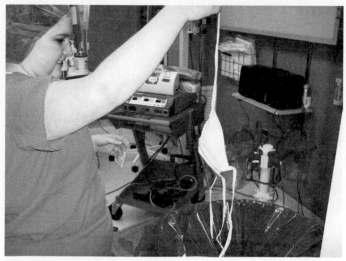

FIGURE 23.14 Remove and hold mask by tie ends.

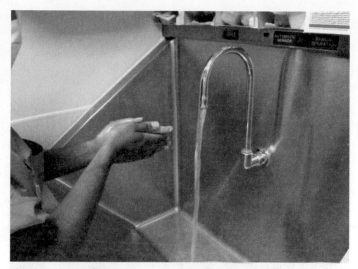

FIGURE 23.15 Perform basic hand hygiene.

7. Remove your face mask by grasping only the ties, and remove eye protection, or goggles.

- Pull and break the tie strings on your face mask. Do not grasp the face mask portion. It is contaminated.
- Remove your eye protection, discard or clean according to your hospital policy.
- Discard the mask in the appropriate bag. Refer to Chapter 3 (see Figure 23.14).

Environmental Stewardship

8. Promote recycling and support environmental stewardship, as appropriate.

- Typically the OR produces a tremendous amount of trash each day; recycling can significantly decrease that amount.
- Many facilities are accepting the challenge to reduce the amount of trash that is incinerated or buried in landfills.
- Sort paper and plastic trash for recycling.
- Disposables that are contaminated with blood or body fluids may not be recycled.
- You may find numerous bags and color-coding options.

9. Perform basic hand hygiene after removing your mask.

- Use the waterless hand solution or wash your hands at the scrub sink. Refer to Chapter 2.
- Use soap and water if your hands are visibly soiled (see Figure 23.15).

Transport Covered Items to the Decontamination Room

10. Transport items for disposal or decontamination.

- Place covered, labeled items on a cart for transportation to the disposal area (soiled utility room).
- Dispose of bagged items in the disposal area.
- Transport the cart in the semirestricted hallway, away from sterile supplies, to the decontamination room.
- Close the doors to the decontamination room to maintain the negative pressure. This vacuum-type pressure prevents room particles from flowing into the hallways; it exhausts to the outside.
- Spray an instrument cleaner onto the instruments, in the decontamination room, while they await the cleaning process. By keeping the instruments moist, the cleaning process is enhanced and entrapment of biofilm colonies under debris is prevented.
- Producing clean instruments is the first step in the sterilization process. The processing department will wash, disinfect, and sterilize the instruments based on a strict protocol (see Figures 23.16 and 23.17).

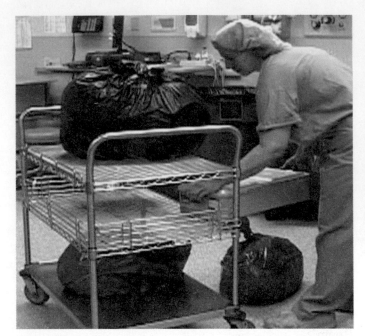

FIGURE 23.16 Transport covered trays to the decontamination area.

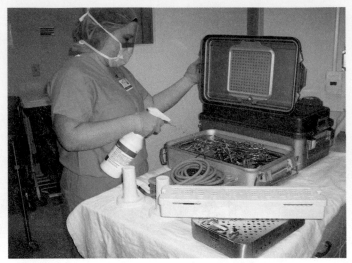

FIGURE 23.17 Moisten instruments with cleaner.

Eyewash Station

11. Locate the eyewash station for emergency use.

- OSHA requires placement in areas where chemicals or cleaners are used.
- Read the directions. Know how to use it in case of an accidental splashing of chemicals, blood, or body fluids (see Figure 23.18).

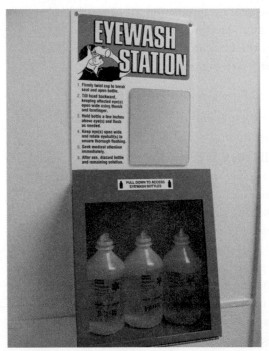

FIGURE 23.18 Locate the eyewash station in case of accidental contamination.

COMPETENCY ASSESSMENT

STUDENT'S NAME: _____

CHAPTER 23 DISMANTLE STERILE FIELD AND DISROBE

PERFORMANCE RANK:

> S or √ = Satisfactory: Competent—safe, accurate, sequential, and timely
> U = Unsatisfactory: Unsafe—inaccurate and unprepared

PERFORMANCE RATING:

> 5   Independent: Expert—safe, confident, seamless performance; mentors others
> 4   Minimally monitored: Intermediate—safe, self-corrects few errors
> 3   Competent: Novice—safe, revises with evaluator cues, few errors
> 2   Remedial: Unsafe—critical errors, unable to implement evaluator cues consistently
> 1   Dependent: Unsafe—unacceptable, requires multiple evaluator interventions

PERFORMANCE CRITERIA	Performance Rank	Performance Rating
1. Perform Mutual Professional and Scholastic Criteria as appropriate (see the Preface or Appendix A).		1 2 3 4 5
2. State rationale for point-of-use cleaning of instruments.		1 2 3 4 5
3. Secure and dispose of all sharps.		1 2 3 4 5
4. Sort and prepare all instruments and equipment for disinfection; open box locks, irrigate lumens, and pack up delicate instruments separately.		1 2 3 4 5
5. Sort and bag all disposables and reusable textiles or supplies.		1 2 3 4 5
6. Dispose of liquid waste such as solutions and secretions.		1 2 3 4 5
7. Remove your gown, gloves, mask, and eye protection; dispose, as appropriate		1 2 3 4 5
8. Perform hand hygiene.		1 2 3 4 5
9. Transport items for disposal and decontamination.		1 2 3 4 5
10. State the location of the eyewash station in your facility.		1 2 3 4 5

ADDITIONAL COMMENTS _____

PERFORMANCE EVALUATIONS AND RECOMMENDATIONS

❑ PASS: Satisfactory Performance
     ❑ Demonstrates professionalism
     ❑ Exhibits critical thinking
     ❑ Demonstrates proficient clinical performance appropriate for time in the program
❑ FAIL: Unsatisfactory Performance
     ❑ Critical criteria not met (**see Performance Rank or Rating above**)
     ❑ Professionalism not demonstrated.
     ❑ Critical thinking skills not demonstrated.
     ❑ Skill performance unsafe or underdeveloped.
❑ REMEDIATION:
     ❑ Schedule lab practice. Date: _____
     ❑ Reevaluate by instructor. Date: _____
❑ DISMISS from lab or clinicals today.
❑ Program director notified. Date: _____

SIGNATURES

Date _____   Evaluator _____   Student _____

ACTIVITIES AND DISCUSSION QUESTIONS

Activities

1. View the Complete Perioperative Process and Focus on Skills video, Skill #23 (video can be found at www.myhealthprofessionskit.com).
2. Observe the instructor perform the skill.
3. Practice this skill with your lab partner. Maintain sharps safety.
4. Select and teach one skill to your lab partner, such as removing your gown, gloves, and mask, then observe and critique the performance.
5. Refer to your ST textbook and this lab manual to answer the Discussion Questions (see next column).
6. Review the video and the information in this lab manual when you prepare for your certification examination.

Discussion Questions

1. Discuss the relationship between point-of-use cleaning and the development of biofilms.
2. Which is more appropriate to perform: a waterless hand hygiene or washing with water at the sink?
3. Name at least three practices that OSHA requires.
4. What will you do if your bloody gloves touch your bare skin when you are removing them?
5. Define environmental stewardship. Why is this important in the operating room setting?
6. Note here any questions that you need your instructor to clarify.

PEARSON
myhealthprofessionskit™

Use this address to access the Companion Website created for this textbook. Simply select "Surgical Technology" from the choice of disciplines. Find this book and log in using your username and password to access interactive activities, videos, and much more.

24 Facilitate Room Turnover and Confidentiality

INTRODUCTION

The surgical technologist continues to support the principles of aseptic technique by collaborating with other team members to clean and disinfect the room in between procedures. Each patient enters an environment that is clean, with new supplies. The Health Insurance Portability and Accountability Act (HIPAA) requires health care workers to respect the private information of the patient. The ST uses professional communication and acts responsibly by maintaining the patient's confidentiality. Information about the patient and the procedure may not be shared with family or friends, or through electronic social networking.

- Before performing the following skill, your lab instructor will discuss some of the principles for practice and objectives involved in this chapter as well as the importance of following the skill sequence and instructions.
- Practice with your lab partner. Encourage and critique each other. Your instructor will offer strategies for success. Appendix E highlights the value of teaching others as a component of active learning strategies. Refer to Appendix C for an overview of the chapter.
- The lab instructor will advise you of any additional criteria to be evaluated. At a designated time, demonstration of these skills will be evaluated and graded by your lab instructor using the competency assessment tool.
- When in the clinical setting, your instructor may once again assess your performance using the same tool. Refer to Appendix A for clinical evaluation and documentation.

Team Member	Type of Role		Timing		
	Nonsterile	Sterile	Preop	Intraop	Postop
Surgical Technologist	X				X
Assistant Circulator	X				X
Operating Room Team	X				X

OBJECTIVES

The learner will demonstrate this skill with 100 percent accuracy each time the operative environment is entered.

1. Define confidentiality and relate it to the ST role.
2. Apply HIPAA guidelines to the ST role.
3. Apply appropriate PPE.
4. Disinfect, or clean, the OR at the end of a case.
5. Participate in daily terminal cleaning.
6. Prepare the OR bed for a surgical procedure.

Principles for Practice

The foundation and rationale for our practice, in the perioperative environment, stem from evidence provided by professionals, organizations, and governmental agencies. Refer to the Bibliography, Glossary of Terms, and the following documents or developmental agencies:

- Hospital policy
- Material Safety Data Sheets (MSDS)

- Environmental Protection Agency (EPA)
- U.S. Department of Health and Human Services (DHHS)
- Health Insurance Portability and Accountability Act of 1996 (HIPAA)
- Occupational Safety and Health Administration (OSHA)
- Centers for Disease Control and Prevention (CDC)
- Association of Surgical Technologists (AST)
- Association of periOperative Registered Nurses (AORN)

SKILL SEQUENCE AND INSTRUCTIONS

Room Turnover Disinfection

1. Provide all patients with a clean environment.

    - Prevent surgical site infections and save lives.
    - Uphold the OR disinfection policies and procedures. Perform these essential but comparatively mundane tasks conscientiously.
    - Recognize dust in the room as a source for infection. Dust is composed of microbes, skin particles, hair, fibers, pollen, mold, and paper particles.
    - Use recommended cleaning techniques and schedules because microorganisms can thrive on surfaces, or fomites, for long periods of time—weeks and months. Examples include, methicillin-resistant Staphlococcus aureus and epidermidis (MRSA, MRSE), vancomycin-resistant Enterococcus (VRE), hepatitis B, and Pseudomonas aeruginosa.
    - Participate in end-of-the case cleaning during "room-turnover" and terminal cleaning, performed once every 24 hours.

2. Disinfect and clean between each surgical procedure, "end-of-case."

    - Perform hand hygiene and don appropriate PPE.
        - Don gloves made of nitrile, rubber latex, chloro-prene blends, or butyl rubber. Vinyl gloves are contraindicated because they lose their protective barrier when exposed to cleaning chemicals.
    - Wear eye protection if splashing is expected.

- Use a lint-free cloth moistened with an EPA-registered solution to clean surfaces and equipment, which are noncritical items in the Spaulding's classification system.
    - Refer to Table 24.1.
    - Use commercially prepared FDA-approved towelettes when supplied.

- Wipe off all flat surfaces, including the OR bed frame and padding, overhead lights, Mayo stands, instrument tables, and equipment.
- Mop the floor surrounding the OR bed. Include a wider margin to remove spilled blood or secretions.
    - Use a new mop head and bucket of fresh detergent-disinfectant for each use.
- Fit the disposal receptacles with new bags.
    - Follow your OR policy for sorting OR waste. Prepare red bags for biohazard incineration, green or clear bags for recycling, blue bags for laundry, and black bags for trash.
- Visually inspect the room for cleanliness before new bedding, padding, supplies, or equipment are brought into the room (see Figures 24.1 through 24.6).

TABLE 24.1 CDC Uses Spaulding's Classification System to Decrease SSI Risk

Classification of Supplies/ Equipment	Risk of SSI	Contact	Examples	Prevent SSI
Critical	High	Sterile body tissue Cardiovascular system Neurological system	Instruments Medications IV catheters Urinary catheters	Sterilize
Semicritical	Significant	Mucus membranes Nonintact skin	Thermometers Scopes: oral, rectal, GI, respiratory	High-level disinfect
Noncritical	Low	Intact skin	B/P cuffs Tourniquets	Intermediate-level disinfect
Noncritical	Low	No contact	Furniture	Low-level disinfect

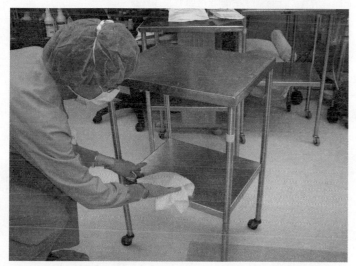

FIGURE 24.1 Disinfect surfaces.

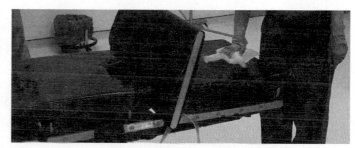

FIGURE 24.2 Disinfect the OR bed and accessories.

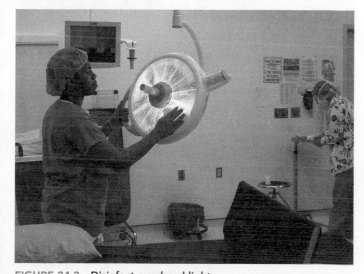

FIGURE 24.3 Disinfect overhead lights.

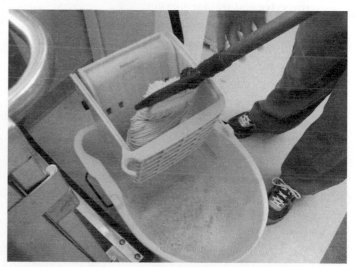

FIGURE 24.4 Use a new mop and detergent after each procedure.

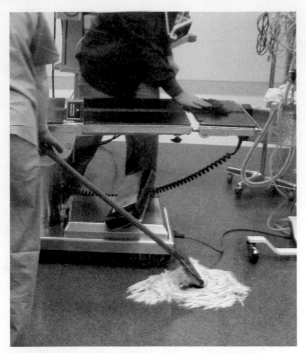

FIGURE 24.5 Clean the floor around the OR bed.

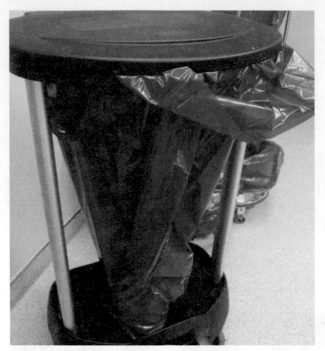

FIGURE 24.6 Place new bags to sort for recycling, incineration, trash, and laundry.

3. Make up the OR bed.
   - Apply fresh linens to the mattress and a folded sheet for a central draw sheet.
   - Prepare positioning aids, as appropriate, such as a head rest and ulnar pads (see Figure 24.7).

4. Prepare the wound suction device, as appropriate for your facility.
   - Insert a new liner into the suction canister.
   - Evaluate the canister for proper function. Turn on the valve and feel for suction.
   - Position an automated drainage storage device, if used, near the OR bed (see Figure 24.8).

5. Arrange furniture and obtain equipment required for the next procedure.
   - Disinfect equipment brought into the room from surrounding storage areas (see Figure 24.9).

6. Participate in terminal cleaning every 24 hours—traditionally performed in the late evening when the procedure schedule is low.
   - Clean the room more extensively according to your OR policy and schedule.
   - Wet-vacuum the floors.
   - Wash walls, ceilings, equipment, and furniture.

   - Clean duct work and filters to remove dust and trapped microorganisms—performed by the engineering department according to a schedule.
   - Evaluate the ventilation systems for air-exchange cycles and positive pressure inside the rooms—performed by the engineering department.

Confidential Patient Information
7. Maintain confidentiality and professionalism.
   - Apply the HIPAA guidelines.
     ◦ Maintain patient confidentiality.
     ◦ Discuss pertinent patient information with OR team members—identification, allergies, NPO status, and procedural information.
     ◦ Know your hospital's policy and system for granting permission to disclose private information.
     ◦ Do not discuss patient information in person or over the phone unless the patient has given permission to release this.
     ◦ Do not fax or email patient information unless you are authorized by the hospital. Verify numbers and addresses.

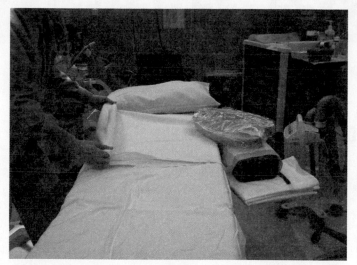

FIGURE 24.7 Apply new bed linens.

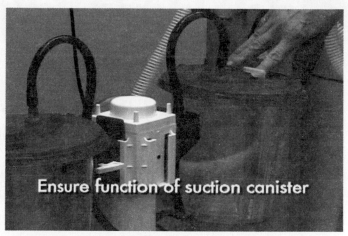

Ensure function of suction canister

FIGURE 24.8 Insert a new liner or canister; assess function.

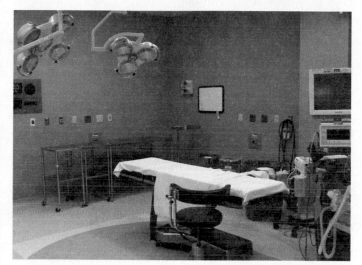

FIGURE 24.9 The room is ready to accept new surgical supplies and packs.

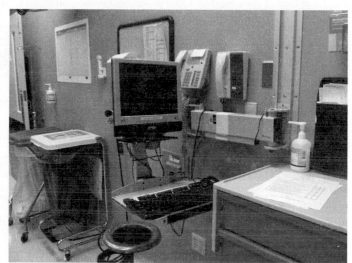

FIGURE 24.10 Honor confidentiality.

○ Begin and end computer documentation on the "desktop-computer screen." Do not leave patient information visible on an unattended computer screen, in a public setting.

○ Do not access patient information on anyone other than your assigned patient. You may not access information pertaining to family, friends, neighbors, or classmates if they are not your assigned patient.

○ Do not discuss confidential patient information in the lunch room, elevator, or in any public location. You may not post pictures or video, or participate in discussions on social networking websites.

○ Do not remove any printed materials containing any patient information, such as a surgery schedule, from the hospital.

• Promote professionalism.

○ Use good judgment, professionalism, and discretion.

○ Do not discuss details of any surgical procedure or mention team members or surgeons by name in any public location (see Figure 24.10).

STUDENT'S NAME: _____

CHAPTER 24 FACILITATE ROOM TURNOVER AND CONFIDENTIALITY

PERFORMANCE RANK:

S or √ = Satisfactory: Competent—safe, accurate, sequential, and timely
U = Unsatisfactory: Unsafe—inaccurate and unprepared

PERFORMANCE RATING:

5   Independent: Expert—safe, confident, seamless performance; mentors others
4   Minimally monitored: Intermediate—safe, self-corrects few errors
3   Competent: Novice—safe, revises with evaluator cues, few errors
2   Remedial: Unsafe—critical errors, unable to implement evaluator cues consistently
1   Dependent: Unsafe—unacceptable, requires multiple evaluator interventions

PERFORMANCE CRITERIA	Performance Rank	Performance Rating
1. Perform Mutual Professional and Scholastic Criteria as appropriate (see the Preface or Appendix A).		1 2 3 4 5
2. Don appropriate PPE; minimally, nonsterile gloves.		1 2 3 4 5
3. Place EPA-registered disinfectant into a nonlint cloth and wipe off all equipment and flat surfaces.		1 2 3 4 5
4. Mop the floor surrounding the OR bed.		1 2 3 4 5
5. Replace disposable bags and canisters.		1 2 3 4 5
6. Make up the OR bed with new linens.		1 2 3 4 5
7. Participate in daily, terminal cleaning; wet-vacuum the floors, and wash walls, ceilings, and equipment.		1 2 3 4 5
8. Remove PPE; perform hand hygiene.		1 2 3 4 5
9. Define HIPAA and confidentiality.		1 2 3 4 5
10. List four examples of the ST role with electronic, oral, and printed patient data.		1 2 3 4 5

ADDITIONAL COMMENTS _____

PERFORMANCE EVALUATIONS AND RECOMMENDATIONS

❑ PASS: Satisfactory Performance
  ❑ Demonstrates professionalism
  ❑ Exhibits critical thinking
  ❑ Demonstrates proficient clinical performance appropriate for time in the program
❑ FAIL: Unsatisfactory Performance
  ❑ Critical criteria not met (see Performance Rank or Rating above)
  ❑ Professionalism not demonstrated.
  ❑ Critical thinking skills not demonstrated.
  ❑ Skill performance unsafe or underdeveloped.

❑ REMEDIATION:
  ❑ Schedule lab practice. Date: _____
  ❑ Reevaluate by instructor. Date: _____
❑ DISMISS from lab or clinicals today.
❑ Program director notified. Date: _____

SIGNATURES

Date _____   Evaluator _____   Student _____

ACTIVITIES AND DISCUSSION QUESTIONS

Activities

1. View the Complete Perioperative Process and Focus on Skills video, Skill #24 (video can be found at www.myhealthprofessionskit.com).
2. Observe the instructor perform the skill.
3. Practice this skill with your lab partner.
4. Develop a small script in which you will give an example of HIPAA violations or a breach of patient confidentiality. Ask your lab partner to identify the errors and discuss how to prevent those errors. For example, make up a conversation between two ST students in the public cafeteria where the patient's family member overhears their conversation.
5. Refer to your ST textbook and this lab manual to answer the Discussion Questions (see next column).
6. Review the video and the information in this lab manual when you prepare for your certification examination.

Discussion Questions

1. When disinfecting or wiping off equipment and flat surfaces in the OR, what PPE will you wear?
2. What is the rationale for periodically changing the filters and cleaning the ventilation ductwork in the OR rooms (performed by the engineering department)?
3. Give three examples of fomites in the operating room.
4. You are preparing to clean the OR furniture and the only box of gloves in the room is vinyl; what should you do next?
5. Note here any questions that you need your instructor to clarify.

PEARSON
myhealthprofessionskit™

Use this address to access the Companion Website created for this textbook. Simply select "Surgical Technology" from the choice of disciplines. Find this book and log in using your username and password to access interactive activities, videos, and much more.

Unit IV

Minimally Invasive Surgery

CHAPTER 25
Facilitate Minimally Invasive Surgery: Laparoscopic and Robot-Assisted

Facilitate Minimally Invasive Surgery: Laparoscopic and Robot-Assisted

25

INTRODUCTION

Minimally invasive surgery (MIS) can enhance surgical precision and provide greater patient satisfaction. The surgical technologist identifies, assesses, and prepares all components and instrumentation on the sterile field for MIS, including robot-assisted procedures. The second assisting, or second scrub, ST manipulates the endoscopic camera and assists the surgeon with retracting, suctioning, sponging, or cutting suture when the robot is not utilized.

- Before performing the following skill, your lab instructor will discuss some of the principles for practice and objectives involved in this chapter as well as the importance of following the skill sequence and instructions.
- Along with a lab partner, practice setting up the supplies and equipment used for a laparoscopy procedure. Practice until you are comfortable

with the mechanics of the equipment. Use a timer to improve your efficiency. Simulate the second assisting or second scrub role by manipulating the endoscopic camera in a pelvic trainer or manikin. Encourage and critique each other. Your instructor will offer strategies for success. Appendix E highlights the value of teaching others as a component of active learning strategies. Refer to Appendix C for an overview of the chapter.

- The lab instructor will advise you of any additional criteria to be evaluated. At a designated time, demonstration of these skills will be evaluated and graded by your lab instructor using the competency assessment tool.
- When in the clinical setting, your instructor may once again assess your performance using the same tool. Refer to Appendix A for clinical evaluation and documentation.

Team Member	Type of Role		Timing		
	Nonsterile	Sterile	Preop	Intraop	Postop
Surgical Technologist	X	X	X	X	X
Assistant Circulator	X		X	X	X
Second Assisting ST, (Second Scrub)		X	X	X	X
Operating Room Team	X	X	X	X	X

OBJECTIVES

The learner will demonstrate the following with 100 percent accuracy each time performed in the operative environment.

1. Apply the principles of aseptic technique.
2. Discuss team member roles during MIS, laparoscopic, and robot-assisted surgeries.
3. Name at least five measures that protect the patient and staff from injury.
4. Gather instrument trays and supplies for conversion to an open procedure.
5. Perform a basic Mayo stand and back table set-up for a laparoscopic procedure.
6. Demonstrate the process for inspecting cables, endoscopes, and instruments.
7. Identify and prepare laparoscopic supplies and equipment on the sterile field.
8. Perform in the first scrub role.
9. Manipulate the endoscopic camera in the second assisting, or second scrub role.
10. Discuss the rationale for robot-assisted surgery.
11. List the three main components of the robot-assisted system.
12. Discuss roles in preparing instruments and equipment for cleaning and sterilization.

Principles for Practice

The foundation and rationale for our practice, in the perioperative environment, stem from evidence provided by professionals, organizations, and governmental agencies. Refer to the Bibliography, Glossary of Terms, and the following documents or developmental agencies:

- Manufacturers' product instructions
- Operating room policies
- Occupational Safety and Health Administration (OSHA)
- Centers for Disease Control and Prevention (CDC)
- Association of Surgical Technologists (AST)
- Association of periOperative Registered Nurses (AORN)

SKILL SEQUENCE AND INSTRUCTIONS
LAPAROSCOPIC SURGERY: FIRST SCRUB ROLE

Laparoscopic Surgery: First Scrub ST

1. Gather and arrange laparoscopic surgery components (nonsterile role). The major components include:

- Cart housing control units
- Video monitor screens
- Surgical site instrumentation
- Back-up instrumentation and supplies for conversion to an open procedure (see Figure 25.1).

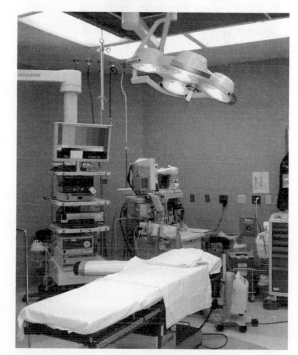

FIGURE 25.1 **Laparoscopic components.**

2. Position the cart or tower (mobile or ceiling-mounted) in an accessible location. It stores:

- Light source unit
- Camera control unit
- Image manager and printer
- Insufflation monitor
- Electrosurgery unit (also available as a separate unit)
  - Wall-mounted control units may be located near the circulator's desk.
- Anticipate traffic patterns; keep equipment and cords out of the path.
- Locate replacement lightbulbs for the light source and cable adaptors, as needed.
- Assess and replace the carbon dioxide tank for insufflation. Piped-in gas may be used and a tank is not needed (see Figure 25.2).

3. Position and turn on the video monitor screens (mobile, wall or ceiling mounted) so that the displays are visible to the surgeon. The video monitors display the endoscope's view during the procedure.

- Position two mobile or ceiling-mounted screens on opposite sides of the patient bed, if these options are used in your facility.

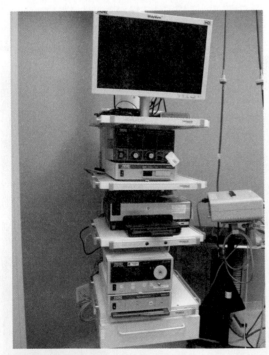

FIGURE 25.2 Storage cart or tower.

4. Perform preoperative nonsterile skills.

- Perform hand hygiene and don PPE. Refer to Chapters 2 and 3.
- Obtain and open sterile supplies and packs. Refer to Chapter 4.
- Obtain positioning aids.
- Gather leg sleeves for the sequential compression device (SCD), used to prevent deep vein thrombosis (DVT).
- Open laparoscopic and general instrument trays, and assess filters and any visible sterilization indicators.

5. Demonstrate the preoperative sterile role:

- Perform a traditional or waterless surgical hand scrub. Refer to Chapter 5.
- Gown and glove self with the closed gloving technique. Refer to Chapter 6.
- Drape the Mayo stand. Refer to Chapter 7.
- Identify and arrange the surgical site equipment:
  - Instrumentation
  - Camera and cord
  - Light source cord
  - Insufflation tubing
  - Suction-irrigation tubing
  - Electrosurgical cord
- Inspect sterilization indicators in the instrument trays.
- Inspect instruments for cleanliness: instruments containing debris are contaminated and may not be used.
- Inspect instruments for intended function: cutting or grasping.
- Inspect instruments for mechanical ability: aligned, all parts present, sharp, no defects, and insulation intact.
- Label any malfunctioning items to be sent out for repair.
- Recognize nuances in set-up styles in the practice setting. Autonomy may be allowed in some facilities, but standardization may be the rule in others.
- Verify, label, and receive medications and solutions on the sterile field. Refer to Chapter 9.
- Perform pre-procedure counts with the circulator. Refer to Chapter 8 (see also Figures 25.3 through 25.5).

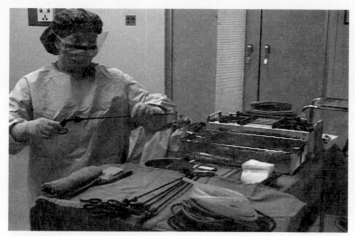

FIGURE 25.3   Inspect all instruments.

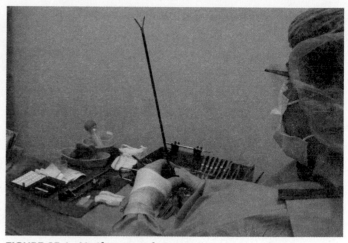

FIGURE 25.4   Verify proper function.

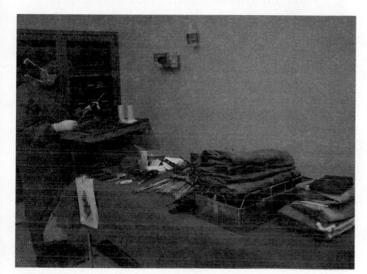

FIGURE 25.5   Plan for a standardized set-up.

6. Examine all cords found in the sterilization trays: camera cord, light source cord, and ESU cord. Refer to Table 25.1.

- Inspect insulation. Cracked insulation can cause unintended burns to the patient, including direct coupling burns (instrument to instrument) or stray capacitative coupling burns.
- Do not use damaged cords. Obtain new ones.
- Control the cords, recoil but not too tightly, and arrange them on the Mayo stand, back table, or in a basin. Due to cord memory, handle them carefully; they may spring in an undesired direction.
- Recoil and arrange plastic tubing for the insufflation, irrigation, and suction onto the Mayo stand, back table, or in a basin (see Figures 25.6 through 25.8).

TABLE 25.1   Component Assessment

Component	Assess				
	Clean	Integrity	Function	Moisture	Clear View
Camera/cord and camera mount	X	X	X	X	
Light source cord	X	X	X		X
Endoscope	X	X		X	X
ESU cord (reusable)	X	X			
Instruments	X	X	X		

7. Prepare the endoscope.

- Obtain the endoscope from the sterile processing container.
- Endoscopes and other delicate items are not sterilized with saturated steam. Paracetic acid or gas plasma is used, and items may be moist when brought to the OR suite.
- Dry the endoscope with a lint-free cloth if it is moist from the sterilization process, according to the manufacturer's instructions.
- Verify the field of vision requested: 0°, 30°, or 45°.
- The 0° is the natural view of your eye. The others, 30° and 45°, aid the surgeon's field of vision around an organ or structure.

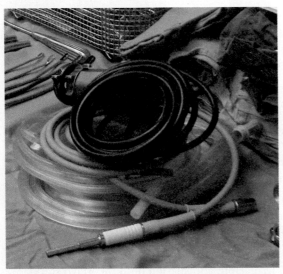

FIGURE 25.6   Examine and prepare all cords and tubes.

8. Evaluate the endoscope and fiber-optic light cord for integrity.

- Examine the shaft of the endoscope for dents, indicating potential damage to the interior.
- Examine the interior, viewing quality of the endoscope. Hold the distal shaft end of the endoscope towards the ceiling light.
  - Look for a solid "yellow glow" at the light post indicating a clear view for the surgeon. (View Figure 25.9, endoscope on right.)
  - Obtain a new endoscope if the original has 25 percent or more fogging, "peppery," or blind spots in view.
- Examine the fiber-optic light cord for integrity.
  - Hold the fiber-optic light cord connector end towards the ceiling light. (View Figure 25.9, light cord on left).
  - Look for a solid "yellow glow" at the opposite end.
  - Dark spots in the view indicate damaged fiber-optic cords.
  - Replace when 25 percent of the view is foggy.
- Do not use a damaged endoscope or light cord.
- Use an endoscope warmer, if available, to prevent fogging of the lens during introduction into the warm abdomen.

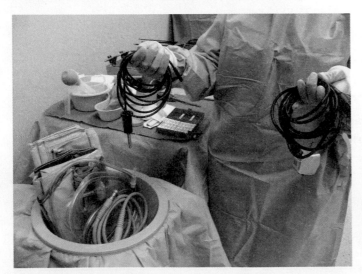

FIGURE 25.7   Purposefully sort and maneuver all cords.

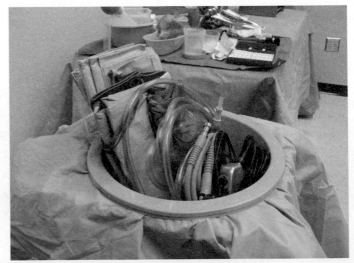

FIGURE 25.8   Arrange cords in the order of use.

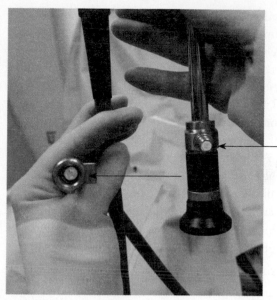

FIGURE 25.9 A solid yellow glow indicates a clear view for the surgeon.

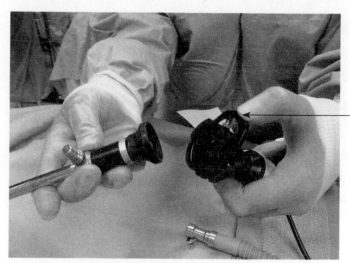

FIGURE 25.10 Attach endoscope to the camera head; lever example shown.

9. Assess the camera head and cord for integrity and connection.

- Remove the camera from the Steris container.
- Dry the inside of the camera lens with a lint-free cloth or sterile cotton-tipped applicator before placing it on the endoscope.
- Verify the connections. Maneuver the lever on the mounting end.
  - Attach the endoscope to the camera head by squeezing the lever or coupler on the camera side over the eyepiece of the endoscope.
  - Use a screw mechanism for the connection, depending on the manufacturing variations.

- Disassemble. You will assemble for use later: the camera cord, endoscope, and light cord.
- Locate the endoscope and camera head on a stable surface (see Figure 25.10).

10. Identify the cord ends that you will pass off the sterile field to the circulator.

- Refer to Table 25.2 and Figure 25.11.

TABLE 25.2 Identify Cords and Tubes for Laparoscopic Surgery (see Figure 25.11)

Name of Cord or Tubing		Identification			
		Color Example	Color Options	Reuse	Dispose
1	Light source cord	Grey	Green, White	X	
2	Camera /cord & mount	Black		X	
3	ESU cord	Green	Black	X	X
4	Suction/irrigation tubing	Clear			X
5	Insufflation tubing	Clear			X

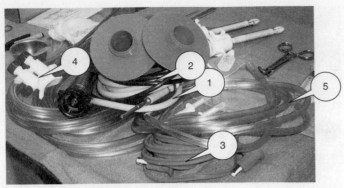

FIGURE 25.11 Laparoscopic cords and tubing arranged on a Mayo stand (see Table 25.2).

In Table 25.3, list the name, color, and disposition during room turnover of the laparoscopic cords and tubes that you will use.

TABLE 25.3 Cord and Tube Information

Tube or Cord	Color	Save or Dispose

11. Prepare the trocar-cannula (port) units.

- Trocars are available in 5–15 mm sizes.
- Routinely used for adults are (1 or 2) 10 mm, (2) 5 mm, and (1) 12 mm.
- Facilities are using single-port cannulas, according to the surgeon's preference. Refer to the manufacturer's instructions. Your instructor will discuss appropriate variations.
- Insert the trocar into the cannula. View the red-color change. Red signals potential puncture danger due to a sharp item.

- Be vigilant, focused, and respectful of the sharp instruments to prevent unintended injury. Do not handle the sharp ends.
- Place the stopcock into the off position (perpendicular to the attachment port for the insufflations tube), thereby preventing insufflation gas from moving into or out of the trocar-cannula unit or body cavity.
- Note: After the surgeon places the trocar-cannula into the abdomen, the trocar will be removed and the cannula portion or port will remain. It provides a seal around the skin borders for protection during introduction of the instruments (see Figures 25.12 through 25.16).

12. Prepare the Veress needle; attach a saline filled syringe.

- The surgeon inserts the Veress needle into the intraabdominal cavity, attaches the insufflation tubing, and expands the cavity with carbon dioxide gas, similar to filling a balloon. The increased space is beneficial to the surgeon's work.
  - Alternately, the surgeon may access the peritoneum using the Hasson technique. Refer to the Glossary of Terms.
- Carbon dioxide gas is used because it does not present a fire hazard and is tolerated by the patient's body (see Figure 25.17).

13. Arrange the Mayo stand with instruments and equipment needed by the surgeon to begin the procedure.

- Select scalpel, sponges, sharp towel clip, and laparoscopic specific instrumentation.
- Plan to rotate instruments and supplies to coordinate with the progression of the procedure (see Figures 25.18 through 25.22).

14. Validate the pre-procedure check list and identify the patient in the OR room. Anticipate the following procedures: anesthesia administration, patient positioning, the skin prep, and draping. Refer to Chapters 12 through 17.

- Be attentive and verbally validate, along with all OR team members, the pre-procedure checklist, or intraoperative pause
- Prevent loud noises during induction into anesthesia.
- Break scrub to assist any team member who requires your help during a patient emergency.

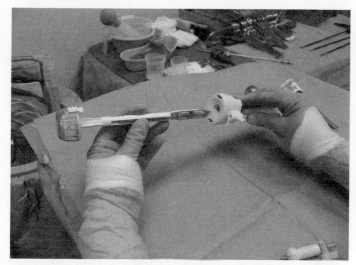

FIGURE 25.12 Assemble trocar-cannula unit.

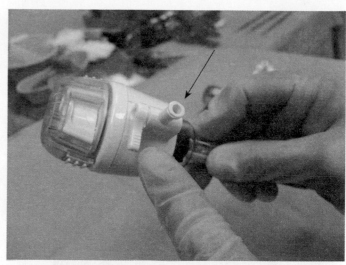

FIGURE 25.13 Flow to the unit is off when the stopcock is in the perpendicular position.

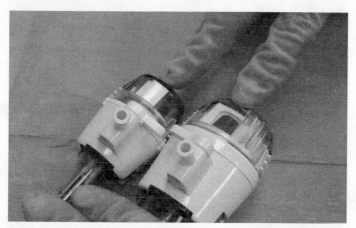

FIGURE 25.14 Color change from white to red indicates this unit has a sharp trocar in place.

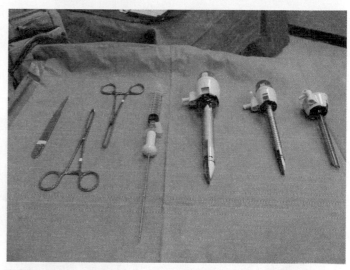

FIGURE 25.15 Prepare the Mayo stand with the instrumentation to begin the procedure.

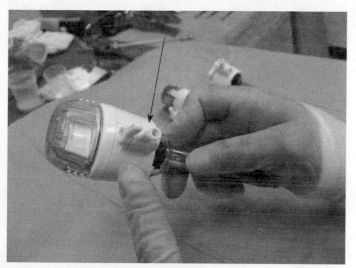

FIGURE 25.16 Parallel stopcock position indicates an open port allowing inflow or exhaust of carbon dioxide gas.

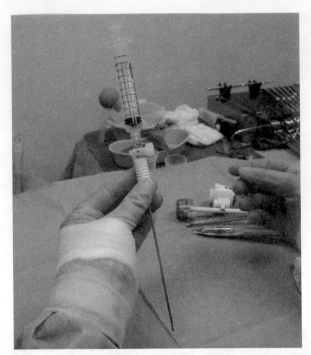

FIGURE 25.17 Veress needle with syringe attached.

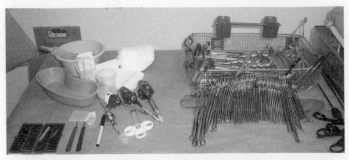

FIGURE 25.18 Select items from the back table.

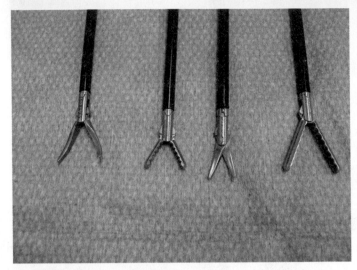

FIGURE 25.20 Laparoscopic instrument tips.
Left to right
- Maryland dissecting forceps
- Toothed or biting graspers
- Scissors
- Atraumatic graspers

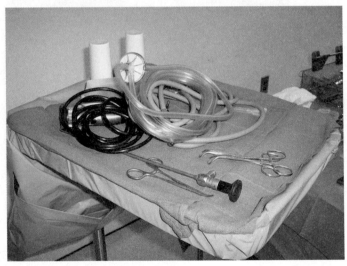

FIGURE 25.19 Arrange Mayo stand.

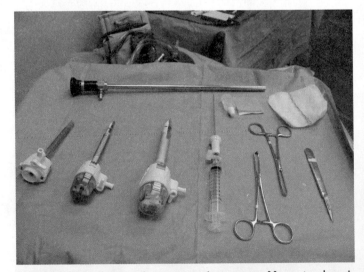

FIGURE 25.21 Arrange instrumentation on your Mayo stand; variations are numerous.

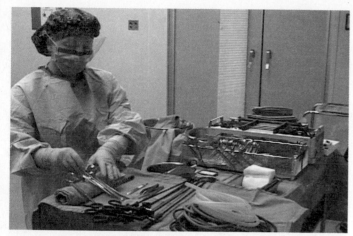

FIGURE 25.22   Mayo stand prepared for laparoscopic procedure.

15. Pull the Mayo stand and back table to the sterile field. Refer to Chapter 18.

- Adjust the height of the stand and protect the patient's abdomen or legs from external pressure from an improperly positioned Mayo stand.
- Place light handle covers on the overhead lights.
- Grasp and move the cords and tubes to prevent uncoiling and contamination.
- Locate the cords and tubes onto the drapes according to the location of the control monitors and the surgeon (see Figure 25.23).

16. Attach all cords to the patient's drapes.

- Use the Velcro tabs on disposable drapes for attaching, and for textile drapes use an Allis clamp or non-penetrating towel clamp.

- Do not wrap cords around the metal clamps; prevent stray electricity and fires.
- Do not use penetrating clamps; prevent a breech in the sterile field.
- Work with other sterile team members to attach the cords and tubes: the surgeon, assistant, and ST perform multiple tasks simultaneously on the sterile field.

17. Assemble the viewing components, and perform a white balance (camera).

- Connect the endoscope eyepiece to the camera head (coupler or screw) mechanism.
- Anticipate holding the endoscope and camera securely.
- Do not drop the endoscope or camera. They are expensive to repair or replace (see Figure 25.24).
- Attach the light cord to the endoscope; light is on standby until ready for use. You may need an adaptor to connect equipment from different manufacturers.
- Pass off the camera cord to the circulator who will connect it to the power source.
- Perform a white balance for the camera-endoscope unit. The circulator will take the light off standby and turn it on. The ST will hold a sterile, solid white item such as a sterile glove wrapper to the endoscope so that the control unit will balance the color and contrast. Gauze sponges are frequently used, but may not be appropriate for some cameras.
- Place the light source on standby mode or off until ready for use by the surgeon. Prevent unintended fires associated with lights left lying on the drapes (see Figures 25.25 through 25.27).

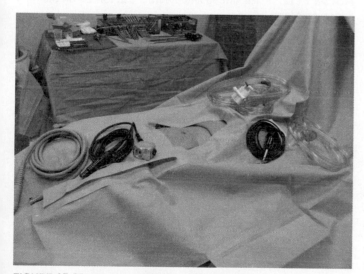

FIGURE 25.23   Locate cords and tubes for use.

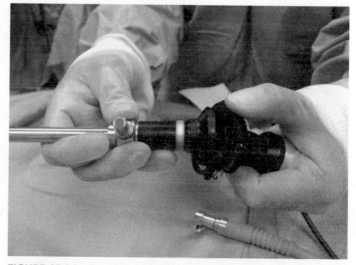

FIGURE 25.24   Connect with a lever or screw mechanism.

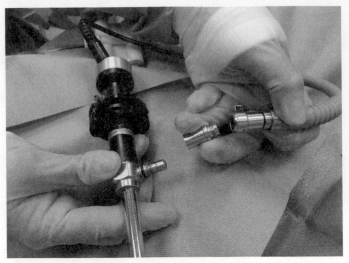

FIGURE 25.25   An adaptor may be used.

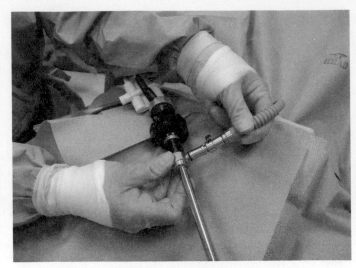

FIGURE 25.26   Connect camera cord to the endoscope.

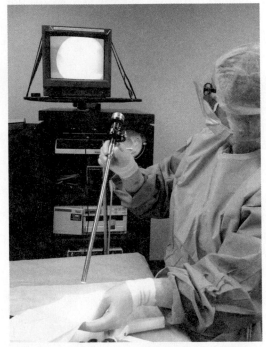

FIGURE 25.27   White balance the endoscopic camera.

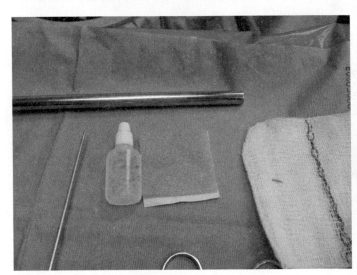

FIGURE 25.28   Place antifog liquid onto a pad for use on the endoscopic lens.

18. Promote a clear view through the endoscope.

   • Squeeze antifog liquid from a plastic bottle onto a sponge pad; the pad is routinely adhered onto the patient drape near the working area for the surgeon. The antifog or "Fred" is used to prevent fogging of the endoscope when it is placed into the warm abdomen (see Figure 25.28).

   • Use an endoscope warmer if available at your facility.

19. Assemble the electrocautery.

   • Attach the electrosurgery instrument to the ESU cord. The instrument will coagulate or cut when the electricity is activated by the surgeon. The example cord shown in black will be reprocessed at the end of the case (see Figure 25.29).

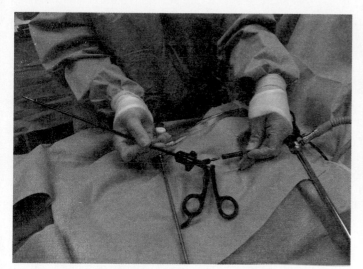

FIGURE 25.29 Connect electricity for coagulation and cutting.

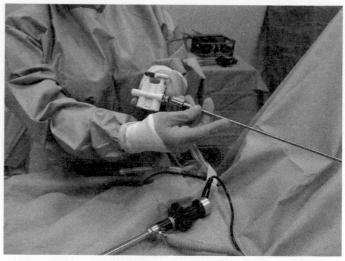

FIGURE 25.30 Attach suction wand to suction-irrigation tubing.

20. Assemble the suction and irrigation equipment.

- Attach a suction wand to the suction side of the dual tubing for suction and irrigation.
- The surgeon operates the control buttons to deliver irrigation solutions or suction.
- Depending on your facility, you may use two separate tubes for individual suction and irrigation.
- The irrigation solution is contained off the sterile field and hangs on a pole at the patient's side. Once used, irrigation solution is collected in the suction canister through the suction wand and tubing.
- Notify the circulator when the irrigation solution bag is nearly empty. A nonsterile team member will hang a replacement bag as needed (see Figure 25.30).

21. Pass off the connecting ends of each cord or tube to the circulator, one at a time.

- Plan to pass off about 3 feet of each. Once passed off, the cords and tubes cannot be retrieved. The circulator will grasp the ends and plug them into the control units (see Figures 25.31 through 25.33).

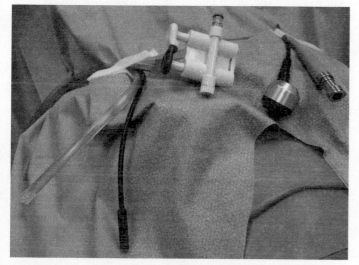

FIGURE 25.31 Keep appropriate ends on the sterile field.

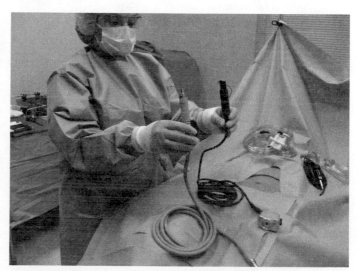

FIGURE 25.32 Pass off connecting ends to the circulator.

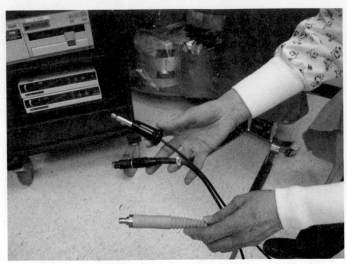

FIGURE 25.33 Circulator connects ends to the nonsterile units.

22. Pass instruments for the skin incisions and establishment of the pneumoperitoneum.

- Pass a loaded knife handle (#7 handle with #11 blade, for example) and two countable sponges to the surgeon to make the first subumbilical incision for the Veress needle.
- Pass two towel clamps to grasp and elevate the skin at the abdomen, thereby increasing the working area and preventing puncture of internal organs.
- Verify the proper preparation of the Veress needle, if used, which will prevent injury to the patient's internal organs during insertion by the surgeon. The sharp tip will be sheathed, once penetration of the skin is complete.
- Observe the surgeon perform a saline test to verify needle placement then carbon dioxide may be instilled.
- Connect the insufflation tubing to the needle so that pneumoperitoneum will be established.
- Return the Veress needle to the back table after use.

23. Begin the flow of carbon dioxide safety, which is performed by the circulator:

- Prefill the insufflation tubing with filtered carbon dioxide before attachment to the patient; room air will be displaced from the tubing.
- Position the control unit above the patient's hip-level to prevent retrograde flow (from patient to the insufflation unit) and monitor the 12–18 mm Hg pressure flow.
- Maintain the audible pressure alert alarms on the unit and confirms unit settings.

24. Pass the trocar-cannula unit for umbilical insertion.

- The surgeon will insert the unit.
  - Return the sharp trocar portion of the unit to the back table. The cannula will keep the port open.
  - Pass the endoscope, with the camera and light cords connected, for insertion into the port.
- Reconnect the insufflation tubing onto the cannula stopcock for additional instillation of carbon dioxide to maintain distension, as requested by the surgeon (see Figures 25.34 through 25.37).

25. Assist with additional port placement.

- Pass selected cannula-trocar units for additional port placement. Pass a scalpel and sequentially pass the two or three remaining trocar-cannula units so that additional ports for instruments can be established.
- Return the scalpel and sharp trocars to the back table in a safe location intended for sharps; place near the needle mat or in an unused container for safety.
- The cannula will self-seal to prevent carbon dioxide from leaking out when the instrument is removed.

26. Pass instruments from the Mayo stand or back table during the procedure.

- Maintain the cleanliness and function of the instruments. Use sterile water to rinse or clean off the instruments.
- Exchange and pass laparoscopic instruments based on the course of the procedure.
- Switch between locking and unlocking handles, according to the surgeon's preference.

27. Facilitate the collection and care of tissue specimens.

- Pass a specimen pouch, as requested, for tissue removal through the port.
- Connect a specimen trap on the suction line for collection of tissue fragments produced by morcellation.
- Manage (hydrate and label) the specimen on the back table until the surgeon verifies that it may be passed off the field to the circulator.
- Specimens intended for frozen section examination must be verified and attended to immediately. Pass into a dry container, or on a dry nonstick pad. Do not immerse this specimen. Follow your hospital's policy. Refer to chapter 21.
- Pass the tissue to the circulator using the utmost caution. Use an acceptable method of transfer.
- Label the specimen container, and place it into a biohazard bag for the laboratory, which is the circulator's role (see Figures 25.38 and 25.39).

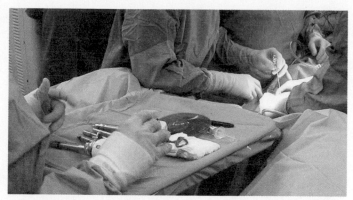

FIGURE 25.34 Surgeon inserts Veress needle into the abdomen.

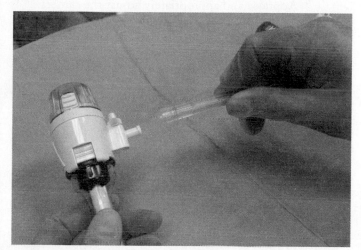

FIGURE 25.36 Connect insufflation tube to cannula, later.

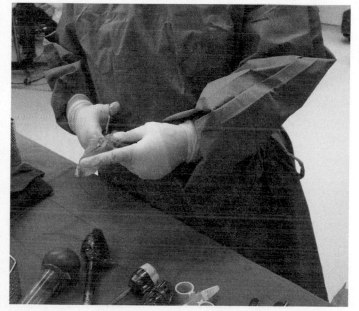

FIGURE 25.38 Remove specimen from endoscopic collection-pouch.

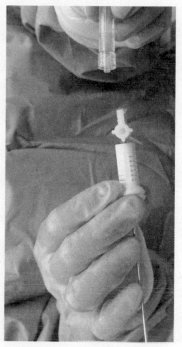

FIGURE 25.35 Connect insufflation tube to Veress needle, first.

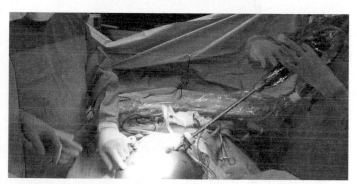

FIGURE 25.37 Endoscope in umbilical port, with camera and light source.

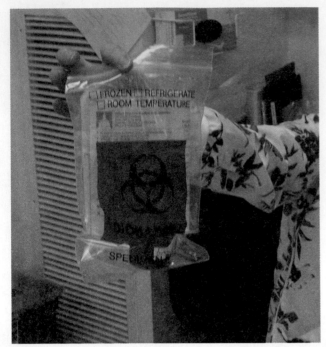

FIGURE 25.39 Biohazard bag used to transport specimens to the lab.

Laparoscopic Second Assisting or Second Scrub Role

32. Perform in the second assisting, or second scrub, ST Role

- Manipulate the endoscopic camera during the surgical procedure instead of performing in the first scrub role, as previously discussed.
- Capitalize on your eye-hand coordination in this skill.
- Remain attentive to the surgeon's instructions for the required navigation and view.
- Maintain a view of the laparoscopic instrument tips used by the surgeon.

  ○ Center the field of vision by maneuvering the endoscope.

  ○ Appraise and appropriately adjust the camera's internal view as you look at the monitor screen in the room.

  ○ Use steady, controlled movements of the endoscopic camera. Quick movements may cause motion-sickness or distract the surgeon.

  ○ With the surgeon's acknowledgement, retract the endoscope and clean off the lens tip when clouded.

  ○ Frequently requested views are provided with a 0° or 30° endoscope.

  ○ The 0° endoscope provides a direct, natural, or forward view. Coordinating this view is less complex.

  ○ The 30° endoscope requires additional practice due to its construction so that an angled view is provided for the surgeon.

  ○ Use the external light cord attachment port to help maintain orientation.

  ○ The light cord port is positioned opposite of the endoscope view, in all planes.

  ○ The orientation is 180° apart. For example, when the light cord port points to the left, the view is to the right.

  ○ Use a laparoscopic trainer, or manikin, in the lab setting to practice.

28. Assist with procedure completion.

- Transfer instruments and equipment to the back table.
- Pass prepared suture or wound adhesive to approximate the port incisions. Refer to Chapter 20.
- Prepare and Pass Steri-strips or Band-Aids for dressings.
  Refer to Chapter 22.
- Perform skin care (see Figures 25.40 and 25.41).

29. Transport the patient to the PACU for recovery from anesthesia.

- Assist with transfers and transportation, in the nonsterile role. Refer to Chapters 11 and 22.

30. Dismantle the back table and Mayo stand (see Figures 25.42 through 25.45).

- Sort instruments and equipment for disposal or reprocessing.
- Dispose of sharps and biohazardous waste per policy. Refer to Chapter 23.
- Wipe off and handle all laparoscopic instruments and equipment with care.
- Return them to their original cases.
- Arrange cases securely onto your cart.

31. Clean and prepare the room for the next procedure. Refer to Chapter 24 (see also Figure 25.46).

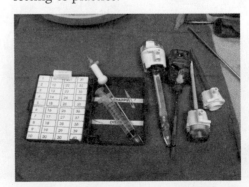

FIGURE 25.40 Return sharps and instruments to the back table.

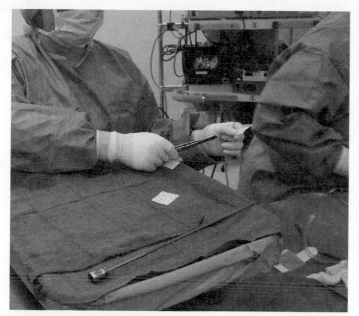

FIGURE 25.41 Pass Steri-strips to cover the abdominal incisions.

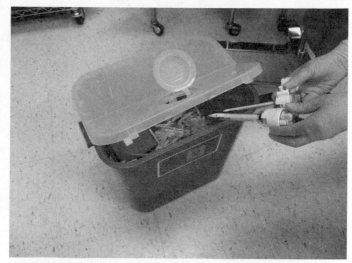

FIGURE 25.42 Dispose of sharps appropriately.

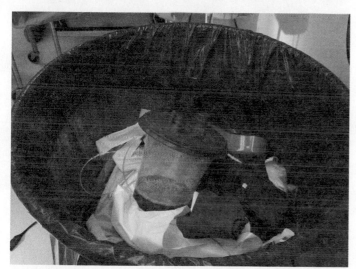

FIGURE 25.43 Solidify drainage and place into biohazard disposal.

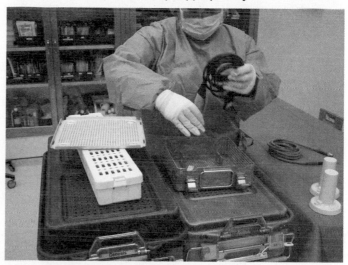

FIGURE 25.44 Repack cords with care.

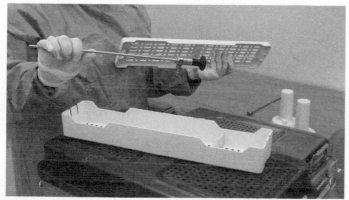

FIGURE 25.45 Protect the endoscope.

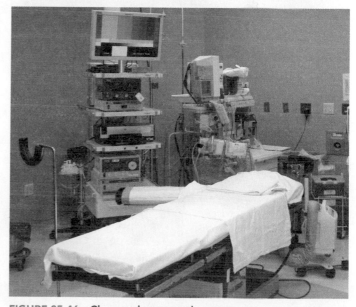

FIGURE 25.46 Clean and prepare the room.

SKILL SEQUENCE AND INSTRUCTIONS

Robot Assisted Surgery: Introduction

Robot-assisted minimally invasive surgery involves a panoply of technology which augments the skill of the surgeon. In the United States, the da Vinci Si HD Surgical System is being used in operating rooms. Extensive training must precede working with complex, robotic systems.

1. View three main components of the robotic surgical system, left to right, manufactured by Intuitive Surgical, Inc. (see Figure 25.47).

   • Surgeon's console
   • Patient-side cart
   • Vision system

2. Patient-side cart (see Figure 25.48).

   • Movable cart with interactive robotic arms
   • Two or three motion arms for removable instruments: Endo-wrist
   • One camera arm
   • Touch screen monitor

3. Surgeon's console (see Figure 25.49).

   • Ergonomically designed
   • Hand controls, foot pedals
   • Scales, filters, and precisely translates surgeon's hand movements
   • Real-time movement

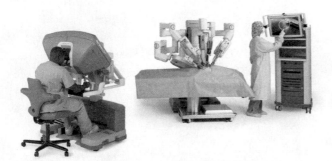

FIGURE 25.47 Main robotic components (© 2010 Intuitive Surgical, Inc.).

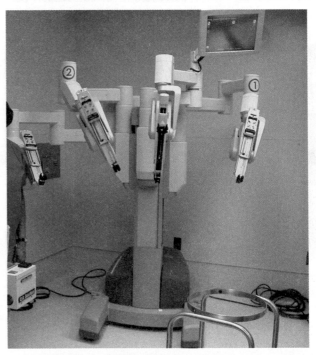

FIGURE 25.48 Patient-side cart. Also known as the "robot."

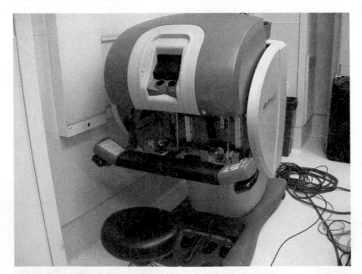

FIGURE 25.49 Surgeon's control console in the OR.

4. Vision system (see Figure 25.50).
   - High resolution viewing
   - 3-D endoscope integration
   - Image processing
5. Preoperative preparation (see Figures 25.51 through 25.60).
   - Position components for communication and safety in the OR suite.
   - Use and maintain aseptic technique. Refer to Chapter 4.
   - Set up the equipment; anticipate 1 to 1½ hours.
   - Monitor the robotic counting system. The life span of each cartridge is 10 uses. Dispose of an expired cartridge per your facility's policy.
   - Set up an endoscope warmer and two endoscopes.
   - Keep one endoscope in the warmer filled with sterile water as a backup.
   - Obtain endoscope heat packs for placement and warming at the field.
   - Drape camera and all cords; coordinator will attach to control units.

- Set up the back table and ring stand basin. Refer to Chapter 7.
- Set up the Mayo stand first for the surgeon (trocars-cannulas) and later for the assistant (robotic instruments or cartridges). Refer to Chapter 10.
- Anticipate the surgeon's preferences, for example, placement of five cannulas or ports: three for robotic instruments, one for a robotic endoscope, and one for the assistant to use.
- Prepare one 12 mm cannula for the endoscope and four 8 mm or 10 mm cannulas for the remaining ports.
- Prepare at least two sets of sterile attire for the surgeon: one set for trocar placement and one set for wound closure.
- Precut suture to about 6½ inches to accommodate the robot cartridge.
- Patient-side cart will be part of the sterile field: drape arms and the display monitor. Move cart to the patient, then complete draping.
- Surgeon makes calculations and adjustments at the console, then scrubs in to place the trocar-cannulas. The surgeon will break scrub and return to the console.

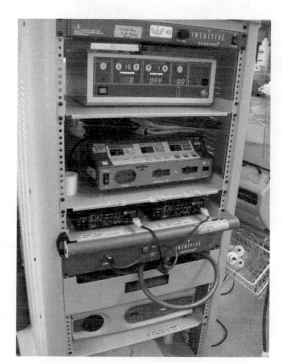

FIGURE 25.50 Robotic vision system.

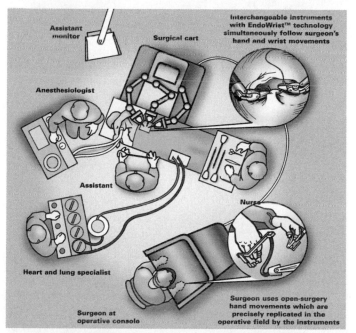

FIGURE 25.51 Anticipate placement of equipment (© 2010 Intuitive Surgical, Inc.).

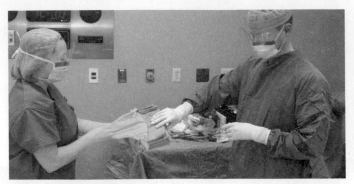

FIGURE 25.52 Maintain aseptic technique.

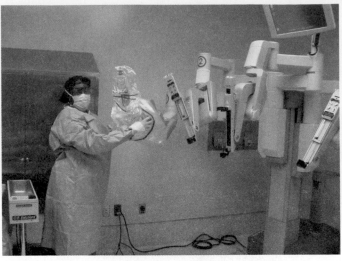

FIGURE 25.53 Drape patient-side cart arms individually.

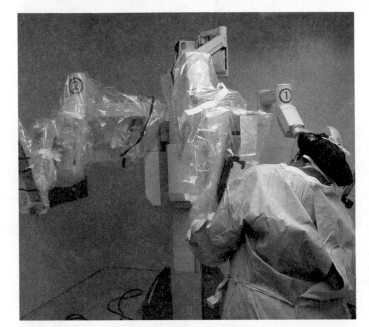

FIGURE 25.54 Drape and maintain sterile.

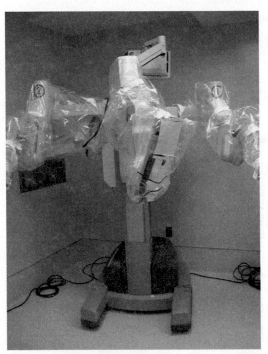

FIGURE 25.55 Patient side cart will be near patient, once draped.

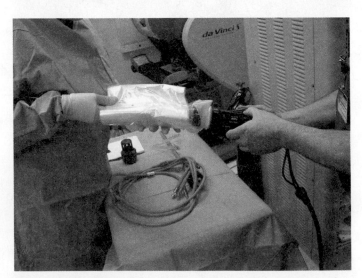

FIGURE 25.56 Drape the endoscopic camera with a clear, sterile drape.

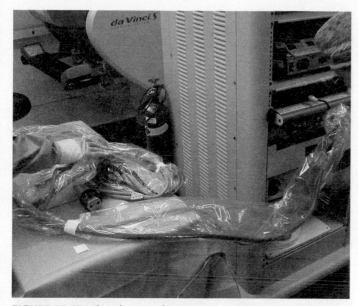

FIGURE 25.57   Circulator, right, connects camera cord to the vision cart.

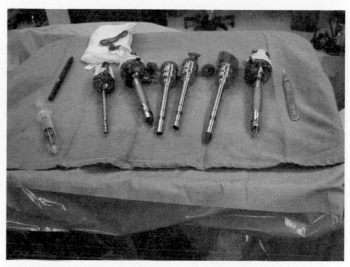

FIGURE 25.58   Mayo stand prepared for the surgeon.

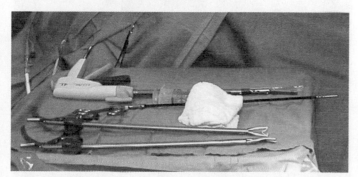

FIGURE 25.59   Mayo stand prepared for the patient-side assistant.

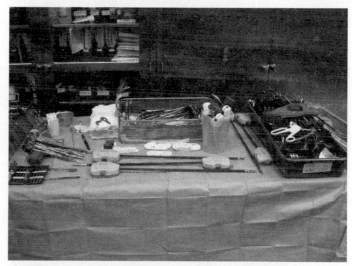

FIGURE 25.60   Back table set-up.

6. Patient preparation (see Figures 25.61 through 25.66).

- Participate in a safe surgery checklist and time-out; patient receives anesthesia, and is prepped and draped. Refer to chapters 12 through 18.
- Surgeon places cannulas.
- Move patient-side cart into position over patient; minimum of two needed to place the cart, nonsterile circulator, and sterile ST or surgical assistant.

- Complete sterile draping.
- Dock the sterile robotic instruments and camera-endoscope into the robotic arms. Performed by the surgeon, ST, and first assistant.
- Refer to the preprinted instrument names on each robotic instrument or "cartridge."

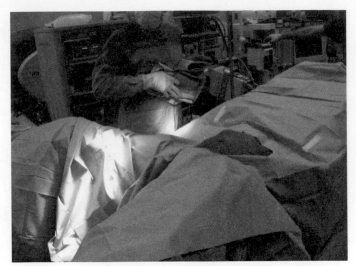

FIGURE 25.61 The patient is prepped and draped.

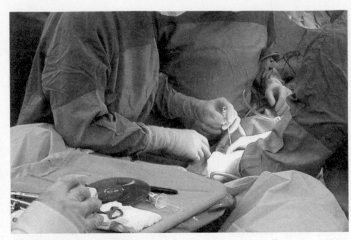

FIGURE 25.62 The surgeon inserts the Veress needle.

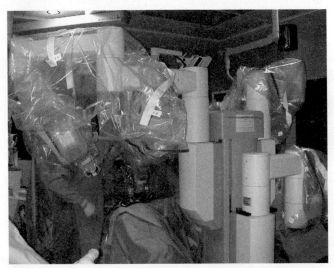

FIGURE 25.63 Use at least two team members to position the patient-side cart.

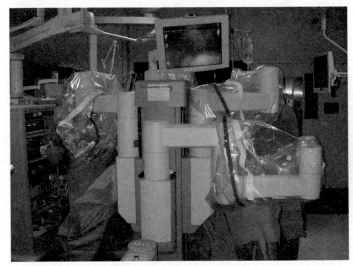

FIGURE 25.64 Complete sterile draping.

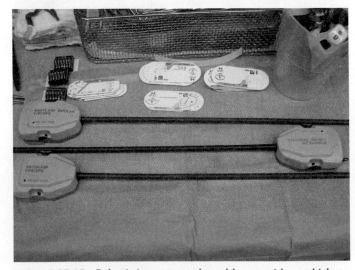

FIGURE 25.65 Robotic instruments have blue cartridges which connect to arms on the patient-side cart.

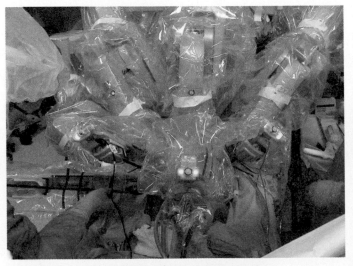

FIGURE 25.66 ST manages robotic instrumentation.

7. Minimally invasive surgery, robot-assisted (see Figures 25.67 through 25.71).

- The surgeon breaks scrub, directs the procedure from the console, and uses 3-D vision, hand controls, and foot-operated controls.
- The surgical assistant or RNFA holds graspers or other pelviscopy-type instruments through the fifth cannula/port.
- View anatomy and instruments on the room monitor. Adjust the room monitor as instructed.
- Circulator and robotic coordinator perform in the nonsterile role for assessment, safety, problem resolution, and case management.
- Circulator performs inventory and documents.
- Exchange instruments (cartridges) or the endoscope during the procedure, as instructed by the surgeon, and manage the sterile components.

- Manipulate the urinary catheter or uterus to facilitate the work of the surgeon, as instructed.
- Monitor your aseptic technique boundaries. If you perform a skill, such as manipulating the uterus, which causes contamination of your gloves or gown, you may not return to a sterile body area until you reglove and regown.
- Maintain organization and function of the surgical instruments.

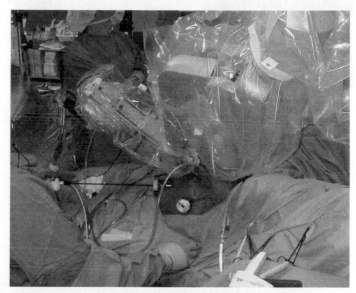

FIGURE 25.68 **The patient and the equipment are prepared and the first assistant is seated on the left.**

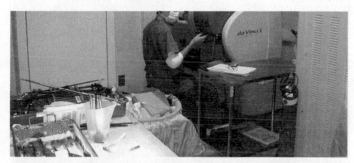

FIGURE 25.67 **The surgeon directs the procedure while seated at the control console.**

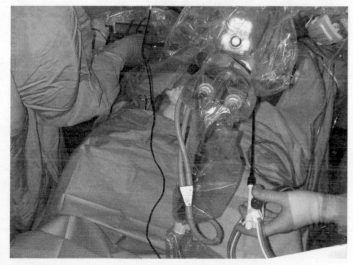

FIGURE 25.69 **Insert suction-irrigation wand, right.**

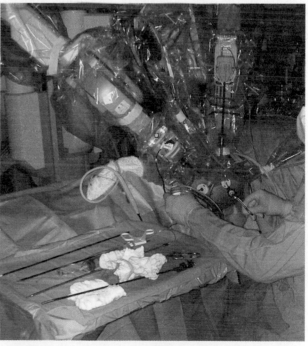

FIGURE 25.70 **First assistant follows instructions from the surgeon.**

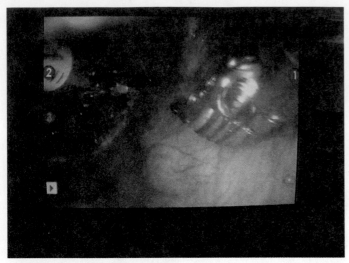

FIGURE 25.71   Room monitor view.

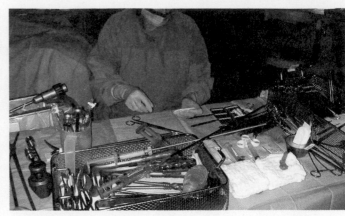

FIGURE 25.72   ST prepares closing suture at the back table.

8. Postoperative responsibilities (see Figure 25.72).

- Receive permission from the surgeon to remove and secure the endoscopic camera and instruments.
- Assist the surgeon to gown and glove for wound closure. Refer to Chapter 14.
- Work with the surgeon and first assistant during wound closure and dressing application.
- Remove the patient-side cart.
- Transport the patient to PACU, for recovery from anesthesia, nonsterile role. Refer to Chapter 22.
- Dismantle the back table and remove drapes from the patient-side cart.
- Remain attentive and sort items according to life span: disposable or reuseable. Refer to Chapter 23.
- Lubricate the robot-instruments.
- Prepare all instruments for decontamination per the manufacturer's instructions; robotic instruments have the added feature of a predetermined life-span (10 uses); check electronic monitor for display.
- Store the robotic technology components.

9. Surgical teams have developed proficiency and confidence in these complex procedures. Attend staff development opportunities and vendor demonstrations (Figure 25.73). Refer to the Intuitive Surgical, Inc. website for additional information at http://www.intuitivesurgical.com/index.aspx.

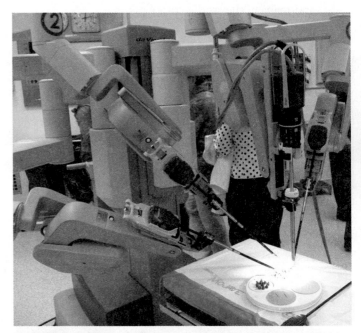

FIGURE 25.73   Robotic demonstration for students. See red training robotic instruments.

COMPETENCY ASSESSMENT

STUDENT'S NAME: _____

CHAPTER 25 FACILITATE MINIMALLY INVASIVE SURGERY

PERFORMANCE RANK:

    S or √ = Satisfactory: Competent—safe, accurate, sequential, and timely
    U = Unsatisfactory: Unsafe—inaccurate and unprepared

PERFORMANCE RATING:

    5   Independent: Expert—safe, confident, seamless performance; mentors others
    4   Minimally monitored: Intermediate—safe, self-corrects few errors
    3   Competent: Novice—safe, revises with evaluator cues, few errors
    2   Remedial: Unsafe—critical errors, unable to implement evaluator cues consistently
    1   Dependent: Unsafe—unacceptable, requires multiple evaluator interventions

PERFORMANCE CRITERIA	Performance Rank	Performance Rating
1. Perform Mutual Professional and Scholastic Criteria as appropriate (see the Preface or Appendix A).		1 2 3 4 5
2. Perform sterile role skills sequentially found in Chapters 1 through 9, laparoscopy example.		1 2 3 4 5
3. Prepare Veress needle and trocars per preference card.		1 2 3 4 5
4. Verify sterilization indicators; place instruments, camera, equipment cords, and endoscope on the back table.		1 2 3 4 5
5. Assess each laparoscopic component or instrument for cleanliness, integrity, function, moisture, or clear view.		1 2 3 4 5
6. Identify all laparoscopic equipment cords and tubes: sterile field ends and unit-connection ends.		1 2 3 4 5
7. Organize all tubes and cords in a specified location.		1 2 3 4 5
8. Protect the endoscope and camera in a designated location; handle with a firm grip.		1 2 3 4 5
9. Prepare Mayo stand, refer to Chapter 10, laparoscopy example.		1 2 3 4 5
10. Perform sterile role skills in Chapters 12 through14, 17, and 18, laparoscopy example.		1 2 3 4 5
11. Assemble laparoscopic components; attach all equipment cords and tubes to patient drape.		1 2 3 4 5
12. Pass equipment cord and tubing ends to the circulator: Camera cord, light cord, ESU cord, suction-irrigation tubing, and insufflation tubing.		1 2 3 4 5
13. Assist to white balance the camera system.		1 2 3 4 5
14. Place antifog solution and pad in designated area.		1 2 3 4 5
15. Perform sterile first scrub role skills found in Chapters 19 through 24, laparoscopy example.		1 2 3 4 5
16. Perform second assisting, or second scrub skills; use steady movements to manipulate the endoscopic camera; coordinate hand position with the monitor views; use a 0° and 30° endoscope.		1 2 3 4 5
17. Robot-assisted MIS: list the three major components of this surgical system and any affiliated ST skills.		1 2 3 4 5
18. Demonstrate draping the patient-side cart (robot arms) with a clear drape or sheath; maintain aseptic technique (lab simulation).		1 2 3 4 5

ADDITIONAL COMMENTS _____

PERFORMANCE EVALUATIONS AND RECOMMENDATIONS

❑ PASS: Satisfactory Performance
   ❑ Demonstrates professionalism
   ❑ Exhibits critical thinking
   ❑ Demonstrates proficient clinical performance appropriate for time in the program
❑ FAIL: Unsatisfactory Performance
   ❑ Critical criteria not met (see Performance Rank or Rating above)
   ❑ Professionalism not demonstrated.
   ❑ Critical thinking skills not demonstrated.
   ❑ Skill performance unsafe or underdeveloped.
❑ REMEDIATION:
   ❑ Schedule lab practice. Date: _____
   ❑ Reevaluate by instructor. Date: _____
❑ DISMISS from lab or clinicals today.
❑ Program director notified. Date: _____

SIGNATURES

Date _____   Evaluator _____   Student _____

ACTIVITIES AND DISCUSSION QUESTIONS

Activities

1. View the Complete Perioperative Process, the Laparoscopic Process, and Focus on Skills video, Skill #25 (video can be found at www.myhealthprofessionskit.com).
2. Observe the instructor perform the skill.
3. Practice preparing for a laparoscopic procedure with your lab partner.
4. Use a laparoscopic trainer as you manipulate the endoscopic camera with a 0° and 30° endoscope. Refine your eye-hand coordination skills and projection of the view onto the room monitor.
5. Select and teach one skill to your lab partner, such as inspecting and identifying all laparoscopic components, then observe and critique the performance.
6. Refer to your ST textbook and this lab manual to answer the Discussion Questions (see next column).
7. Review the video and the information in this lab manual when you prepare for your certification examination.

Discussion Questions

1. When will aseptic technique be difficult to maintain during laparoscopy? Give three examples.
2. Discuss one advantage and one disadvantage of MIS compared to open procedures.
3. Name two similarities and two differences between laparoscopic and robot-assisted surgery.
4. What evidence will indicate that you may not use the endoscope in your tray? the light cord? a laparoscopic instrument?
5. How is the patient protected from potential injury during MIS?
6. Where will you place supplies for an emergency conversion to an open case?
7. Identify three main components of a robotic system.
8. Why is an endoscope warmer used for at least two endoscopes?
9. How does the ST anticipate the needs of the surgeon for sterile attire during a robot-assisted procedure?
10. What would you say to a friend who asks you if a robot can perform surgery?
11. Note here any questions that you need your instructor to clarify.

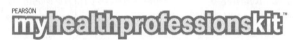

PEARSON

Use this address to access the Companion Website created for this textbook. Simply select "Surgical Technology" from the choice of disciplines. Find this book and log in using your username and password to access interactive activities, videos, and much more.

Glossary of Terms

AAMI: The Association for the Advancement of Medical Instrumentation. Advocates for safety in medical technology. http://www.aami.org/

Absorbable or nonabsorbable: The body's chemical processes can break down absorbable suture whereas nonabsorbable suture remains intact, usually indefinitely.

Accountability: To promote patient safety and prevent a retained instrument, all team members are able to account for or know the location of all surgical instruments.

Active electrode: The working end of the handheld device. Also known as a pencil, Bovie, or "tip."

Alcohol-based hand rubs or waterless agents: Applied as an acceptable alternative to the traditional hand scrub methods. Supplemental water is not used. Follow manufacturer's guidelines for application.

American Academy for Orthopaedic Surgeons (AAOS): Professional organization serving members and providing educational information to the public. http://www.aaos.org/.

American College of Surgeons (ACS): Professional organization serving members and providing public information. http://www.facs.org/.

American Heart Association (AHA): Provides public and professional education. Referenced for CPR skills for the healthcare provider. https//www.aha.org/

American Patient Safety Foundation (APSF): Promotes training and education for patient safety. www.APSF.org.

American Society of Heating, Refrigerating, and Air Conditioning Engineers (ASHRAE): Founded in 1894, this society is an international organization of over 50,000 members. ASHRAE fulfills its mission of advancing heating, ventilation, air conditioning, and refrigeration to serve humanity and promote a sustainable world through research, standards writing, publishing, and continuing education. Refer to the website. http://www.ashrae.org/aboutus/.

American Society of PeriAnesthesia Nurses (ASPAN): Guides professional practice for nurses in preanesthesia, postanesthesia, and pain management specialties. http://www.aspan.org/.

Aseptic technique, sterile technique, or Principles of Asepsis: Note: The terms may be used interchangeably. Identify and use the appropriate terms related to your geographical region. Aseptic technique is defined as: Actions that prevent microbial contamination of sterile, patient body areas during invasive surgical procedures. The guidelines are summarized here. Only sterile touches sterile; protect the surgical site; respect spatial boundaries; when in doubt, throw it out; and use the same technique for all patients. Aseptic means free from microbes and spores; a series of processes that are conducted to reduce, eliminate, or confine microbes and, therefore, reduce the risk of an infection.

Assistant circulator: The ST acting in the nonsterile role; performs circulating duties as defined by both state practice acts for licensed and nonlicensed personnel and OR policy. Refer to the AST's Core Curriculum for Surgical Technology, 6th edition, for additional information. (The circulator may be a registered nurse or a surgical technologist, depending on individual state laws. An ST cannot perform duties that are legally the function of a licensed nurse.)

Association of periOperative Registered Nurses (AORN): A professional organization that develops, enriches, and supports the role of the registered nurse in the perioperative environment. Refer to www.AORN.org.

Back table or Instrument table: Large stainless steel table, one- or two-tiered, approximately 3' × 5', on wheels. This table holds large quantities of supplies and instruments.

Bioburden: Organic debris on surfaces.

Biofilm: Thin layer of active or nonactive microbes that adhere firmly to surfaces; may become trapped under debris.

Biohazard: Biological materials (blood or body fluids) that are potentially infections; the biohazard label means to be cautious and to wear appropriate PPE; may also refer to chemicals or solutions that may be harmful.

Bipolar: An electrosurgical mode using two electrodes so a dispersive pad is not required.

Blunt needle: Noncutting tip that pushes tissue aside; used on friable, delicate tissue such as the liver.

Braided: Strands of suture connected in an interlaced pattern.

Cannula-trocar device: This two-piece device is used to place 5 mm to 15 mm sized openings into the abdomen for laparoscopic surgery. The trocar is sharp and is pulled out of the opening, keeping the outer hollow cannula in place. The device forms a seal around the cannula and skin margins. The endoscope and instruments will be inserted into cannulas during the procedure.

Carbon dioxide, insufflation gas: Used to inflate the abdomen to increase visibility and safety during laparoscopic procedures. Flammable gases in containers in the OR should not be confused with carbon dioxide, which is nonflammable.

Circulator: Team member functioning in the nonsterile role; may be a registered nurse, practical nurse, or surgical technologist depending on the required legal qualifications in the state of employment.

Clamp-Clamp-Cut-Tie-Cut: An example of a pattern related to the progression of the procedure. In this example, the surgeon will need two clamps, followed by tissue scissors to cut, then a tie to occlude, followed by suture scissors to cut the tie.

Closed-eye and French split needle eyes: Suture material is threaded onto the needle by the ST.

Closed-gloving: Sterile skill sequence in which the hands do not extend through the gown cuff until the gloves are on. Refer to Chapter 6.

Coagulate: To firm up or congeal.

Communication etiquette: A protocol which demonstrates an appreciation for professional methods of communication by using appropriate and timely oral, written, or nonverbal interchanges among colleagues; professional manners and diplomacy. Demonstrates a commitment to professionalism, cultural norms, learning, being a team player, discussing facts and not hearsay, seeking appropriate assistance, showing time management, and striving to perform as an outstanding team member.

Confidentiality: Maintain the privacy of the patient and any information related to the surgical procedure, surgeon, and hospital. You may only use the computer to access confidential health information related to your assignment. You may not share information, photography, or videos verbally or visually, nor through any web-based social media. Refer to the U.S. Department of Health and Human Services for information concerning the Health Insurance Portability and Accountability Act of 1996 (HIPAA). http://www.hhs.gov/ocr/privacy/hipaa/understanding/index.html.

Contamination: Touching a sterile item with something nonsterile, thereby rendering the item as unusable on the sterile field. Occurs when a sterile person or sterile item touches a surface that is not sterile—outside of the sterile boundaries or not covered with sterile drapes.

Counted brush-stroke method: Strokes are counted and performed for each plane beginning at the fingertips and moving proximally to 2 inches above the elbow.

Critical thinking: Ability to anticipate the needs of the surgical team, to prioritize one's own actions, and to convert thoughts into appropriate actions; based on preparation and experience.

Cross-contamination: The movement of microorganisms from one location to another; contaminating multiple persons or surfaces.

Cutting needle: Incises or cuts through dense tissue such as skin.

Degrees of freedom: Rotations and translations in the Cartesian coordinate system, also known as the x–y–z planes; six degrees are routinely referenced. Robotic instruments are said to have seven degrees of freedom, or movement, the seventh being the addition of the pivoting or wristlike maneuver.

Dispersive electrode: Prevents burns during monopolar electrosurgery. It is also a grounding pad or return electrode.

Disposable drapes: Supplied sterile from the manufacturer; will be incinerated after one use.

Distal to proximal: Movement that starts at a location farthest away from the body and moves towards the midline of the body; begins at the fingers and moves toward the shoulder.

Doff: To remove or take off.

Don: To apply, put on, or wear.

Drape: A sterile cloth (disposable or reusable) used to cover nonsterile surfaces. Manufactured as a barrier and to resist puncture or moisture penetration (also known as *strike-through*).

The metal Mayo stand is covered with a sterile drape. The sterile gloves of the scrub person are cuffed with the drape as it is manipulated over the stand to prevent self-contamination with the metal stand.

Drug-resistant microbes: Microorganisms with the ability to thrive even though the patient is taking antibiotics. The fear is that eventually there will be no antibiotics that can effectively kill the microbes. People may not be able to survive a disease caused by drug-resistant microbes.

Economy of time and motion: By planning and practicing, supplies and equipment will be prepared for the case in the least amount of time and with the least amount of movement.

Electrosurgery: Electrical energy is used to assist the surgeon to perform the procedure through various devices. Also known as ES or ESU.

Emergency Care Research Institute (ECRI): Organization that promotes activities, including education, to improve patient care. http://www.ECRI.org.

Environmental distractions: The OR environment can be noisy with intercom voices or music playing, and with multiple people performing specific tasks simultaneously.

Environmental stewardship: Recycling; a plan is implemented to reduce the amount of trash that is generated, incinerated, or is disposed of at a landfill. Operating rooms may use more reusable gowns and drapes and may sort disposables for recycling.

Ergonomics: The science of adapting the job and/or the equipment and the human body to each other for optimal safety and productivity. Health care workers need to protect their backs from injury. Information concerning ergonomics is available in print and on the Internet, published by organizations such as the Occupational Safety and Health Administration (OSHA), the National Institute of Occupational Safety and Health (NIOSH), the National Safety Council, and the Human Factors and Ergonomic Society.

Eschar: Coagulated, dark, or charred tissue; builds up on the active electrode during the procedure. It must be routinely removed to prevent fires, and ensure safe function.

Excoriate: To strip or remove skin.

Exogenous pathogens: Microbes can live on fomites or inanimate objects; damp-dusting or disinfecting establishes a clean, safe environment for the patient. Hospital-acquired infections are associated with contaminated surfaces. Dust contains microbes, shed human skin and hair, molds, fungi, fibers, pollens, and other particles that contribute to SSIs.

Expiration date: End or final date determined by the company when the characteristics of products are guaranteed to be ideal and reliable.

Facility Guidelines Institute (FGI): *The Guidelines for Design and Construction of Health Care Facilities:* The institute develops best practices used in 42 states. Refer to the website. http://fgiguidelines.org/.

FDA (Food and Drug Administration): A U.S. federal agency that studies and regulates items that enter or contact our body.

Fenestrated drape: Drape with a window or opening designed to expose the incision site.

Fire Safety: AORN collaborated on many joint ventures, including a comprehensive safe surgery checklist with a fire safety component. Refer to Fire Safety Information and Training. www.AORN.ORG/Toolkits.

Five rights of medication administration: Prior to administration of a drug, health care practitioners verify the correct patient, the correct medication, the correct time, the correct dose, and the correct route. These are the traditional indicators of correctness. There are multiple other indicators that are also verified, including the correct label, expiration date, correct documentation, and no known drug allergies.

Fomites: Nonliving surfaces that harbor microorganisms.

Friction: A force created when rubbing the surfaces of hands and fingers together with pressure and movement.

Generator: Known as the electrosurgical unit, or ESU; powers the active electrode, produces an audible tone when the unit is activated, and is part of the circuit.

Granulation tissue: Forms during healing; containing capillaries and fibrous tissue. If granulation continues in excess, the protruding tissue is called *proud flesh.*

Hands-free transfer (HFT): Use of a basin, mat, or designated area for passing sharp instruments or suture between sterile team members; the item is not passed hand to hand. This is also referred to as using a neutral zone, or as the no-touch technique.

Hasson, or Fielding technique: Due to previous abdominal surgeries, scar or adhesion formation, surgeons may open the periumbilical area using sharp and blunt dissection; the Veress needle will not be used.

High-risk exposure category: Health care workers in the OR environment are at a greater risk of contracting a blood-borne communicable disease, such as Hepatitis B, due to the greater chance of blood exposure during invasive procedures.

Holster, Bovie Box, or Bovie Holder: Synonymous names for the storage container for the active electrode when it is not in use. Refer to http://www.aami.org/.

Hospital-acquired infection. See noscomial infection.

Ignaz Semmelweis: The origins of infection control in the form of hand hygiene or hand washing dates to 1847. The director of an obstetrics ward in Vienna,

Austria, Dr. Ignaz Semmelweis associated hand-washing practices of nurse-mid-wives with a low rate of maternal post-partum infection and deaths. Conversely, Dr. Semmelweis' interns did not wash their hands in between duties, such as performing autopsies and delivering babies. The interns' patients experienced higher infection and mortality rates. Dr. Semmelweis mandated hand washing with a chlorinated lime solution before patient contact. Hand washing in between patients and duties resulted in a drastic decrease in infection and deaths. Today, hand hygiene remains a critical component of infection control.

Impedance: The flow of current is blocked. Loss of contact between the return electrode and the skin can result in tissue injury or a burn when using monopolar electrocautery.

Incident report: When an error in a process occurs in the hospital, a report is completed and submitted to the quality assurance department. The incident report is not a part of the patient's record.

Instruments: Included in this category are metal or plastic instruments designed to be extensions or aids for the surgeon's hand. Examples include scissors, forceps, and retractors.

Intact skin: Skin that is free of cuts, lesions, or exudates. Impaired skin integrity puts the patient and worker at a greater risk of acquiring an infection.

International Sharps Injury Prevention Society (ISIPS): Organization promotes education to decrease the number of accidental sharps injuries; promotes the use of safety-engineered products and services. http://www.isips.org.

The Joint Commission: Founded in 1951, it is an independent, not-for-profit organization which accredits and certifies more than 18,000 health care organizations and programs in the United States. This organization strives to promote safe patient care of the highest quality and value, in collaboration with other stakeholders. http://www.jointcommission.org.

Laparotomy: Incision into the abdomen.

Left-handed surgeon: The surgeon will suture using his/her left hand. The curved needle will need to be reoriented by the ST before passing it to the left-handed surgeon. Refer to chapter 20.

Lithotomy drape: Draping sheets for a gynecological or perineal procedure. Includes a fenestrated lithotomy drape and two triangular drapes for the legs. The patient will be in a lithotomy position—legs in stirrups.

Low-linting drapes: Used to prevent SSIs; lint or cloth fuzz can carry microbes from the OR environment into the surgical wound. These can be a source of a postoperative infection and adhesions.

Material Safety Data Sheets (MSDS): Information available to staff members related to chemicals, disinfectants, and other products used in the environment; health hazards and countermeasures postexposure are listed.

Maximum dosages: Each medication has a safe dosage range. Dosages outside of this range produce untoward side effects and can harm the patient. Everyone involved with medications must know the safe dosage range and upper, or maximum, limit.

Mayo stand: A tray, approximately 16×20 inches, on a movable, adjustable stand. Instruments are moved to and from the back table onto the draped Mayo stand according to the progression of the surgical procedure.

Microorganisms: Endogenous: microbes that are part of our normal flora and reside with us. Exogenous: microbes that are not part of our normal flora.

Microorganisms that cause SSIs: Staphylococcus aureus, Coagulase-negative staphylococci (CoNS), Enterococcus species (E. faecalis, E. faecium), Escherichia coli, Pseudomonas aeruginosa, Enterobacter species, Klebsiella pneumoniae, Candid species, Acinetobacter baumannii, and Klebsiella oxytoca.

Minimally invasive surgery (MIS): Procedures performed with minimal tissue disruption and little blood loss; the patient will return to daily activities in less time than with open procedures.

Monofilament: One strand of suture material.

Monopolar: A mode for electrosurgery; looks like a pencil and requires the use of a dispersive electrode. This is the most common mode of electrosurgery in use.

Moral compass: The application of aseptic technique in all situations is the compass which guides actions in the OR. This concept is also known as a *surgical conscience.*

Multifilament: More than one strand, supplied as braided or twisted.

Multiple care providers and hand-off: The patient is taken care of by multiple caregivers during their perioperative experience. Errors can occur due to a lack of clear communication when the patient is "handed off" or care giving is begun by the next employee. Prevent with precise communication.

Multiple dose forms and concentrations: The same drug can have different concentrations or be supplied in various forms. For example, Bupivacaine solution can be supplied in various concentrations such as 0.5% or 0.25% (plain), or it can contain epinephrine (with epi.).

Multiple dose forms with epinephrine: Epinephrine (epi) may be added to local anesthetics, for injection, to prolong the effect of the anesthetic due to vasoconstriction. The vial will have a RED label which serves as a visual cue to be alert to this additive. The ST and RN must verify the correct strength or concentration of the epinephrine. For example, Epinephrine 1:100,000 is a stronger dose than Epinephrine 1:200,000. Medications with epinephrine added are not used routinely in anatomical areas that are located in the extreme distal areas of the body: fingers, toes, penis, or nose.

National Fire Protection Agency (NFPA): Advocates for fire prevention; develops and publishes codes and standards, such as the Standards for Health Care Facilities used by The Joint Commission.

National Highway Traffic Safety Administration (NHTSA) and Fatality Analysis Reporting System (FARS): Dedicated to achieving the highest standards of excellence in motor vehicle and highway safety, NHTSA works to help prevent crashes and their attendant costs, both human and financial. The FARS reports data related to motor vehicle accidents, fatalities, and trends. www.NHTSA.org.

National Institute for Occupational Safety and Health (NIOSH): https//www.cdc.gov/niosh/. Dedicated to the prevention of workplace illness and injury.

National Pain Foundation: Dedicated to providing information and education. http://www.nationalpainfoundation.org.

Natural or synthetic: Natural materials are found in nature; synthetic are engineered and manufactured.

Needle curvature: The size of the needle curve is stated as a relationship to the circumference around a full circle. For skin, muscle, or vessels, a 3/8 circle needle may be used.

Needlestick Prevention Act of 2000 (NSPA): Law promoting employee safety and prevention of injury due to sharp devices. OSHA revised the Bloodborne Pathogen Standard in 2001 in response to this Clinton law.

Nitrous oxide: N_2O; anesthetic gas; when heated, this compound releases oxygen.

Normothermia: Body temperature within defined parameters, approximately 98.6°F. Hypothermia, significantly lower than 98.6°F initiates shivering and infections. Shivering shunts oxygen to the muscles, reduces the amount of oxygen available to the heart muscle, and may precipitate a heart attack in susceptible patients. Promotes hemostasis (balanced blood coagulation) and prevents infections.

Nosocomial infection or hospital-acquired infection: An infection that was not present or incubating prior to the hospitalization, or surgery. The most frequently occurring is a urinary tract infection (UTI).

No-touch zone: An area used to pass sharp items between team members. The sharp instrument is placed onto a pad or into a basin, and only one person touches the instrument at a time. Also known as *hands-free transfer (HFT)*.

Occupational Safety and Health Administration (OSHA): Federal agency that establishes guidelines to protect the employee from hazards and injury. Refer to the website for additional information. http://www.osha.gov/.

Open-gloving: Method of donning sterile gloves while in nonsterile attire.

OSHA (Occupational Safety and Health Administration): Part of the U.S. Department of Labor. http://www.osha.gov/.

Package memory: The folded edges of the wrapper recoil and return to the original folded position.

Patterns or sequences: Anticipation and critical thinking are skills used to prepare instruments in advance, based on a plan or regular manner of performance. For example, suture scissors are readied when suture or ties are passed.

Phase I Recovery: Requires ECG and more complex, intensive monitoring; plan to discharge to Phase II or to an in-patient room.

Phase II Recovery: Also called the *step-down*, or *discharge, area;* for patients from an ambulatory surgery area; initial plan is for same-day discharge to home or to an extended care facility.

Phase III, or Extended Observation Recovery: Monitoring patient over a longer period of time with plans for discharge to home or an extended care facility.

Pneumoperitoneum: Distension of the abdomen with carbon dioxide gas so that surgically entering the abdomen is safer. Visualization for the surgeon during laparoscopic surgery is enhanced. Risks include: potential puncture of internal organs, increased intraabdominal pressure, impaired breathing or cardiac function, and air embolism causing death, infection, and severe postoperative shoulder pain due to irritation of nerves.

Postanesthesia Care Unit: Traditionally known as the recovery room, or PACU, and located near the OR for convenience and patient safety; patient is closely monitored while recovering from the effects of anesthesia medications.

PPE: Personal protective equipment is used to place a barrier between the health care worker and potentially infectious or harmful materials. There are various levels of protection available. A cap, surgical mask, eye protection, shoe covers, and a fluid-resistant gown protect the health care worker's skin, mucus membranes, and OR attire from blood-borne pathogens which may splash or spray during invasive procedures. Protection from other hazards requires different barriers, such as a lead apron, dosimeter x-ray badge, or special eyewear to protect the cornea during LASER procedures. OSHA regulations give specific guidelines for protecting workers in many occupations from injury. Follow the guidelines. The surgical mask simultaneously protects the patient from microbial contamination from the mouth and nares of health care workers.

Preference card: A listing of the supplies, equipment, and preferences of the surgeon for a particular procedure.

Primary intention: Ideal closure with suture; edges of skin are approximated; usually yields a small scar and minimal complications.

Privacy: Exposing bare body parts causes embarrassment to many people. Window shades should be closed and private body parts should be covered with blankets while the patient is awake.

Resident flora: Microorganisms that live in the layers of our skin and in the pores. They are not removed entirely by hand antisepsis. The skin cannot be made sterile. Usually reside in a symbiotic relationship.

Retrograde: Flowing backwards; opposite of the usual order.

Reuseable drapes: Made from high quality textiles and may be laundered and sterilized dozens of times, usually at an off-site facility. Quality control is essential.

Right-handed surgeon: The surgeon will close a surgical wound, or suture using his/her right hand. The curved needle will be loaded from the suture pack as oriented in the pack.

Safe Medical Devices Act of 1990 (SMDA): This federal law requires reporting the failure of medical devices including gowns or drapes to perform as intended. The FDA and the manufacturer are also notified of any malfunctions.

Saline test: A saline-filled 10 mL syringe is attached to the hub of the Veress needle. Due to the negative pressure inside of the abdomen, the saline will be automatically pulled into the abdominal cavity if the needle is placed correctly. When placement is confirmed, insufflation can begin.

SCIP (Surgical Care Improvement Project): National partnership of organizations working towards reducing the incidence of surgical complications. Modifiable risk factors include timing prophylactic antibiotics, usually one-hour preincision, only clipping hair if it interferes with the surgical site, and controlling glucose levels in diabetics. Also modifiable is preparing the patient's skin at the surgical site.

Scratch pad: Abrasive pad, 1 × 1 inch. Known as "scratch" and is x-ray detectable. Use to clean the tip of the Bovie pencil.

Secondary intention: Wound heals from the base up by filling in; risk of complications and infection is greater; expect a large scar.

Sentinel event: An event that causes the patient injury or death; it is a reportable event. Frequency is tracked and solutions are devised and implemented.

Sequential compression devices: Automated sleeves that are placed over the lower extremities to prevent formation of a deep vein thrombus (DVT); they alternate squeezing and releasing which mimic the patient's normal muscle movements; venous return of blood to the heart is promoted. A thrombus can form due to pooling of blood in the extremities during inactivity. An embolus or clot can return to the heart, lungs, or brain and cause disability or death.

Sharps and miscellaneous items: included in this category are sharp items and various other supplies that could be retained. Examples include blades, hypodermic needles, suture needles, electrocautery tips, tip scratch pads, vessel loops, and broken parts.

Skin antisepsis (Prep): Cleaning/scrubbing the skin to prevent infections.

Skin squams: Particles of skin shed during the normal life cycle of skin. Humans shed approximately 10 million skin squams per day. Microorganisms can reside on the skin squams and can cause SSIs.

Spatula needle: Shaped like a spatula and aids in excising small amounts of tissue during suturing.

Spaulding's classification system: A grading system that is used to determine the level of disinfection required for an item based on the composition of the item and the intended use. There are three levels: critical, semicritical, and noncritical. Critical items enter sterile body areas such as tissue or the vascular system. Semicritical items contact nonintact skin or mucous membranes, such as endoscopes or laryngoscopes. Noncritical items contact intact skin, such as blood pressure cuffs or bed linens.

Sponges: These textile materials, in various sizes, are designed to be used on tissue during invasive procedures; they are supplied with an x-ray-detectable mark or stripe. Examples include 4 × 8 inch laparotomy sponges, Kittners, and 4 × 4 inch RAY-TEC sponges.

SSI (Surgical site infection): An infection that occurs within 30 days of the surgery and may be superficial, deep, or found in organs or spaces. A standardized surveillance system has been developed by the Center for Disease Control and Prevention, National Nosocomial Infection Surveillance. Manifested as a fever 5 to 30 days postoperatively with heat, redness, pain, or drainage at the wound site and an elevated white blood cell count. See surgical site infections and Staphylococcus aureus.

Standing order: This is an order for a medication that is routinely given for a particular procedure. It will be prepared for each case until the surgeon changes the order.

Staphylococcus aureus: Microscopic organisms or flora that look like bunches of grapes; anerobic, gram-positive cocci; cause a majority of surgical site infections postoperatively. Methacillin Resistant Staphylococcus Aureus (MRSA) is a variation in this category of microbes. It has developed a resistance to the antibiotic Methacillin and is more virulent. http://aaos.org/. Other organisms causing surgical site infections: Coagulase-negative staphylococci (CoNS), Enterococcus species (E. faecalis, E. faecium), Escherichia coli, Pseudomonas aeruginosa, Enterobacter species, Klebsiella pneumoniae, Candid species, Acinetobacter baumannii, and Klebsiella oxytoca.

Sterile attire: Sterile surgical gown, gloves, or other required coverings which have been processed using sterilization methods. May be reusable cloth or disposable paper.

Sterile field: Specially prepared area that is sterile; it includes the patient's surgical site, sterile supplies, sterile equipment, and sterile OR team members.

Sterile transfer device: This is a strawlike item with sterile, capped ends that assists with the sterile transfer of medications contained in a vial into a sterile cup on the back table.

Sterile water: Contained in a labeled, sterile basin on the back table and used to clean blood or tissue off of instruments during the case. Normal saline or salt solutions should not be used because they can pit or damage the surface of the instruments. Sterile water should not be used in the body, so accurate labeling is essential. Immersing body tissue in water, a hypotonic solution, will cause the cells to absorb water and swell. Therefore, sterile normal saline, an isotonic solution, is used for irrigation. Occasionally, sterile water is used during procedures involving cancer cells.

Sterile, aseptic technique: *Aseptic* means "free from microbes and spores"; a series of processes that are conducted to reduce, eliminate, or confine microbes and, therefore, reduce the risk of an infection.

Stoma: Surgically made intestinal opening on the outer surface of the abdomen.

Strike-through: Contamination occurs when the physical barrier of the drape is broken and microbes enter a sterile area via a hole or by wicked moisture.

Subungual areas: Surface under the fingernails; area harbors larger colonies of microbes due to the growth promoting environment.

Surgical conscience: This concept includes the knowledge, commitment, and actions guiding aseptic technique. Also known as a moral compass, where your beliefs are evidenced by a commitment to accountability, honesty, integrity, and self-regulation.

Surgical mask: Specially designed masks cover the mouth and nose and act as a filter for microorganisms exiting from the mouth and nose. The patient is protected from the worker's microbes. The skin of the worker is protected from spraying of tissue and blood during invasive procedures. Wear surgical masks during the surgical hand scrub, when sterile supplies are open, during the operative procedures, and in the center core at some facilities.

Surgical site infection (SSI): Infection occurring in the area where surgery was performed, incisional or organ/space. SSIs are the third most common cause of health care–acquired infections in the United States and account for approximately 500,000 infections per year. For additional information, refer to the Centers for Disease Control and Prevention and the National Nosocomial Infection Surveillance system. http://www.cdc.gov/nhsn/.

Surgical technologist (ST): Health care professional who assists the surgeon during invasive procedures. In this lab manual, "ST" is used to indicate the sterile team member and to differentiate these functions from the nonsterile team member or assistant circulator. The ST cannot perform duties that are legally the function of a licensed individual, according to each state's practice laws.

Suture strand sizes: The diameter or thickness of the strand. Sizes range from very small (12-0) to very large (5). The numbers starting at 2-0 and going backwards to 12-0 are like numbers on a negative scale: the larger the number, the smaller the value, or size.

Swaged or eyeless needle: Suture material is attached or imbedded into the needle.

Tapercut needle: Combination action that will suture and cut without pulling apart dense tissue such as fascia.

Tapered needle: Sharp end punches through tissue, such as muscle or peritoneum.

Tensile strength: The ability to resist rupture; term refers to both suture strands and tissue undergoing healing.

Tertiary intention: Delayed primary closure; wound is left open to correct an infection and sutured later.

Three phases of wound healing: Inflammatory, proliferation, and remodeling; healing begins at the time of the incision with hemostasis; normal healing ends with a small scar; abnormal healing can produce a keloid or very large, raised scar.

Time-out protocol: The Joint Commission's protocol that promotes patient safety by correctly identifying multiple parameters before the surgical procedure begins.

Timed method: The process of performing the surgical hand scrub within 5 minutes or 2½ minutes per hand and arm. The scrub begins at the fingertips and moves proximally to 2 inches above the elbow.

Transient flora: Microorganisms that may be found on our skin, but are not a part of the resident flora. These are acquired as part of our daily routine when touching surfaces, and can be removed by hand hygiene, or antisepsis.

Trendelenburg position: As the OR bed is adjusted, the patient's head is placed downward and the pelvis and legs are positioned higher. The abdominal organs are shifted towards the head by this position using gravity. Position used for surgery in the pelvis.

Twisted: Strands that are turned in a corkscrew pattern.

Unambiguous: A single, clearly defined meaning.

Unclear communication patterns: Surgical masks can make verbal communication difficult to understand. Written orders can be illegible. Surgeon preferences can change but not be documented. Noise in the OR can be distracting or prevent clarity.

United States Environmental Protection Agency (EPA): Studies and makes recommendations for cleaning products and other environments controls. http://www.epa.gov/.

Verbal medication order: This is an order for a medication that is spoken by the surgeon and is received by the circulator. The order is verified and transcribed into the patient's record. Only licensed personnel can accept a verbal order. The surgeon later cosigns the order. This process may occur in writing or through electronic documentation.

Veress needle: Developed in the 1930s; it is a spring-loaded needle with a sharp tip surrounded by a blunt covering; frequently used when creating pneumoperitoneum in laparoscopic surgeries. As the needle is inserted into the subumbilical area, resistance raises the blunt tube and sharp tips are advanced. Once the intraabdominal cavity has been reached, the resistance decreases and the spring allows the blunt tube to quickly cover the sharp tip—the bowel and other organs are protected from puncture. A tube will be connected to a stopcock on the needle for carbon dioxide gas instillation; the abdomen will be distended. Disposable and reusable variations are found.

Vial: Glass bottle that contains liquid or powder medication. The vial should be intact, not cracked, and the top should have an intact (metal) seal. The top of the bottle, under the seal, is closed with a rubber stopper or diaphragm. To access the vial, the circulator removes the metal cap and punctures the stopper with a sterile transfer straw. The liquid medication is poured via the sterile straw into a sterile container or medicine cup. If the vial contains a powder then it will need to be reconstituted with a dilutant, such as normal saline solution, before it is poured.

Water conservation: Turn the water off during nonuse at the scrub sink.

World Health Organization (WHO): The directing and coordinating authority for health within the United Nations system. It is responsible for providing leadership on global health matters, shaping the health research agenda, setting norms and standards, articulating evidence-based policy options, providing technical support to countries, and monitoring and assessing health trends. http://www.WHO.org.

Wound classification: The Centers for Disease Control and Prevention (CDC) developed the four class schema; it is an adaptation from the American College of Surgeons. The classification score is assigned at the end of the surgical procedure; it predicts the risk of contracting a surgical site infection; also used to compile data and to influence best practices. The divisions are I. Clean; II. Clean-contaminated; III. Contaminated; and IV. Dirty or Infected.

Written medication order: This is the traditional method used by a surgeon to order a medication. The order for the drug is listed in the patient's chart. For example, the surgeon may order an antibiotic to be given 1 hour preoperatively: Ancef 1 Gm. I.V., administer 1 hour preincision.

Yankauer suction wand: A curved hollow instrument that may be plastic or metal; it is used as a sterile or nonsterile tool. The metal wand has two parts, the curved wand and a detachable cap or tip. The plastic wand is disposable and supplied as one unit. The anesthesia care provider will use the unsterile suction wand to clear the mouth and upper airway of secretions to maintain a patent airway. The surgeon or assistant will use a separate sterile wand to suction blood from the operative site to maintain visualization. Occasionally, the wand will be held over the operative site to evacuate smoke plume when the ESU active electrode (pencil) is used for cutting tissue. The Yankauer has nicknames such as "tip," or "suction."

Bibliography

1. AAMI Standards. AAMI. http://www.aami.org/. Accessed October 15, 2011.

2. About the WHO. World Health Organization. http://www.who.int/about/en/. Accessed April 5, 2010.

3. AFP. Lysacek wins men's figure skating gold. http://www.vancouver2010.com/. Accessed May 2, 2010.

4. Alexander, S.M. & Rothrock, J.C. (2011). *Alexander's surgical procedures*. St. Louis, MO: Mosby.

5. American Academy of Orthopaedic Surgeons. http://www.aaos.org/. Accessed April 18, 2011.

6. American College of Surgeons. http://www.facs.org/. Accessed April 18, 2011.

7. American Society of Heating, Refrigerating, and Air Conditioning Engineers. http://www.ashrae.org/. Accessed October 4, 2010.

8. AORN Comprehensive Surgical Checklist. AORN, Inc. http://www.aorn.org/Practice Resources/ToolKits/CorrectSiteSurgery ToolKit/Comprehensivechecklist/. Accessed May 22, 2010.

9. Aronson, S. (March, 2010). *Surgical fire safety: the best response is prevention*. Presentation at the annual congress of the Association of periOperative Registered Nurses, Denver, CO, March, 2010.

10. Association of periOperative Registered Nurses. (2011). *Perioperative standards and recommended practices*. Denver, CO: AORN.

11. Association of periOperative Registered Nurses. (2010*). Perioperative competencies, position descriptions, and evaluation tools*. Denver: AORN.

12. Association of Surgical Technologists. (2011). *Core curriculum for surgical technology* (6th ed.). Centennial, CO: Author.

13. AST, Inc. (2010). MRSA leads to worse outcomes, staggering expenses for surgical patients. *The Surgical Technologist, 42* (2), 87.

14. AST, Inc. (2008). *Surgical technology for the surgical technologist*. Clifton Park, NY: Delmar Cengage Learning.

15. Bloodborne pathogens and needlestick prevention. Occupational Safety and Health Administration; US Department of Labor. http://osha.gov/SLTC/bloodbornepathogens/index.html. Accessed February 20, 2010.

16. Borak, T. (2009). Where in the world to go? *The Surgical Technologist, 41* (9), 410–416.

17. Boivin, J. (2010, May 3). Tea and empathy: the power of one. *Nursing Spectrum*, 24–25.

18. Brand, S. (2011, April). *Going from good to great*. Presentation conducted at a gathering of surgical technology students at Frederick Community College, Frederick, Maryland.

19. Brown-Brumfield, D., and DeLeaon, A. (2010). Adherence to a medication safety protocol: current practice for labeling medications and solutions on the sterile field. *AORN Journal, 91* (5), 610–617.

20. Career Services. Frederick Community College. http://www.frederick.edu/student_services/CareerCenter/index.cfm?CCPage =Tutorials_Text&TC=1001|Job%20Search. Accessed April 17, 2010.

21. Career Services: Pointing you towards tomorrow. http://careers.d.umn.edu/cs_handbook/cshandbook_portfolio.html. Accessed April 17, 2010.

22. Carney, B., West, P., Neily, J., Mills, P., and Bagian, J. (2010). Differences in nurse and surgeon perceptions of teamwork: implications for use of a briefing checklist in the OR. *AORN Journal, 91* (6), 722–729.

23. Centers for Disease Control and Prevention. National Nosocomial Infection Surveillance. http://cdc.org. Accessed August 2, 2010.

24. Council on Surgical & Perioperative Safety. (2009). Statement on violence in the workplace. *The Surgical Technologist Journal, 91,* 113–115.

25. Dankanich, N., Santelli, J., and Schellenberg, R. (Producers). (2008). *General surgery instruments* [CD]. Available from www.surgeryessentials.com.

26. Dankanich, N., Santelli, J., and Schellenberg, R. (Producers). (2010). *General surgery instruments* [iPod Application]. Available from www.surgeryessentials.com.

27. da Vinci® Si System. Intuitive Surgical. http://www.intuitivesurgical.com/index.aspx. Accessed April 2, 2010.

28. Facility Guidelines. Facility Guidelines Institute. http://fgiguidelines.org/. Accessed October 4, 2010.

29. Fires. Emergency Care Research Institute. www.ecri.org/surgical_fires. Accessed March 29, 2010.

30. Fuller, J. (2010). *Surgical technology principles and practices* (5th ed.). St. Louis, MO: Saunders.

31. Gawande, A. (2009). *The checklist manifesto: how to get things right*. New York: Metropolitan Books.

32. Goldman, M. A. (2008). *Pocket guide to the operating room* (3rd ed.). Philadelphia: FA Davis Co.

33. Hospital survey on patient safety culture: 2008 comparative database report. Agency for Healthcare Research and Quality. http://www.ahrq.gov/qual/hospsurvey08. Accessed March 30, 2010.

34. Hemingway, M., Freehan, M., and Morrissey, L. (2010). Expanding the role of nonclinical personnel in the OR. *AORN Journal, 91* (6), 753–761.

35. Stoker, R. Making a difference in sharps safety. ISIPS. http://www.isips.org/reports/Articles/mic1209r50.pdf. Accessed January 15, 2011.

36. Jagger, J., Berger, R., Kornblatt-Phillips, E., Parker, G., and Gomaa, A. (2010). Increase in sharps injuries in surgical settings versus nonsurgical settings after passage of national needlestick legislation. *Journal of the American College of Surgeons, 210* (4), 496–502.

37. Kaplan, K., Mestel, P., and Feldman, D. (2010). Creating a culture of mutual respect. *AORN Journal, 91* (2), 495–510.

38. Laundry Accreditation. Healthcare Laundry Accreditation Council. www.hlacnet.org/laundries.php. Accessed June 13, 2010.

39. Learning Pyramid and Cone of Learning. http://www.google.com/search?client=firefox-a&rls=org.mozilla%3Aen-US%3Aofficial&channel=s&hl=en&source=hp&q=Learning+Pyramid&btnG=Google+Search. Accessed April 24, 2010.

40. Lewis, S., Dirksen, S., Heitkemper, M., Bucher, L., & Camera, I. (2011). *Medical surgical nursing: assessment and management of clinical problems* (8th ed.). St. Louis, MO: Mosby.

41. Lippincott, Williams & Wilkins. (2007). *Surgical care made incredibly visual.* Ambler, PA: Lippincott, Williams & Wilkins.

42. Rothrock, J. (2011). *Alexander's care of the patient in surgery* (14th ed.). New York: Mosby, Inc.

43. National Fire Protection Agency. NFPA 99. Proposal 99–409, section 13.4.1.2.2.3. http://www.nfpa.org/Assets/Files/PDF/ROP/99-A2009-ROP.pdf. Accessed October 15, 2010.

44. National Highway Traffic Safety Administration. Fatality analysis reporting system (FARS). http://www-fars.nhtsa.dot.gov/Main/index.aspx. Accessed September 26, 2010.

45. National Patient Safety Goals. Joint Commission. http://www.jointcommission.org/PatientSafety/NationalPatientSafetyGoals/. Accessed March 24, 2010.

46. National Time Out Day. AORN. www.aorn.org/nationaltimeoutday. Accessed June 13, 2010.

47. Needlestick Prevention Act. United States Department of Labor. http://www.osha.gov/SLTC/bloodbornepathogens/index.html. Accessed April 18, 2011.

48. New clinical guide to surgical fire prevention. (2009). *Health Devices, 38* (10) 314–332.

49. Phippen, M., Ulmer, B., and Wells, M. (2009). *Competency for safe patient care during operative and invasive procedures.* Denver, CO: Competency & Credentialing Institute.

50. Position Statements. ASPAN. https://www.aspan.org/ClinicalPractice/PositionStatements/tabid/3253/Default.aspx. Accessed May 15, 2010.

51. Poston, B., (2009). Maslow's hierarchy of needs. *The Surgical Technologist, 41* (8), 347–353.

52. Ratner, T. (2006, October 23). Communication in the OR. *Nursing Spectrum,* 10–11.

53. Recent initiatives. Emergency Care Research Institute. ECRI. https://www.ecri.org/Press/Pages/default.aspx. Accessed March 29, 2010.

54. Recommended practices for a safe environment of care. In: *Perioperative standards and recommended practices.* Denver, CO: AORN, Inc; 2010: 217–236.

55. Recommended practices for sponge, sharp, and instrument counts. In: *Perioperative standards and recommended practices.* Denver, CO: AORN, Inc; 2010: 207–216.

56. Recommended practices for surgical attire. In: *Perioperative standards and recommended practices.* Denver, CO: AORN, Inc; 2011: 57–71.

57. Roesler, R., Halowell, C., Elias, G., and Peters, J. (2010). Chasing zero: our journey to preventing surgical site infections. *AORN Journal, 91,* 224–235.

58. Rogers, E., Boegli, E., and LaRue, K. (2013). *Pearson's surgical technology exam reveiw* (3rd ed.). Upper Saddle River, NJ: Pearson.

59. Rothrock, J. (2011). *Alexander's care of the patient in surgery.* St. Louis, MO: Elsevier Mosby.

60. Phillips, N. (2007). *Berry and Kohn's operating room technique.* St. Louis, MO: Elsevier Mosby.

61. Shepherd, A. (2009). The role of the surgical technologist in wound management. *The Surgical Technologist, 41* (6), 255–261.

62. Smith, S. (2010). Managing up can improve teamwork in the OR. *AORN, Journal, 91* (5), 576–582.

63. Standards. Association for the Advancement of Medical Instrumentation. AAMI. http://www.aami.org/. Accessed February 27, 2010.

64. Sentinel Events. The Joint Commission. http://www.jointcommission.org/SentinelEvents/SentinelEventAlert/sea_6.htm. Accessed November 20, 2009.

65. Surgical Fire Victims. SFO. http://surgicalfire.org/index.cfm?fuseaction=63. Accessed March 30, 2010.

66. Veress Needle. Get A Note From Your Doctor (ganfyd). http://www.ganfyd.org/index.php?title=Veress_needle. Accessed April 3, 2010.

67. Webster, D.P. (2003). *Handbook of general surgical instruments.* Westminster, MD: Dan-Mar Medical Publishing.

68. World Health Organization Guidelines for Safe Surgery 2009. Safe Surgery Saves Lives. FARS. http://www-fars.nhtsa.dot.gov/Main/index.aspx. Accessed September 26, 2010.

69. Wound Classifications. Centers for Disease Control and Prevention. http://wonder.cdc.gov/wonder/prevguid/p0000420/p0000420.asp. Accessed March 27, 2010.

70. Yewell, T., Knowlden, E., and Corcoran, C. (2009, April). *Robot-assisted surgery.* Presentation conducted at a meeting of surgical technology students at Frederick Community College, Frederick, Maryland.

71. Yewell, T. (2009, April). *Robot-assisted surgery—a student surgical technologist's perspective.* Presentation conducted at a gathering of surgical technology students at Frederick Community College, Frederick, Maryland.

Index

Note: Page numbers with *f* indicate figures; those with *t* indicate tables.